M. Nakashima, N. Takamura, K. Tsukasaki,
Y. Nagayama, S. Yamashita (Eds.)
Radiation Health Risk Sciences

M. Nakashima, N. Takamura, K. Tsukasaki,
Y. Nagayama, S. Yamashita (Eds.)

Radiation Health Risk Sciences

Proceedings of the First International Symposium
of the Nagasaki University Global COE Program
"Global Strategic Center for Radiation Health
Risk Control"

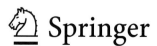

Masahiro Nakashima M.D., Ph.D.
Associate Professor, Tissue and
 Histopathology Section, Atomic Bomb
 Disease Institute
Nagasaki University Graduate School of
 Biomedical Sciences
1-12-4 Sakamoto, Nagasaki 852-8523, Japan

Noboru Takamura M.D., Ph.D.
Associate Professor, Department of
 Radiation Epidemiology, Atomic Bomb
 Disease Institute
Nagasaki University Graduate School of
 Biomedical Sciences
1-12-4 Sakamoto, Nagasaki 852-8523, Japan

Kunihiro Tsukasaki M.D., Ph.D.
Associate Professor, Department of
 Molecular Medicine and Hematology,
 Atomic Bomb Disease Institute
Nagasaki University Graduate School of
 Biomedical Sciences
1-12-4 Sakamoto, Nagasaki 852-8523, Japan

Yuji Nagayama M.D., Ph.D.
Professor, Department of Medical Gene
 Technology, Atomic Bomb Disease
 Institute
Nagasaki University Graduate School of
 Biomedical Sciences
1-12-4 Sakamoto, Nagasaki 852-8523, Japan

Shunichi Yamashita M.D., Ph.D.
Professor, Department of Molecular
 Medicine
Atomic Bomb Disease Institute
Nagasaki University Graduate School of
 Biomedical Sciences
1-12-4 Sakamoto, Nagasaki 852-8523, Japan

Library of Congress Control Number: 2008937558

ISBN 978-4-431-88658-7 Springer Tokyo Berlin Heidelberg New York
e-ISBN 978-4-431-88659-4

This work is subject to copyright. All rights are reserved, whether the whole or part of the material is concerned, specifically the rights of translation, reprinting, reuse of illustrations, recitation, broadcasting, reproduction on microfilms or in other ways, and storage in data banks. The use of registered names, trademarks, etc. in this publication does not imply, even in the absence of a specific statement, that such names are exempt from the relevant protective laws and regulations and therefore free for general use.
Product liability: The publisher can give no guarantee for information about drug dosage and application thereof contained in this book. In every individual case the respective user must check its accuracy by consulting other pharmaceutical literature.

Springer is a part of Springer Science+Business Media
springer.com
© Springer 2009
Printed in Japan
Typesetting: SNP Best-set Typesetter Ltd., Hong Kong
Printing and binding: Kato Bunmeisha, Japan
Printed on acid-free paper

Acknowledgments

The publication of this volume was supported by the Ministry of Education, Culture, Sports, Science and Technology of Japan through the Nagasaki University Global COE (center of excellence) Program "Global Strategic Center for Radiation Health Risk Control."

Organizing Committee

Honorary Chairman
Hiroshi Saito, *President, Nagasaki University*

Chairman
Shunichi Yamashita, *Professor, GCOE Program Leader, Nagasaki University*

Program Committee
Naoki Matsuda, *Professor, Nagasaki University*
Yuji Nagayama, *Professor, Nagasaki University*
Masahiro Nakashima, *Associate Professor, Nagasaki University*
Akira Ohtsuru, *Associate Professor, Nagasaki University*
Hiroki Ozawa, *Professor, Nagasaki University*
Keiji Suzuki, *Associate Professor, Nagasaki University*
Noboru Takamura, *Associate Professor, Nagasaki University*
Kunihiro Tsukasaki, *Associate Professor, Nagasaki University*
Koh-ichiro Yoshiura, *Associate Professor, Nagasaki University*

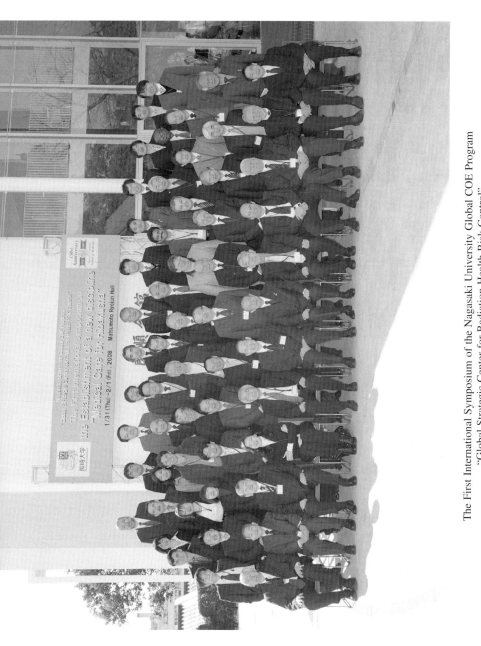

The First International Symposium of the Nagasaki University Global COE Program
"Global Strategic Center for Radiation Health Risk Control"
Matsumoto Ryojun Hall, Nagasaki University School of Medicine, 31 January–1 February 2008

Preface

Ionizing radiation is a recognized and a well-documented human cancer risk factor, based on a remarkably consistent body of information from epidemiological studies of exposed populations in the world. The atomic bomb survivors study in Hiroshima and Nagasaki remains the single most important study on excess cancer risk and also, recently, on noncancer risk. The youngest atomic bomb survivors, considered to be the most radiosensitive, have now reached the "cancer age."

A continuous endeavor in the field of radiation health risk sciences is critical and important especially for the Nuclear Age of the twenty-first century from the standpoint of radiation safety and risk management. Besides the atomic bomb studies in Japan, lessons from the Chernobyl accident also tell us about various health effects in several population categories directly affected by the accident, such as emergency workers and people living in radio-contaminated areas. Among the latter, there has been a dramatic increase in thyroid cancer in those who were children at the time of the accident; their risk of disease is expected to be long-lasting. We are now facing the most difficult part in the follow-up of the long-term health consequences in individuals who were exposed at a young age, either externally or internally. An additional source of information on radiation health effects in humans is the data obtained and accumulated from occupational, medical, and other exposure scenarios. Along with studies in human populations, it is also essential to promote basic radiation life sciences at the molecular, cellular, tissue, and laboratory animal levels, particularly as they address exposure to low dose and low dose-rate radiation, to further understand and apply these findings to future regulatory guidance and public health policy.

Another important issue of the Nuclear Age is to prepare for emergency radiation medicine against nuclear disasters and any radiological accident. The global radiation health initiative should be taken under the auspices of an international consortium on emergency radiation medicine, focusing on regenerative medicine and related regulatory sciences. Here we would like to re-emphasize to the world our mission and task of Nagasaki University in the field of radiation health risk sciences.

On the basis of our previous achievements of the 21st century COE program entitled "The International Consortium for Medical Care of Hibakusha and Radiation Life Science" selected by the Japanese Ministry of Education, Culture, Sports,

Science and Technology from FY 2002 to FY 2006, a new Global COE program termed "Global Strategic Center for Radiation Health Risk Control" has been newly selected for the coming five years starting in FY 2007.

As an inaugural meeting of the new GCOE Program, we held the First International Symposium from 31 January–4 February 2008, at Matsumoto Ryojun Hall, during the special occasion of the 150th anniversary of the founding of the Nagasaki University School of Medicine. More than 130 scientists, including 20 scientists from 10 countries in addition to Japan, participated in the symposium and satellite meetings and were engaged in intensive discussions of the issues mentioned above. New and revised academic cooperation agreements were signed with several sister universities, and a number of prospective joint research projects were successfully negotiated. The future direction of the GCOE Program in Nagasaki University thus has been clearly manifested during the symposium.

The present proceedings is a compilation of papers presented at the First International Symposium on the Establishment of a New Discipline, "Medical Care for Hibakusha," including two-day satellite symposia. The symposia featured presentations by international experts on the topics of 1) atomic bomb disease medicine, 2) international radiation health sciences, and 3) radiation basic life sciences. Furthermore, special issues of radiation risk management including mental health care and cancer research were included.

We would like to express our sincere gratitude to all contributors for their fascinating and valuable papers. Through continuous academic cooperation and concerted efforts in further investigations of the deleterious effects of ionizing radiation on human health, especially at low dose and low dose-rate, we greatly hope to create a new disciplinary research field of comprehensive radiation health risk control.

The Editors

Greetings

It is a great honor and pleasure for me to extend my cordial greetings on the occasion of the First International Symposium on the Establishment of a New Discipline, "Medical Care for Hibakusha." As the President of Nagasaki University, I consider this symposium very important for the following three reasons.

First of all, this is the remarkable result of a continuous endeavor in Radiation Medical Sciences by the research project leader, Professor Shunichi Yamashita, and his trusted staff of the Graduate School of Biomedical Sciences. Their study received the highest rating in the interim assessment of the "21st COE Program" from 2002 to 2006, and its high standard has already been widely recognized. I am very proud that they have established a global research network in Radiation Medical Sciences with research institutes around the world, including Chernobyl and Kazakhstan and internationally renowned organizations such as WHO, and that their various achievements in international medical initiatives have come to be appreciated with the help of this strong network.

The second reason for the significance of our symposium is that our subject in this field of research was "Interdiscipline, Combination, and New Area." Although Nagasaki University consists of eight faculties and one research institute, it has no departments in basic subjects such as literature, law, and science, in contrast to other large-scale national university corporations. Its undergraduate and graduate schools concentrate mainly on applied science. However, we have never taken this fact to be a negative factor. Rather, we have always thought of this as an opportunity and have tried to create new disciplines crossing the borders between established learning fields, thus taking up the challenge to develop Nagasaki's unique and traditionally fostered "forever enterprising spirit." I believe that our mission is to put into practice our philosophy as a "center for the transmission of intellectual information" by creating the cutting edge in science and continuously conveying our achievements to the world. Winning the "FY 2007 Global COE Program" will certainly be one of the driving forces to promote that mission. The Japan Society for the Promotion of Science pointed out that "Research needs to be reinforced in both its social science aspect and its physical chemistry aspect by an interdisciplinary point of view, and it also needs further elaboration and deliberation to become a firmer base for educational research." With this advice, I have realized that there are still more issues in which we have to make improvements.

Finally, this research originated in the self-sacrificing efforts of our seniors and forerunners who devoted themselves to the treatment of radiation victims during the terrible devastation by the atomic bomb. Nagasaki University first lost 897, and then up to 1000, precious lives of faculty and administrative staff and students in Nagasaki Medical College and various predecessor schools, respectively. The University lived through this together with the people of Nagasaki and supported them or was supported by them when the whole city was trying to recover from the atomic disasters. The research field "Global Strategic Center for Radiation Health Risk Control" emerged from Nagasaki's recovery and development. In that sense, we must be grateful to the citizens of Nagasaki.

Yet, it is also true that we cannot feel genuine "joy" because we all know the background from which this research subject was born. We are fully aware of our responsibilities as a university in Nagasaki, having experienced and inherited the tragedy of the atomic bomb. On winning the "Global COE Program" in the year of the 150th anniversary of the School of Medicine, Nagasaki University remains determined to make further contributions to local society and the world, ever recalling the calamity of 62 years ago.

I sincerely hope that you will all take advantage of this invaluable opportunity and spend your spare time during and after the symposium enjoying Nagasaki, the only city that was open to the world throughout Japan's period of isolation.

Hiroshi Saito, M.D., Ph.D.
President of Nagasaki University
January 2008

Addresses

National Institute of Radiological Sciences, Chiba, Japan

Yoshikaru Yonekura, President

President Saito, Professor Yamashita, distinguished guests, ladies, and gentlemen. It is indeed my great pleasure and honor to address these congratulatory remarks to Nagasaki University and all members of the global COE program at the opening session of this symposium. This global COE program, "Global Strategic Center for Radiation Health Risk Control," is an extension of the previous program, which concluded last year with great success.

Nagasaki University has accumulated outstanding scientific results on atomic bomb survivors in Japan and gained extensive experience in providing medical aid for people exposed to radiation. Meanwhile, the National Institute of Radiological Sciences (NIRS) was initially founded in 1957 to conduct comprehensive research on radiation and human health. During the past half-century, we have devoted our major efforts in two important research fields: medical use of radiation in different areas from diagnosis to treatment of the patient for human health and health protection from radiation. Because of the common interest in these research fields, Nagasaki University and NIRS reached a comprehensive agreement 2 years ago for mutual collaboration and cooperation in research and education as well as for information exchange.

Because of the increasing demand for uses of radiation, health risk assessment and medical care of radiation injury will be the most important problems in modern society. The proposed program by Nagasaki University is definitely the means to solve these problems. We strongly support the activities of Nagasaki University to establish an international network for radiation medical sciences.

I believe this symposium will lead the initiative toward the aim of the program, and we look forward to continuing our collaborative efforts to realize our common mission.

Thank you for your attention.

Radiation Effects Research Foundation, Hiroshima and Nagasaki, Japan

Toshiteru Okubo, Chairman

I would like to start my speech by offering sincerest congratulations on the national government's approval of the Nagasaki University Global Center of Excellence (COE) program, which will embark on a second 5-year term starting this year, following the first term, which lasted through 2007. Nagasaki University and the Radiation Effects Research Foundation (RERF) enjoy a close relationship and have entered into an agreement on comprehensive collaboration in research and education. Therefore, RERF will make every effort to cooperate with this Global COE program.

The year 2007 marked RERF's 60th anniversary, starting with the 1947 establishment of Atomic Bomb Casualty Commission ABCC. I would like to use this opportunity to speak about the current status and future projections of our cohorts, which have been continuously followed up from the days of ABCC, as well as about RERF's future.

Of the lifespan follow-up cohort (LSS cohort), established in 1950 and consisting of approximately 120 000 persons, 50 000 are still alive, with a mean age of 74 years. According to age at time of bombing (ATB), the follow-up of those over age 40 ATB was virtually completed as of 2003. However, more than 80% of those who were under the age of 10 ATB are still alive, and estimation based on 2005 life tables indicates that in this young age group 20% of the men and 40% of the women will still be alive in 2030, or around 20 years from now, requiring more than 40 years to complete the observations.

Approximately 24 000 subjects were selected from the LSS cohort and assigned to undergo biennial health examinations starting in 1958 (thus making up the AHS cohort). The participation rate has been high, and more than 70% of those eligible and still alive continue to participate 50 years after initiation of the study. Completion of this AHS cohort's lifetime follow-up will clarify the lifetime incidence of diseases and associated death information, which will enable RERF to study mechanisms of onset of specific diseases using the blood samples obtained from the cohort members during their health examinations and thereby reaching back over their entire lifetimes.

The study on death causes and cancer incidence among the 77 000 children of atomic bomb survivors is ongoing, and it is estimated that more than 60 years will be required to complete the lifetime follow-up of all such individuals. RERF also just completed the first cycle of its clinical study in 2006, with the examination of 12 000 of the atomic bomb survivor children. RERF plans to continue the follow-up of these participants. When realized, the planned lifetime follow-up of the health effects in this population will mark the first such achievement in human history, and it will be of great value in that there will likely never be another, similar opportunity.

As already stated, there will be a gradual natural decrease in the number of surviving cohort members with the passage of time. If we adhere to our current organizational objective of conducting research on the health effects in atomic bomb survivors (and their children), the controversy over the abolishment of RERF could become a very real possibility in light of personnel strength and other issues within 30 years at maximum, even if some cohort members were still alive. Moreover, considering that an organization without future plans cannot attract outstanding human resources, RERF is now standing at a crossroads. Within the next 10 years or so, we will have to determine the nature of a succeeding organization to RERF that can continue operating on a permanent basis. To accomplish this, consideration should be paid to the following requirements:

- To become a "Center of Excellence" that is capable of providing training to researchers/practical specialists in the field of radiation effects research.
- To conduct research on both radiation and nonradiation effects for many years to come that utilizes the longitudinal, stored biospecimens from the AHS cohort in the clinical study lasting more than 50 years.
- To conduct research and educational programs that utilize epidemiological research data accumulated by ABCC/RERF.
- To create close affiliations with the activities of other international organizations.

RERF's scientific achievements, including its efforts toward the establishment of radiation protection standards, are highly acclaimed as a significant contribution to all of humanity. Such achievements are the fruits of cooperation between the people of the United States and Japan and, above all, would not have been possible without cooperation from the atomic bomb survivors. This long-lasting radiation effects research in Nagasaki and Hiroshima, which has been supported by many people, therefore, should never be discontinued, as it has become a symbol of the everlasting hopes of the atomic bomb survivors and people of the two countries for world peace and the abolition of nuclear weapons.

To seek the most appropriate pathway to the future directions just mentioned, RERF will continue to keep this good collaboration and would like to expand it to a new area with the University of Nagasaki in which both parties will benefit. We are particularly interested in the start of the Global COE program of University of Nagasaki from this future perspective. Finally, I would like to conclude my talk with sincere congratulations to the new Global COE program.

Sasakawa Memorial Health Foundation, Tokyo, Japan

Kenzo Kiikuni, Chairman

It is a great pleasure for me to be here, for the second time, to participate in this Symposium celebrating the selection of Nagasaki University as one of the Japan's Center of Excellence (COE) Programs of the Japanese Government. I would like to congratulate the University, for this is the second time for them to be selected. It is clear evidence of continuous efforts on the part of the University in the fields of scientific research, human resource development, and international collaboration, following the previous COE program.

Historically, Nagasaki was the only Japanese city that was allowed to open windows to foreign countries during the period of national isolation, *Sakoku*. Since the opening of Japan to the world, Japan has spent much energy to collect information from the outside world. It stands to reason that a university in the city with such a historical background now aims for global activity and plans to build a global strategic center for radiation risk control. Nagasaki University is today ready to transmit information to the world.

In 1990, our foundation was asked by the then Soviet government to help people affected by the Chernobyl accident. Our foundation had no experience in radiation medicine and did not know much about Chernobyl and its aftermath. But we thought perhaps we would be able to help somewhat based on Japan's experiences of Hiroshima and Nagasaki. Being laypeople in this field, we consulted Dr. Itsuzo Shigematsu, then the Chairman of Radiation Effects Research Foundation, a world-prominent scientist and leading figure in this field. He introduced us to the experts of RERF, Hiroshima University and Nagasaki University.

In this project, our primary aim was to carry out the health screening of children living in the areas affected by the Chernobyl Nuclear Power Station Accident, because we witnessed unnecessary anxiety among mothers in these areas and we hoped to alleviate them by determining the actual health status of the children. Five cities in Russia, Ukraine, and Belarus were chosen as our screening "centers."

In starting the project, we had two principles. First, it should be such a cooperation that our counterpart(s) (that is, the Soviet Union, or later, Russia, Ukraine, and Belarus) would be able to continue the activities on their own in the following years. We thought one-way assistance was not sufficient. Second, our Chernobyl project needed to be carried out with scientifically solid methods. For this, we were privileged to have the collaboration of professors from Nagasaki University as well as Hiroshima University.

The project ended in 2001, achieving the health screening of more than 200 000 children. One of the important findings was an extraordinary high prevalence, compared to Japan or Western countries, of thyroid cancer among young children, as made clear also by IAEA. This finding was made possible by the continuous efforts of Professor Nagataki and Professor Yamashita. We had immeasurable cooperation from Nagasaki University. More than 100 scientists from Russia, Belarus, and Ukraine had training at this University.

After the screening project, our Foundation joined in establishing the Chernobyl Tissue and Data Bank with EC, NCI, and WHO. Professor Yamashita, who chairs this opening ceremony, is acting as our representative in this project.

It is my great joy to witness that some projects our Foundation had initiated, such as the health screening of children in Russia, Ukraine, and Belarus in 1990, or the Chernobyl Tissue Bank project, have produced seed and are thus well incorporated in the Global COE program of Nagasaki University.

In closing, I wish you all success for the continued global activities of this program.

Thank you.

Japan Radiation Research Society, Hiroshima, Japan

Kenji Kamiya, Chairman

On behalf of the Japan Radiation Research Society, I would like to say a few words of greeting. First of all, I would like to extend my heartfelt congratulations on the success of the G-COE program and this international symposium.

Nagasaki University achieved remarkable results on a health survey of the Chernobyl nuclear power plant victims and residents living in the area of Semipalatinsk nuclear test site in the 21st Century COE Program. In particular, Nagasaki University is taking on a role as a world leader in studies of childhood thyroid cancer that occurred after the accident at the Chernobyl nuclear power plant. Also, their medical services for exposed residents have been highly appreciated around the world. I am excited that Nagasaki University was newly chosen as one of the GCOE programs in recognition of their distinguished efforts and results.

The Japan Radiation Research Society is the nation's largest academy in the studies of radiation effect. We are internationally active as a core member of IARR, including acting as chairman and vice-deputy chairman of IARR. Japan has taken a key role in studies of radiation effects to the human body as the only country that has experienced nuclear bombings, and Nagasaki and Hiroshima have been the hubs of these studies. I am proud that both Nagasaki and Hiroshima Universities, which belong to the Japan Radiation Research Society, have played an active part together as one of the COE programs, which is a significant governmental policy for education and research in Japan.

Considering the fact that radiation research enter a new phase through progress in science of "genome damage and cellular response," I believe that as the distinguished leader, Nagasaki University has embarked on new activities now with just the right timing. I hope your activities become an accelerator for fostering young researchers of Japan Radiation Research Society and increasingly develop our country's radiation research.

I would like you to accept my message of good wishes on the occasion of this memorable international symposium.

Thank you very much.

Research Institute for Radiation Biology and Medicine, Hiroshima University, Hiroshima, Japan

Fumio Suzuki, Director

Professor Tomonaga, Professor Yamashita, distinguished guests, ladies, and gentlemen, it is my great honor to be invited to the First International Symposium on the Establishment of a New Discipline "Medical Care for Hibakusha." On behalf of the Research Institute for Radiation Biology and Medicine, Hiroshima University,

I would like to express my sincere congratulation on the foundation of the Nagasaki University Global COE program entitled "Global Strategic Centre for Radiation Health Risk Control."

The Research Institute for Radiation Biology and Medicine was established as a key research organization of Hiroshima University in April 1961. Since then, the Institute has consistently focused on research such as radiation damage and related diseases, and the analysis and development of medical treatment of diseases and injuries of atomic bomb survivors.

In 2002, the Institute underwent a drastic organizational reform so as to clarify the mechanisms of radiation injuries that cause diseases using various new techniques of genome science, as well as to develop the new methods of tissue regeneration using pluripotent stem cells for acute radiation injury.

Based on a policy of the Japanese Ministry of Education, Culture, Sports, Science and Technology, the 21st Century COE Program was established in 2002 to cultivate a competitive academic environment among universities by giving targeted support and to create world-class research and education centers. Hiroshima University has five programs that have been adopted as COE research projects during the past 3 years. As one of the current programs, our 21st Century COE Program entitled "Research Center for Advanced Radiation Casualty Medicine" was adopted in 2003 in the field of medical sciences, and has been highly praised for its uniqueness in being created based on the research property of Hiroshima. Our ultimate goal is the achievement of a comprehensive medical system that is capable of dealing with all types of radiation injury on the basis of radiation dose estimated from the information of the genome damage.

The Global COE Program should be prepared to provide crucial aid to 21st Century COE Programs that produce excellent results to create centers of excellence of the world's highest order. To create a world center in the integrative promotion of radiation medical research, we are currently planning a program with the members of the 21st Century COE Program. The aim of our plan is to establish the COE as a world-leading research program through the further development of the studies that have been extensively carried out for 5 years.

Hiroshima University has been working in close cooperation with Nagasaki University on various research subjects regarding the biological effects of radiation and its application for prevention of health disorders induced by radiation. However, the Global COE Program seeks to build core education and research center in cooperation with more related universities and research institutions, and we believe that our plan has not yet fully been able to fulfill the role demanded by the Program.

I am convinced that the Global COE Program of Nagasaki University will make a great contribution to the medical care of Hibakusha and to radiation life science.

I hope that you continuously exchange knowledge during the symposium for further collaboration and encourage us to achieve our common goals.

Thank you for your attention.

Nagasaki University Graduate School of Biomedical Sciences, Nagasaki, Japan

Masao Tomonaga, Dean and *Former Leader of 21st Century COE Program*

On behalf of the Graduated School of Biomedical Sciences, Nagasaki University, I would like express my sincere congratulation to all members and participating doctors and scientists of the new G-COE program for its success to have been selected by the second phase of the Japanese Government's COE Program Budget.

The concept of the new G-COE Program and the title "Global Strategic Center for Radiation Health Risk Control" were generated by the newly selected COE members, being based on the outcome of the previous 21st Century COE Program "International Consortium for Radiation Life Science and Medical Care for Hibakusha."

Here as the former leader of 21st Century COE, I am most grateful to all member institutions, professors, and investigators for participating the International Consortium and conducting intensive collaborations for 5 years since 2002 to 2006 with Nagasaki University investigators. I am very glad to see most of them also participating in the new Global COE Program and attending this symposium.

Long-lasting radiation-induced cancer risks were clearly demonstrated by the first COE Projects in two epidemiological fields, namely, the atomic bomb and the Chernobyl accident. This most important observation provides a number of questions concerning radiation-related carcinogenesis or leukemogenesis: (1) what is the mechanism of the lifelong risk for cancer? (2) how low a dose is meaningful? (3) what molecular mechanisms are responsible for the early genetic instability and cancer development as the end result? (4) what kind of medical system is suitable for the early diagnosis and curative treatment of Hibakushas' cancers? (5) how should we handle multiple cancers in a single Hibakusha? and (6) how can we introduce molecular targeting drugs to refractory cancers? And, finally, there is a serious, but reasonable, question raised by radiation victims: Is cancer development preventable?

Conventional and molecular epidemiology is still an important tool for us; however, we need to develop new strategic systems to give answers to these questions. Actual medical relief from many types of cancer and leukemia is a real goal of the next Global COE Program.

Finally, I believe that with strong leadership by Professor Yamashita and a high level of collaboration by new, young COE members, participating scientists, and graduate students, we will see enormous progress in understanding the long-term effects of radiation on the human body and psychology and in developing the methodology to overcome radiation risk.

Contents

Acknowledgments V
Organizing Committee VI
Group photograph VII
Preface IX
Greetings XI
Addresses XIII
Contributors XXVI

Overview of the Global COE Program

Global Strategic Center for Radiation Health Risk Control
    S. Yamashita 3

Overview of the Lectures

Discussion on Points of Radiation Safety and the Scope of
The University of Tokyo Global COE Program
    T. Kosako and T. Iimoto 13

Network System for Radiation Emergency Medicine in Japan and
the Role of Hiroshima University
    K. Kamiya... 23

Non-DNA-Targeted Effects and Low-Dose Radiation Risk
    B.D. Michael... 29

Update from the Chernobyl Tissue Bank: Effect of Latency on
Different Types of Thyroid Cancer Post-Chernobyl
    G.A. Thomas.. 34

Current Risk Estimate of Radiation-Related Cancer and Our Insight
into the Future
    M. Kai and N. Ban 43

Atomic Bomb Disease Medicine

Introduction of Atomic Bomb Disease Medical Research
in Global COE Program
   K. Tsukasaki, M. Nakashima, and N. Matsuda 51

The Offspring of Atomic Bomb Survivors: Cancer and
Non-Cancer Mortality and Cancer Incidence
   A. Suyama, S. Izumi, K. Koyama, R. Sakata, N. Nishi, M. Soda,
   E.J. Grant, Y. Shimizu, K. Furukawa, H.M. Cullings, F. Kasagi,
   and K. Kodama 57

Ischemic Heart Disease Among Atomic Bomb Survivors:
Possible Mechanism(s) Linking Ischemic Heart Disease
and Radiation Exposure
   M. Akahoshi.. 63

Leukemia, Lymphoma, and Multiple Myeloma Incidence
in the LSS Cohort: 1950–2001
   W.-L. Hsu, M. Soda, N. Nishi, D. Preston, S. Funamoto,
   M. Tomonaga, M. Iwanaga, A. Suyama, and F. Kasagi............. 69

Follow-Up Study of 78 Healthy Exposed Atomic Bomb Survivors for
35 Years in Hiroshima, with Special Reference to Multiple Cancers
   N. Kamada 74

International Radiation Health Sciences

Research Activities and Projects Within a Framework of
International Radiation Health Sciences Research
   N. Takamura, A. Ohtsuru, H. Ozawa, and S. Yamashita 81

Age and Prognosis: Do Adjuvant Therapies Influence the Real
Prognosis?
   R.C.F. Leonard, M. Morishita, and G.A. Thomas 90

Mortality of the Chernobyl Emergency Workers: Analysis of
Dose Response by Cohort Studies Covering Follow-Up Period of
1992–2006
   V.K. Ivanov, S.Y. Chekin, V.V. Kashcheyev, M.A. Maksioutov,
   and A.F. Tsyb... 95

Twenty Years After Chernobyl: Implications for Radiation Health
Risk Control
   Y. Shibata.. 103

Fallout Exposure of the Population and Thyroid Nodular Diseases
Z.S. Zhumadilov and A.M. Orymbaeva 113

Radiation Basic Life Sciences, Part 1

Higher-Order Chromatin Structure and Nontargeted Effects
K. Suzuki, M. Yamauchi, Y. Oka, and S. Yamashita 123

p53 Dependency of Delayed and Untargeted Recombination in
Mouse Embryos Fertilized by Irradiated Sperm
O. Niwa 127

The Yin and Yang of Low-Dose Radiobiology
T.K. Hei, H. Zhou, and V.N. Ivanov............................ 135

Induction and Persistence of Cytogenetic Damage in Mouse Splenocytes
Following Whole-Body X-Irradiation Analysed by Fluorescence In Situ
Hybridisation. V. Heterogeneity/Chromosome Specificity
M.P. Hande and A.T. Natarajan 143

Cancer Research

Molecular Understanding of RET/PTC-Mediated Thyroid Carcinogenesis
Y.S. Jo, D.W. Kim, M.H. Lee, S.J. Kim, J.H. Hwang, and M. Shong ... 153

Molecular Prediction of Therapeutic Response and Adverse Effect of
Chemotherapy in Breast Cancer
Y. Miki.. 177

Multiple Roles of NBS1 for Genotoxic and Nongenotoxic Stresses
K. Komatsu, M. Shimada, K. Tsuchida, K. Nakamura, H. Yanagihara,
and J. Kobayashi 183

Radiation Basic Life Sciences, Part 2

The DNA Damage Response in Nontargeted Cells
K.M. Prise, G. Schettino, and S. Burdak-Rothkamm 193

The Role of Telomere Dysfunction in Driving Genomic Instability
S.M. Bailey, E.S. Williams, and R.L. Ullrich 199

Secretory Clusterin Is a Marker of Tumor Progression Regulated
by IGF-1 and Wnt Signaling Pathways
Y. Zou, E.M. Goetz, M. Suzuki, and D.A. Boothman 204

Target of Radiation Carcinogenesis Is Protein: Becoming Triploid Is
Proximate Cause of Cell Transformation
    M. Watanabe and H. Yoshii.................................... 212

Adult Stem Cells, the Barker Hypothesis, Epigenetic Events,
and Low-Level Radiation Effects
    J.E. Trosko and K. Suzuki..................................... 216

Combined Effect of Ionizing Radiation and N-Ethyl-N-Nitrosourea
on Mutation Induction and Lymphoma Development
    K. Yamauchi, S. Kakinuma, A. Nakata, T. Imaoka, T. Takabatake,
    M. Nishimura, and Y. Shimada................................. 227

γ-Ray-Induced Mouse Thymic Lymphomas: Bcl11b Inactivation and
Prelymphoma Cells
    R. Kominami, H. Ohi, K. Kamimura, M. Maruyama, T. Yamamoto,
    K. Takaku, S. Morita, R. Go, and Y. Mishima 232

Radiation Risk Management

Framework of Radiation Safety Management in Japan:
Laws, Administrative Agencies, and Supporting Associations
    N. Matsuda, M. Yoshida, H. Takao, and M. Miura 243

Background Radiation Dose to the Population Around
the Kudankulam Nuclear Power Plant
    S. Selvasekarapandian, J. Malathi, G.M. Brahmanandhan, and
    D. Khanna 248

International Cooperation in Radiation Emergency Medical Preparedness:
Establishment of a Medical Network in Asia
    M. Akashi... 254

Disaster and Mental Health

Long-Term Biopsychosocial Consequences of Disaster: Focus
on Atomic Bomb Survivors
    N. Shinfuku 263

Health Status of Children Exposed to the Chernobyl Accident In Utero:
Observations in 1989–2003 and the Implications for Prioritizing
Prophylactic Programs
    N.A. Korol and Y. Shibata 271

Psychological Consequences More Than Half a Century After the
Nagasaki Atomic Bombing
  Y. Suzuki, A. Tsutsumi, T. Izutsu, and Y. Kim 277

Radiation and Cancer

Significance of Oncogene Amplifications in Breast Cancer in
Atomic Bomb Survivors: Associations with Radiation Exposure
and Histological Grade
  S. Miura, M. Nakashima, H. Kondo, M. Ito, S. Meirmanov,
  T. Hayashi, M. Soda, and I. Sekine 285

Paracrine Interactions Between Normal, but Not Cancer, Epithelial
and Normal Mesenchymal Cells Attenuate Radiation-Induced
DNA Damage
  V.A. Saenko, Y. Nakazawa, T.I. Rogounovitch, K. Suzuki,
  N. Mitsutake, M. Matsuse, Y. Oka, and S. Yamashita 294

Chernobyl and Semipalatinsk Nuclear Test Sites: Related Issues

Thyroid Cancer in Ukraine After the Chernobyl Accident: Incidence,
Pathology, Treatment, and Molecular Biology
  M. Tronko, T. Bogdanova, I. Likhtarev, I. Komisarenko,
  A. Kovalenko, V. Markov, V. Tereshchenko, L. Voskoboynyk,
  L. Zurnadzhy, V. Shpak, L. Gulak, R. Elisei, C. Romei,
  and A. Pinchera 305

Current Trends in Incidence and Mortality from Thyroid Cancer
in Belarus
  P.I. Bespalchuk, Y.E. Demidchik, E.P. Demidchik, V.A. Saenko,
  and S. Yamashita 317

The Health Status of the Population in the Semey Region and
Scientifically Proven Measures to Improve It
  T.K. Rakhypbekov 322

Nuclear Explosions and Public Health Development
  A. Akanov, S. Meirmanov, A. Indershiev, A. Musahanova,
  and S. Yamashita 328

Subject Index 335

Contributors

Akahoshi, Masazumi
Radiation Effects Research Foundation, Nagasaki, Japan

Akanov, Aikan
Institute of Public Health, Almaty, Kazakhstan

Akashi, Makoto
National Institute of Radiological Sciences (NIRS), Chiba, Japan

Bailey, Susan M.
Cancer SuperCluster, Colorado State University, Fort Collins, CO, USA
Colorado State University, Fort Collins, CO, USA
College of Veterinary Medicine and Biological Sciences, Colorado State University, Fort Collins, CO, USA

Ban, Nobuhiko
Oita University of Nursing and Health Sciences, Oita, Japan

Bespalchuk, Pavel I.
Belarusian State Medical University, Minsk, Belarus

Bogdanova, Tetyana
Institute of Endocrinology and Metabolism of Academy of Medical Sciences of Ukraine, Kyiv, Ukraine

Boothman, David A.
Simmons Comprehensive Cancer Center, University of Texas Southwestern Medical Center Dallas, TX, USA

Brahmanandhan, Gopalganapathi M.
Bharathiar University, Coimbatore, India

Burdak-Rothkamm, Susanne
Centre for Cancer Research and Cell Biology, Queen's University Belfast, Belfast, UK

Chekin, Sergey Yu
Medical Radiological Research Center of Russian Academy of Medical Sciences, Obninsk, Kaluga Region, Russia

Cullings, Harry M.
Radiation Effects Research Foundation, Hiroshima, Japan

Demidchik, Eugene P.
Belarusian State Medical University, Minsk, Belarus
Thyroid Cancer Center, Minsk, Belarus

Demidchik, Yuri E.
Belarusian State Medical University, Minsk, Belarus
Thyroid Cancer Center, Minsk, Belarus

Elisei, Rossella
Pisa University, Pisa, Italy

Funamoto, Sachiyo
Radiation Effects Research Foundation, Hiroshima, Japan

Furukawa, Kyoji
Radiation Effects Research Foundation, Hiroshima, Japan

Go, Rieka
Graduate School of Medical and Dental Sciences, Transdisciplinary Research Center, Niigata University, Niigata, Japan

Goetz, Eva M.
Simmons Comprehensive Cancer Center, University of Texas Southwestern Medical Center Dallas, TX, USA

Grant, Eric J.
Radiation Effects Research Foundation, Hiroshima, Japan

Gulak, Lyudmyla
Institute of Oncology and Radiology of Academy of Medical Sciences of Ukraine, Kyiv, Ukraine

Hande, M. Prakash
Yong Loo Lin School of Medicine, National University of Singapore, Singapore

Hayashi, Tomayoshi
Nagasaki University Hospital, Nagasaki, Japan

Hei, Tom K.
Center for Radiological Research, College of Physicians and Surgeons
Mailman School of Public Health, Columbia University, New York, USA

Hsu, Wan-Ling
Radiation Effects Research Foundation, Hiroshima, Japan

Hwang, Jung Hwan
Laboratory of Endocrine Cell Biology, Chungnam National University School of Medicine, Daejeon, Korea

Iimoto, Takeshi
The University of Tokyo, Tokyo, Japan

Imaoka, Tatsuhiko
Experimental Radiobiology for Children's Health Research Group, National Institute of Radiological Sciences, Chiba, Japan

Indershiev, Arslan
Institute of Public Health, Almaty, Kazakhstan

Ito, Masahiro
National Hospital Organization Nagasaki Medical Center, Nagasaki, Japan

Ivanov, Victor K.
Medical Radiological Research Center of Russian Academy of Medical Sciences, Obninsk, Kaluga Region, Russia

Ivanov, Vladimir N.
Mailman School of Public Health, Columbia University, New York, USA

Iwanaga, Masako
Atomic-Bomb Disease Institute, Nagasaki University Graduate School of Biomedical Sciences, Nagasaki, Japan

Izumi, Shizue
Faculty of Engineering, Oita University, Oita, Japan

Izutsu, Takashi
National Center of Neurology and Psychiatry, National Institute of Mental Health, Tokyo, Japan

Jo, Young Suk
Laboratory of Endocrine Cell Biology, Chungnam National University School of Medicine, Daejeon, Korea

Kai, Michiaki
Oita University of Nursing and Health Sciences, Oita, Japan

Kakinuma, Shizuko
Experimental Radiobiology for Children's Health Research Group, National Institute of Radiological Sciences, Chiba, Japan

Kamada, Nanao
Hiroshima Atomic Bomb Survivors Relief Foundation (HABREF), Hiroshima, Japan

Kamimura, Kenya
Graduate School of Medical and Dental Sciences, Transdisciplinary Research Center, Niigata University, Niigata, Japan

Kamiya, Kenji
Research Institute for Radiation Biology and Medicine, Center for the Promotion of Radiation Emergency Medicine, Hiroshima University, Hiroshima, Japan

Kasagi, Fumiyoshi
Radiation Effects Research Foundation, Hiroshima, Japan

Kashcheyev, Valery V.
Medical Radiological Research Center of Russian Academy of Medical Sciences, Obninsk, Kaluga Region, Russia

Khanna, David
Bharathiar University, Coimbatore, India

Kim, Dong Wook
Laboratory of Endocrine Cell Biology, Chungnam National University School of Medicine, Daejeon, Korea

Kim, Soung Jung
Laboratory of Endocrine Cell Biology, Chungnam National University School of Medicine, Daejeon, Korea

Kim, Yoshiharu
National Center of Neurology and Psychiatry, National Institute of Mental Health, Tokyo, Japan

Kobayashi, Junya
Radiation Biology Center, Kyoto University, Kyoto, Japan

Kodama, Kazunori
Radiation Effects Research Foundation, Hiroshima, Japan

Komatsu, Kenshi
Radiation Biology Center, Kyoto University, Kyoto, Japan

Kominami, Ryo
Graduate School of Medical and Dental Sciences, Transdisciplinary Research Center, Niigata University, Niigata, Japan

Komisarenko, Ihor
Institute of Endocrinology and Metabolism of Academy of Medical Sciences of Ukraine, Kyiv, Ukraine

Kondo, Hisayoshi
Atomic Bomb Disease Institute, Nagasaki University Graduate School of Biomedical Sciences, Nagasaki, Japan

Korol, Nataliya A.
Research Center for Radiation Medicine, Academy of Medical Sciences of Ukraine, Kiev, Ukraine

Kosako, Toshiso
School of Engineering, The University of Tokyo, Ibaraki, Japan

Kovalenko, Andriy
Institute of Endocrinology and Metabolism of Academy of Medical Sciences of Ukraine, Kyiv, Ukraine

Koyama, Kojiro
Sanyo Hospital, Fukuyama, Japan

Lee, Min Hee
Laboratory of Endocrine Cell Biology, Chungnam National University School of Medicine, Daejeon, Korea

Leonard, Robert C.F.
Imperial College School of Medicine, Hammersmith Hospital, London, United Kingdom

Likhtarev, Ilya
Research Center for Radiation Medicine of Academy of Medical Sciences of Ukraine, Kyiv, Ukraine

Maksioutov, Marat A.
Medical Radiological Research Center of Russian Academy of Medical Sciences, Obninsk, Kaluga Region, Russia

Malathi, Jeyapandian
Bharathiar University, Coimbatore, India

Markov, Valentyn
Institute of Endocrinology and Metabolism of Academy of Medical Sciences of Ukraine, Kyiv, Ukraine

Maruyama, Masaki
Graduate School of Medical and Dental Sciences, Transdisciplinary Research Center, Niigata University, Niigata, Japan

Matsuda, Naoki
Center for Frontier Life Sciences, Nagasaki University, Nagasaki, Japan
Nagasaki University Graduate School of Biomedical Sciences, Nagasaki, Japan

Matsuse, Michiko
Atomic Bomb Disease Institute, Nagasaki University Graduate School of Biomedical Sciences, Nagasaki, Japan

Meirmanov, Serik
Atomic Bomb Disease Institute, Nagasaki University Graduate School of Biomedical Sciences, Nagasaki, Japan

Michael, Barry D.
University of Oxford, Gray Cancer Institute, Middlesex, United Kingdom

Miki, Yoshio
Medical Research Institute, Tokyo Medical and Dental University, Tokyo, Japan
The Cancer Institute of JFCR, Tokyo, Japan

Mishima, Yukio
Graduate School of Medical and Dental Sciences, Transdisciplinary Research Center, Niigata University, Niigata, Japan

Mitsutake, Norisato
Atomic Bomb Disease Institute, Nagasaki University Graduate School of Biomedical Sciences, Nagasaki, Japan

Miura, Miwa
Center for Frontier Life Sciences, Nagasaki University, Nagasaki, Japan

Miura, Shiro
Atomic Bomb Disease Institute, Nagasaki University Graduate School of Biomedical Sciences, Nagasaki, Japan

Morishita, Mariko
Imperial College School of Medicine, Hammersmith Hospital, London, United Kingdom

Morita, Shin-ichi
Graduate School of Medical and Dental Sciences, Transdisciplinary Research Center, Niigata University, Niigata, Japan

Musahanova, Aigul
Semey Oncology Center, Semey, Kazakhstan

Nakamura, Kyosuke
Radiation Biology Center, Kyoto University, Kyoto, Japan

Nakashima, Masahiro
Atomic Bomb Disease Institute, Nagasaki University School of Biomedical Sciences, Nagasaki, Japan

Nakata, Akifumi
Experimental Radiobiology for Children's Health Research Group, National Institute of Radiological Sciences, Chiba, Japan

Nakazawa, Yuka
Atomic Bomb Disease Institute, Nagasaki University Graduate School of Biomedical Sciences, Nagasaki, Japan

Natarajan, A.T.
University of Tuscia, Viterbo, Italy

Nishi, Nobuo
Radiation Effects Research Foundation, Hiroshima, Japan

Nishimura, Mayumi
Experimental Radiobiology for Children's Health Research Group, National Institute of Radiological Sciences, Chiba, Japan

Niwa, Ohtsura
National Institute of Radiological Sciences, Chiba, Japan

Ohi, Hiroyuki
Graduate School of Medical and Dental Sciences, Transdisciplinary Research Center, Niigata University, Niigata, Japan

Ohtsuru, Akira
Takashi Nagai Memorial International Hibakusha Medical Center, Nagasaki University Graduate School of Biomedical Sciences, Nagasaki, Japan

Oka, Yasuyoshi
Atomic Bomb Disease Institute, Nagasaki University Graduate School of Biomedical Sciences, Nagasaki, Japan

Orymbaeva, Assem M.
Semey State Medical Academy, Semey, Kazakhstan

Ozawa, Hiroki
Nagasaki University Graduate School of Biomedical Sciences, Nagasaki, Japan

Pinchera, Aldo
Pisa University, Pisa, Italy

Preston, Dale
Hirosoft International, Eureka, CA, USA

Prise, Kevin M.
Centre for Cancer Research and Cell Biology, Queen's University Belfast, Belfast, UK

Rakhypbekov, Tolebay K.
Semey State Medical Academy, Republic of Kazakhstan

Rogounovitch, Tatiana I.
Atomic Bomb Disease Institute, Nagasaki University Graduate School of Biomedical Sciences, Nagasaki, Japan

Romei, Cristina
Pisa University, Pisa, Italy

Saenko, Vladimir A.
Atomic Bomb Disease Institute, Nagasaki University Graduate School of Biomedical Sciences, Nagasaki, Japan
Medical Radiological Research Center RAMS, Obninsk, Russian Federation

Sakata, Ritsu
Radiation Effects Research Foundation, Hiroshima, Japan

Schettino, Giuseppe
Centre for Cancer Research and Cell Biology, Queen's University Belfast, Belfast, UK

Sekine, Ichiro
Atomic Bomb Disease Institute, Nagasaki University Graduate School of Biomedical Sciences, Nagasaki, Japan

Selvasekarapandian, Subramaniyan
Bharathiar University, Coimbatore, India

Shibata, Yoshisada
Atomic Bomb Disease Institute, Nagasaki University Graduate School of Biomedical Sciences, Nagasaki, Japan

Shimada, Mikio
Radiation Biology Center, Kyoto University, Kyoto, Japan

Shimada, Yoshiya
Experimental Radiobiology for Children's Health Research Group, National Institute of Radiological Sciences, Chiba, Japan

Shimizu, Yukiko
Radiation Effects Research Foundation, Hiroshima, Japan

Shinfuku, Naotaka
School of Human Sciences, Seinan Gakuin University, Fukuoka, Japan

Shong, Minho
Laboratory of Endocrine Cell Biology, Chungnam National University School of Medicine, Daejeon, Korea

Shpak, Victor
Institute of Endocrinology and Metabolism of Academy of Medical Sciences of Ukraine, Kyiv, Ukraine

Soda, Midori
Radiation Effects Research Foundation, Nagasaki, Japan

Suyama, Akihiko
Radiation Effects Research Foundation, Nagasaki, Japan

Suzuki, Keiji
Atomic Bomb Disease Institute, Nagasaki University Graduate School of Biomedical Sciences, Nagasaki, Japan

Suzuki, Masatoshi
Simmons Comprehensive Cancer Center, University of Texas Southwestern Medical Center Dallas, TX, USA

Suzuki, Yuriko
National Center of Neurology and Psychiatry, National Institute of Mental Health, Tokyo, Japan

Takabatake, Takashi
Experimental Radiobiology for Children's Health Research Group, National Institute of Radiological Sciences, Chiba, Japan

Takaku, Ken-ichi
Graduate School of Medical and Dental Sciences, Transdisciplinary Research Center, Niigata University, Niigata, Japan

Takamura, Noboru
Nagasaki University Graduate School of Biomedical Sciences, Nagasaki, Japan

Takao, Hideaki
Center for Frontier Life Sciences, Nagasaki University, Nagasaki, Japan

Tereshchenko, Valery
Institute of Endocrinology and Metabolism of Academy of Medical Sciences of Ukraine, Kyiv, Ukraine

Thomas, Gerry A.
Hammersmith Hospital, London, United Kingdom, on behalf of the Pathology Panel and the Scientific Project Panel of the Chernobyl Tissue Bank

Tomonaga, Masao
Atomic-Bomb Disease Institute, Nagasaki University Graduate School of Biomedical Sciences, Nagasaki, Japan

Tronko, Mykola
Institute of Endocrinology and Metabolism of Academy of Medical Sciences of Ukraine, Kyiv, Ukraine

Trosko, James E.
College of Human Medicine, Michigan State University, East Lansing, MI, USA

Tsuchida, Ken
Radiation Biology Center, Kyoto University, Kyoto, Japan

Tsukasaki, Kunihiro
Nagasaki University Graduate School of Biomedical Sciences, Nagasaki, Japan

Tsutsumi, Atsuro
National Center of Neurology and Psychiatry, National Institute of Mental Health, Tokyo, Japan

Tsyb, Anatoly F.
Medical Radiological Research Center of Russian Academy of Medical Sciences, Obninsk, Kaluga Region, Russia

Ullrich, Robert L.
Cancer SuperCluster, Colorado State University, Fort Collins, CO, USA
College of Veterinary Medicine and Biological Sciences, Colorado State University, Fort Collins, CO, USA

Voskoboynyk, Larysa
Institute of Endocrinology and Metabolism of Academy of Medical Sciences of Ukraine, Kyiv, Ukraine

Watanabe, Masami
Research Reactor Institute, Kyoto University, Osaka, Japan

Williams, Eli S.
Colorado State University, Fort Collins, CO, USA

Yamamoto, Takashi
Graduate School of Medical and Dental Sciences, Transdisciplinary Research Center, Niigata University, Niigata, Japan

Yamashita, Shunichi
Atomic Bomb Disease Institute, Nagasaki University Graduate School of Biomedical Sciences, Nagasaki, Japan

Yamauchi, Kazumi
Experimental Radiobiology for Children's Health Research Group, National Institute of Radiological Sciences, Chiba, Japan

Yamauchi, Motohiro
Atomic Bomb Disease Institute, Nagasaki University Graduate School of Biomedical Sciences, Nagasaki, Japan

Yanagihara, Hiromi
Radiation Biology Center, Kyoto University, Kyoto, Japan

Yoshida, Masahiro
Center for Frontier Life Sciences, Nagasaki University, Nagasaki, Japan

Yoshii, Hanako
Research Reactor Institute, Kyoto University, Osaka, Japan

Zhou, Hongning
Center for Radiological Research, College of Physicians and Surgeons, Columbia University, New York, NY 10032, USA

Zhumadilov, Zhaxybay Sh.
Semey State Medical Academy, Semey, Kazakhstan

Zou, Yonglong
Simmons Comprehensive Cancer Center, University of Texas Southwestern Medical Center Dallas, TX, USA

Zurnadzhy, Lyudmyla
Institute of Endocrinology and Metabolism of Academy of Medical Sciences of Ukraine, Kyiv, Ukraine

Overview of the Global COE Program

Global Strategic Center for Radiation Health Risk Control

Shunichi Yamashita

Summary. In the framework of the 21st Century Center of Excellence (COE) Program entitled "International Consortium for Medical Care of Hibakusha and Radiation Life Science," a world-class academic research consortium, we intend to establish a pivotal center for education/research, with close focus on local populations in Chernobyl and Semipalatinsk, as well as on atomic bomb survivors. Moreover, in the context of social issues, including the nuclear power plant construction rush in Asia, radioactive waste disposal, and expanding medical exposure, the newly established Global COE Program will emphasize education/research in these three disciplines: (1) international radiation health sciences, (2) atomic bomb disease medicine, and (3) radiation basic life sciences. Interdisciplinary approaches will be employed to enhance the quality of individual educational/research projects and to integrate basic and clinical research. Specifically, we will link bench-scale work at laboratories with world-scale field work unique to Nagasaki University; that is, medical cooperation and academic joint research on the radio-contaminated area and the radiation-exposed populations, with the aim of benefiting the public from the research outcomes. To this end, it is critical to establish a discipline of "Radiation Health Risk Control," based on research in the world's radiation-exposed populations, and to develop human resources who will become leading figures in the field of radiation medical sciences worldwide in cooperation with the research institutes in the Unites States and Europe, WHO, and other international organizations. The COE finally seeks to make Japan-driven, creative, social, and international contributions through a new establishment of Radiation Health and Life Sciences.

Key words GCOE · Radiation risk · International health · Atomic bombing · Chernobyl · Semipalatinsk

---

GCOE Program Leader, Atomic Bomb Disease Institute, Nagasaki University Graduate School of Biomedical Sciences, 1-12-4 Sakamoto, Nagasaki 852-8523, Japan

Introduction

First, based on assessments of the "21st Century COE Program" and verifications of its results to date carried out by Japan's Ministry of Education, Culture, Sports, Science and Technology from FY2002, a decision was made to establish the "Global COE Program." The renewal program has provided funding support for advancing education and research centers that perform at the apex of global excellence to elevate the international competitiveness of the Japanese universities. The program will strengthen and enhance the education and research functions of graduate schools, to foster highly creative young researchers who will go on to become world leaders in their respective fields through experiencing and practicing research of the highest world standard.

Second, based on the highly evaluated achievement of the 21st Century COE Program entitled "International Consortium for Medical Care of Hibakusha and Radiation Life Science" [1], Nagasaki University intends to establish a new Global COE Program, the "Global Strategic Center for Radiation Health Risk Control." The new program has been successfully selected among various competitive applications from all the universities in Japan [2]. The aim of our program is to explore human health risks from radiation on a global scale, to develop measures for overcoming the negative legacies of radiation, and to establish a scientific center for contributing to the safety and security of human beings, thereby pursuing integrated international strategic research and human resource development in the field of radiation medical sciences. To these ends, we will further expand and develop the international consortium comprising research institutes in the radio-contaminated areas of the former USSR and advanced radiation research institutes in the Unites States and Europe, which have been formed over the past 5 years, to address yet-to-be-resolved challenges, such as the physical and mental effects of accidental and environmental radiation exposures, the difference between external and internal exposures, the evaluation of lifelong health risks, and the promotion of comprehensive medical care for Hibakusha (radiation-exposed victims).

Based on the health issues of atomic bomb survivors as well as of Hibakusha that have resulted from nuclear disasters and radiation accidents in the world, we promote high-level studies in the field of radiation effects research to establish a new scientific area named "Assessment and Management of Radiation Health Risk."

To pursue the world's top-level education/research, we plan to newly establish master courses and also a graduate school to foster various human resources who will play an important role in "Radiation Health Risk Control" worldwide under the three main themes described below. Each project leader will take initiative and responsibility for coordination and cooperation of individual research together with members and staff of the Atomic Bomb Disease Institute, Center for Advanced Life Science Research, and Nagasaki University Hospital [3].

Research Projects

International Radiation Health Science Research

We promote comprehensive medical support for and joint research on the effects of low-dose internal exposure as well as external exposure of Hibakusha by the Chernobyl nuclear power plant (NPP) accident, and international research projects for radiation-induced cancer and psychological effects, in collaboration with the established COE centers in the United States and Europe and the World Health Organization (WHO) (Fig. 1). Large-scale molecular epidemiological studies will be performed to clarify health risks of Hibakusha, through linkage with the Chernobyl Tissue Bank, the joint organization of Nagasaki University, USA, Europe, Russia, and Ukraine for collecting radiation-induced thyroid cancer tissue, and newly constructing a cancer research network in Russia and the center for collection of thyroid cancer/breast cancer biological samples and patient information in Belarus. Furthermore, we will improve the basic medical infrastructure in

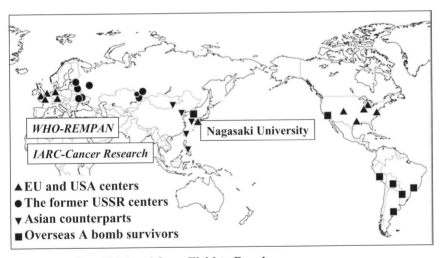

From Bench to Field and from Field to Bench
Based on the highly evaluated achievement of the 21st Century COE Program entitled *"International Consortium for Medical Care of Hibakusha and Radiation Life Science"*, Nagasaki University intends to establish a new Global COE Program entitled the "Global Strategic Center for Radiation Health Risk Control" from 2007 to 2012.

Database establishment for Radiation Health Risk Control
Based on Chernobyl Tissue Bank, international collaborative projects will be promoted.

Fig. 1. Map of the International Consortium on Radiation Health and Life Science network in the world. Nagasaki University has already established close relationships with overseas strongholds as indicated

Kazakhstan, to promote humanitarian aids, scientific collaboration, and radiation health risk management research, not only at the population level but at the individual level as well. Furthermore, we will comprehensively develop a network system to be used during a radiation emergency in preparation for NPP accidents and radiation disasters in Asia. These challenges will bring new ideas from field to bench and, vice versa, from bench to field, and establish a valuable database for radiation health risk control.

Atomic Bomb Disease Medical Research

Comprehensive medical care for late effects of radiation, particularly the still persistent cancer risks in 45 000 aging Nagasaki atomic bomb survivors and also in 2 500 survivors residing overseas, will be pursued. By making use of medical records, of information on individual radiation exposures that have been gathered and managed to date, and of standardized biological tissues, a medical research network will be established to promote studies on molecular pathology and molecular targeted therapy, as well as regenerative medicine for radiation tissue damage. Furthermore, to disseminate our original expertise obtained through medical research on late effects of radiation exposure to the world, particularly to Asia, radiological educational/training programs will be prepared in cooperation with the WHO, International Atomic Energy Agency (IAEA), and worldwide research institutes in this field. At the same time, we will establish the training course for the specialists who will be engaged in medical care of acute and chronic phases of radiation-related health issues and in the establishment of guidelines for use during a radiation emergency.

Radiation Basic Life Science Research

We will elucidate the molecular mechanism of late effects of low-dose (dose rate) radiation exposure. Based on the outcomes obtained from the aforementioned clinical epidemiological population survey and molecular epidemiological study, biological response to radiation will be analyzed at the cellular, molecular, and genetic levels to elucidate the mechanism of cell death escape and genetic variation induction in the process of genetic damage repair. In particular, we will identify the molecules involved in late health effects of radiation exposure including carcinogenesis, to elucidate the mechanism of radiation signature at the gene level. We will further develop the results that we obtain into life sciences research on sensitivity and resistance to radiation exposure at the somatic/stem cell level of individuals. Furthermore, by using the microbeam irradiation system introduced by the 21st Century COE Program at Nagasaki University, we will clarify the mechanism of "bystander" effects to nonirradiated cells adjacent to irradiated cells, to provide

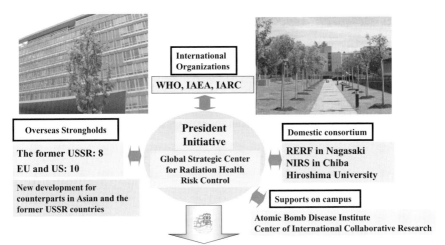

Fig. 2. Structure of the Global Strategic Center for Radiation Health Risk Control according to Nagasaki University President's Initiative

scientific evidence for the guidelines of radiation health risk assessment and management.

Through the abovementioned research activities, we will establish the "Global Strategic Center for the Radiation Health Risk Control," which can train experts who are capable of disseminating obtained research outcomes to the international society in the field of medical care for Hibakusha. Through interdisciplinary attempts to link atomic bomb disease medicine and international medical care for Hibakusha with radiation basic life sciences, we seek to establish a system for risk assessment at both population and individual levels.

Furthermore, a comprehensive educational/research organization for radiation health effects regarding internal and external exposures will be established, as well as the discipline of "Radiation Health Risk Control," which will emphasize risk communications with Hibakusha, thereby developing comprehensive "Medical Care for Hibakusha." Finally, we aim at newly establishing "Radiation Health and Life Sciences" as a core academic research concept in Japan (Fig. 2).

Expected Research Achievements

The achievements will be integrated so as to emerge in 5 years as new interdisciplinary development in the form of "Medical Care for Hibakusha" and "Radiation Health Risk Control." Therefore, concrete targets for achievements in research activities within 5 years are as follows.

Scientific Research Aspect

Goals are (1) identification of signature gene(s) or sensitive gene groups relating to radiation carcinogenesis; (2) molecular biochemical, molecular pathological, and molecular biological characterization of radio-responsive gene groups involved in chromosomal/genetic instability; and (3) elucidation of differences in the molecular mechanism between early and late carcinogenesis in the same organs in young exposed persons.

Medical Aspect

Goals are (1) planning and implementation of international joint research projects for medical care for Hibakusha and establishment of the guidelines for radiation safety for low-dose exposure; (2) establishment of comprehensive holistic medical care for atomic bomb survivors; and (3) development of radiation health risk assessment at individual and population levels.

Sociomedical Aspect

Goals are (1) formulation of the world standard radiation health risk management program and safety guidelines for radiation exposure, as part of joint programs with WHO, IAEA, and COE research centers in the USA and Europe; (2) provision of guidelines in the field of medical radiation exposure and radiation emergency; and (3) implementation of an education/training program in the field of radiation medicine, which thus far has targeted the former USSR, in Asian countries (particularly those with increasing nuclear power plants) so as to establish an Asian network for comprehensive cooperation in medical care for Hibakusha, as well as an Asian network for radiation emergency.

Molecular Epidemiology of Childhood Thyroid Cancers

Among several important research projects in the framework of our GCOE program, such as radiation-associated leukemia and blood disorders and metabolic and psychiatric disorders, here I would like to emphasize, as an important example, the necessity of joint research on radiation-induced thyroid cancers around Chernobyl. Thyroid cancer in children is usually rare, but in the individuals exposed to radiation the risk of this disease increases considerably. The incidence of thyroid cancer in children increased dramatically in the territories affected by the Chernobyl nuclear accident; this increase is probably attributable to short-lived radioactive iodine released into the environment. There was a broad range of latency periods in children who developed thyroid cancer; some periods were less than 5 years. Experience from Chernobyl childhood thyroid cancer has substantially improved our understanding of the disease in several fields of knowledge, including clinical practice, pathology, and molecular carcinogenesis [4,5].

Childhood thyroid cancers have a fairly good prognosis based on early diagnosis and appropriate treatment strategy combining surgery and radioactive iodine therapy [6,7]. The mutational spectrum of childhood thyroid cancers demonstrates that gene rearrangements that lead to the activation of mitogen-activated protein kinase signaling seem to have a pivotal role; point mutations are rare. So far none of the cancer genes or tumor suppressors, or a peculiar gene expression pattern, has been specifically implicated in radiation-induced thyroid carcinogenesis. The frequency of certain oncogenes does, however, vary in tumors that develop after different periods of latency. Such differences in the distribution of gene abnormalities in radiation-related cancers imply that they could possibly be associated with patient age at exposure and diagnosis, clinicopathological manifestations of disease, and an individual's genetic characteristics. Therefore, the large-scale molecular epidemiology studies of thyroid cancer are essentially needed in the framework of the Global COE program, and further strengthening of the Chernobyl Tissue Bank is planned [8].

Future Scope and Planning

Our GCOE program clearly aims at the achievement of a new multidisciplinary academic outcome, an establishment of "Radiation Health and Life Sciences" in cooperation with the leading education/research institutes and universities in Eurasia and developed countries established in our global consortium network. Nagasaki University is simultaneously planning and forwarding its unique education/research activities in the three major research fields: international radiation health science, atomic bomb disease medicine, and radiation basic life science. After the completion of our GCOE program, Nagasaki University plans to newly establish an Integrated Global Education and Research Center for Environmental Health and Life Sciences, joining up with the Global Network of Tropical and Emerging Infectious Disease Risk Control and Environmental Safety Network for Marine Resources Around the Far East China Sea, both of which are very characteristic ongoing programs established in Nagasaki University (Fig. 3).

Finally, radiation effects on human beings are complicated but are always categorized simply into two groups: acute and chronic effects, and high-dose and low-dose effects. The international cooperative projects are, therefore, essential to solve the problems in emergency radiation medicine and identify potential impacts on low-dose and low dose rate radiation effects and models. Risk communication based on established regulatory sciences is really required for maintaining healthy lives and safeguards in the nuclear age of the 21st century.

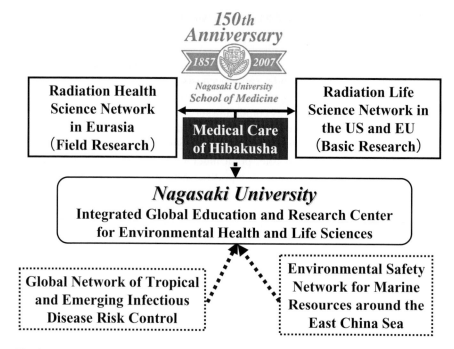

Fig. 3. Future planning of Integrated Global Education and Research Center for Environmental Health and Life Sciences in Nagasaki University

References

1. http://www.jsps.go.jp/english/e-21coe/index.html
2. http://www.jsps.go.jp/english/e-globalcoe/index.html
3. http://www-sdc.med.nagasaki-u.ac.jp/gcoe/index.html
4. Demidchik YE, Demidchik EP, Reiners C, et al (2006) Comprehensive clinical assessment of 740 cases of surgically treated thyroid cancers in children of Belarus. Ann Surg 243: 528–532
5. Yamashita S, Saenko V (2007) Mechanism of disease: molecular genetics of childhood thyroid cancers. Nat Clin Pract Endocrinol Metab 3:422–429
6. Demidchik Y, Saenko V, Yamashita S (2007) Childhood thyroid cancer in Belarus, Russia and Ukraine after Chernobyl and at present. Arq Bras Endocrinol Metab 51:748–762
7. Kumagai A, Reiners C, Drozd V, et al (2007) Childhood thyroid cancers and radioactive iodine therapy: necessity of precautious health risk management. Endocr J 54:839–847
8. http://www.chernobyltissuebank.com/

Overview of the Lectures

Discussion on Points of Radiation Safety and the Scope of The University of Tokyo Global COE Program

Toshiso Kosako[1] and Takeshi Iimoto[2]

Summary. Two topics are presented here. The first is "Discussion Points on Radiation Safety." The scheme of radiation safety in Japan has mainly been based on the International Commission on Radiological Protection (ICRP) recommendation, Publication 60. The new recommendation, Publication 103, replacing Publication 60, was recently published, in January 2008. "Optimization" in the system plays a more important part. The principle of optimization of radiological protection is defined as the source-related process to keep the magnitude of individual doses, the number of people exposed, and the likelihood of potential exposure as low as reasonably achievable below the appropriate dose constraints or reference levels, with economic and social factors being taken into account. The way in which the optimization process should be implemented is now viewed more broadly to reflect the increasing role of individual equity, safety culture, and stakeholder involvement in our modern societies. These points of view will become more important, especially to establish future guidelines and regulations on radiation safety. The second point is the "Scope of the University of Tokyo Global COE (Center of Excellence) Program." We are developing a well-rounded research and education program in response to worldwide nuclear utilization. Our Global COE (GCOE) "Nuclear Education and Research Initiative" will create a comprehensive nuclear engineering discipline, incorporating three different aspects of nuclear engineering: nuclear energy, radiology, and nuclear energy sociology. Radiation safety is mainly categorized under radiology. In the radiation safety area in the GCOE program, we are mainly focusing on the following three subjects: radiation safety system, radiation shielding, and radiation measurement/dosimetry.

Key words Radiation safety · Optimization · Dose constraints · Reference level · The University of Tokyo Global COE Program

---

[1]Department of Nuclear Professional School, School of Engineering, University of Tokyo, Ibaraki, Japan
[2]Division for Environment, Health and Safety, University of Tokyo, 7-3-1 Hongo, Bunkyo-ku, Tokyo 113-8656, Japan

Introduction

Two topics are presented here. The first is "Discussion Points on Radiation Safety." The contents are quoted mainly from the International Commission on Radiological Protection (ICRP) recommendations. The second is "Scope of The University of Tokyo Global COE Program." The contents are quoted mainly from the related web site of The University of Tokyo.

Discussion Points on Radiation Safety

Evolution of Radiological Protection [1]

Around 9 years ago, ICRP embarked on a process of rationalizing and clarifying the system of radiological protection. The new ICRP recommendations [2] were the basis for the new set of recommendations that were approved by the Main Commission in March 2007 at its meeting in Essen in Germany. These recommendations will replace the Commission's previous recommendations from 1990 [3].

The new Recommendations take account of new biological and physical information and trends in setting of protection standards. Although much more information has accumulated since 1990, the overall estimate of the risk of various levels of harmful effects following exposure to radiation remains fundamentally the same. Nevertheless, there are some differences in our understanding of how this risk is distributed across body organs, which result in some changes in the way the quantity of effective dose is calculated. The new recommendations are intended to apply to all radiation sources and exposures, regardless of size or origin. This does not mean, of course, that action has to be taken to protect against all such sources and exposures. In many cases, application of the system of protection will indicate that no action is required, which will be the case for most exposures from natural sources, for example.

The three fundamental principles of radiological protection—justification, optimization, and dose/risk limitation—are retained. In some cases the principles have, however, been developed to make their use more generally applicable. The principle of justification is modified to encompass action to either increase or decrease exposures: any decision that alters the radiation exposure situation should do more good than harm. This change means that by introducing a new radiation source or by reducing existing exposure, one should achieve an individual or societal benefit that is higher than the detriment it causes. For practical purposes, however, particularly in the context of nuclear power, this principle is unchanged from the previous recommendations in Publication 60. The principle of optimization of protection is a cornerstone of radiological protection. Essentially, it means that the level of protection should be the best possible under the prevailing circumstances, maximizing the margin of benefit over harm. In any situation, however, there will be a level of dose or risk that should not be exceeded, if possible. The process of optimization is therefore constrained by restrictions on doses or risks that will be specific to the situation under consideration. The concept of a constraint was introduced in ICRP Publication 60 in the context of practices. Thus, optimization has been applied in this manner in the control of practices and in some cases of exposure to natural sources (e.g., radon). Application to other exposure situations could, however, be viewed as "new." The principles of justification and optimization, with restrictions on doses and risks, represent the fundamental system of protection to be applied to all sources and exposures, the principle of dose or risk limitation applying only to a subset of sources referred to as practices. The manner in which the system of protection should be applied will, however, depend upon the characteristics of the exposure situation; for example, whether exposures are being increased or decreased.

For application of the system of protection, ICRP has divided exposure situations into three categories: planned exposure situations, existing exposure situations, and emergency exposure situations. *Planned exposure situations* are situations involving the planned introduction and operation of sources; this would also include their decommissioning, disposal of associated radioactive waste, and rehabilitation of the previously occupied land in the case of installations. Medical exposures are included in this category of exposures. *Existing exposure situations* are exposure situations that already exist when a decision on control must be taken, including natural background radiation and residues from past practices that have been operated outside the Commission's recommendation, or, long-term exposure situations. *Emergency exposure situations* are unexpected situations that occur during the operation of a planned situation, or from a malicious act, requiring urgent action. One difference between these situations will be the selection of the value for the restriction on dose or risk applied during the optimization. Perhaps confusingly, the ICRP refers to these restrictions as "constraints" in the case of planned exposure situations and as "reference levels" in the case of both existing and emergency exposure situations. ICRP provides guidance on the selection of values for constraints or reference levels (Table 1).

Table 1. Maximum values for dose constraints or reference levels

mSv	Situations
100	Emergencies, high level of existing exposure, no benefit can compensate for higher exposures
20	Situations where there is direct or indirect benefit for the exposed individual but not necessarily from the exposure
1	Situations where there is no direct benefit to the exposed individual

SV, seivert

Optimization of Radiological Protection [4]

The principle of optimization of radiation protection is defined by the ICRP as the source-related process to keep the magnitude of individual doses, the number of people exposed, and the likelihood of potential exposure as low as reasonably achievable below the appropriate dose constraints, with economic and social factors being taken into account. According to the revised recommendations of ICRP [2], this process of optimization below constraint should be applied whatever the exposure situation: that is, planned, emergency, or existing. The previous recommendations for the practical implementation of the optimization process are still valid. Implementation must occur through an ongoing, cyclical process that involves the evaluation of the exposure situation to identify the need for action, the identification of the possible protective options to keep the exposure as low as reasonably achievable, the selection of the best option under the prevailing circumstances, the implementation of the selected option through an effective optimization program, and regular review of the exposure situation to evaluate if the prevailing circumstances call for the implementation of corrective protective actions. However, the way in which the optimization process should be implemented is now viewed more broadly to reflect the increasing role of individual equity, safety culture, and stakeholder involvement in our modern societies.

Dose Constraints and Reference Levels [2]

The concepts of dose constraint and reference level are used in conjunction with the optimization of protection to restrict individual doses. A level of individual dose, either as a dose constraint or a reference level, always needs to be defined. The initial intention would be to not exceed, or to remain at, these levels, and the ambition is to reduce all doses to levels that are as low as reasonably achievable, economic and societal factors being taken into account. For the sake of continuity with its earlier Recommendations [3], the Commission retains the term "dose constraint" for this level of dose in planned exposure situations (with the exception of medical exposure of patients). For emergency exposure situations and existing exposure situations, the Commission proposes the term "reference level" to describe this level of dose. The difference in terminology between planned and other exposure situations (emergency and existing) has been retained by the Commission to express the fact that, in planned situations, the restriction on individual doses can be applied at the planning stage, and the doses can be forecast so as to ensure that the constraint will not be exceeded. With the other situations, a wider range of exposures may exist, and the optimization process may apply to initial levels of individual doses above the reference level. Diagnostic reference levels are already being used in medical diagnosis (i.e., planned exposure situations) to indicate whether, in routine conditions, the levels of patient dose or administered activity from a specified imaging procedure are unusually high or low for that procedure. If so, a local review should be initiated to determine whether protection has been adequately optimized or whether corrective action is required. The chosen value for a constraint or a reference level will depend upon the circumstances of the exposure under consideration. It must also be realized that neither dose and risk constraints nor reference levels represent a demarcation between "safe" and "dangerous" or reflect a step change in the associated health risk for individuals.

An Example of Japanese Guidelines for Reference Levels [5,6]

It is not appropriate to control exposures from natural radiation sources that exist in soil, air, and other surroundings as such control may have little effect on reduction of the exposures. The ICRP specifies that these radioactive sources shall be subject to "Exclusion." However, industrial activities using naturally occurring radioactive materials (NORM) and use of NORM-containing consumer goods can be controlled, cause exposure of workers and the public, and are selected to produce some benefits. Those activities are considered in a category of "planned exposure situations" as the use of artificial radiation sources.

Because exposure to NORM is no different from that from artificial radiation sources, it can be considered that exposure to NORM should be subject to regulation for radiation protection. NORM exist with a wide range of activity concentrations in our surroundings, from very low level to high level, and cause exposure of insignificant to significant levels. For this reason, it is difficult to set an exemption level, which can be considered as one of the reference levels, and to regulate all NORM that exceed the level, based only on a concept of "low doses to the extent which radiation effects are trivial." In addition, raw materials containing NORM that are used for industrial applications are not produced as radioactive substances nor used for the purposes of radioactive substances. Furthermore, various raw materials containing NORM have been used for a long time without taking into consideration the exposure from those substances and have caused exposure pathways; therefore, there are some possibilities that they are subject to "existing exposure situations." In particular, an initial process of raw materials is considered as less artificial, so there are higher possibilities these are subject to "existing exposure situations." The ICRP recommends the different radiation protection criteria for "existing exposure situations" from those for "planned exposure situations." Implementation of more proper regulation is expected to reduce risks in an effective manner. From the foregoing points of view, it is necessary to classify the usage pattern of NORM taking into consideration the artificial aspects and actual exposure potential and possibilities and to regulate these by using the concepts of exemption or intervention exemption according to their features and exposure doses.

It is necessary to classify NORM-containing substances and review the measures for individual regulation, as described in the previous section. Table 2 shows their

Table 2. Categorizing materials containing naturally occurring radioactive materials (NORM)

	Category/exemption level
1	Raw materials such as mineral ore without procedure of enhancing concentration (excluding categories 2, 3, 4, 5 and 6). Exclusion
2	Waste rock residues from past mine or industrial activities. 1–10 mSv/year
3	Ash, scale, etc. produced by industries (concentration of substances treated as raw materials should be exemption level or below). 1–10 mSv/year
4	Soil from mines currently in operation and industrial residues (disposal). 1 mSv/year
5	Raw materials for industrial use (manufacture, energy production and mining) (excluding Category 7). 1 mSv/year
6	Consumer products (usage). 0.01–1 mSv/year
7	Nuclear fuel material refined to intentionally use its natural radioactive emissions and material to be used as radiation source.
8	Radon

categories and the regulation measures proposed. Cases that should be examined in the table represent some substances selected through literature survey and an actual condition survey on substances that contain relatively great amounts of NORM.

Category 1 in Table 2 shows substances that are not adaptable to being regulated and from which the effects of radiation exposure are hardly prevented by regulation. Therefore, the substances shall be subject to "Exclusion."

Category 2 in Table 2 shows substances that should be subject to "existing exposure situations" because long-term exposure from past activities (e.g., mining, surplus soil, and residues generated from industrial use) was not controlled as "planned exposure situations."

NORM in Category 3 includes substances that are used as raw materials in general industries such as energy production. Industrial activities for those NORM are not subject to "planned exposure situations" because their activity concentrations are generally well below the Basic Safety Standards (BSS) exemption levels [7]. Products (coal ash, scale, etc.) generated through the processes of these industrial applications are those that are not intended to contain radioactive substances. The products are not produced for radiation purposes, and their activity concentrations and activities are distributed over a wide range. For this reason, Category 3 should also be subject to "existing exposure situations." However, the products are included in Categories 4 and 5 when being disposed of or reused. In addition, they are included in Category 6 when being used as consumer goods.

The disposal of residues from operating mines and other industrial applications, in case of Category 4, is basically considered to be involved in "planned exposure situations" when exposure dose from the activity is significantly increased. In most cases, however, these residues are not perceived to contain radioactive substances although their activity concentrations vary widely. For this reason, it is difficult to set an exemption level for the residues and regulate them in the same manner as artificial radiation sources. Furthermore, these residues are often disposed of in the same manner as substances from past activities. It may be difficult to distinguish the residues from the substances when they are disposed of. Therefore, there is some possibility that the residues can be subject to "existing exposure situations."

Mining and industrial activities using raw materials in Category 5 are regarded as "planned exposure situations," similar to the use of artificial radiation sources, when exposure dose from those activities is significantly increased. NORM is contained in these raw materials. However, those materials were not produced as radioactive substances and are often used without perception of radioactive substances. In addition, their activity concentrations vary widely. Because the industrial use and mining of these raw materials have a longer history than that of radiation regulation, their exposure pathways may already exist. Therefore, exposure in an initial process where these raw materials are treated becomes subject to "existing exposure situations" in the same manner as that in Category 4.

ICRP Publication 82 proposes about 1 mSv of annual individual dose for exemption criteria on "Intervention" for commodities. An individual dose of 1 mSv/year is suggested also as a dose constraint against "planned exposure situations." Therefore, a dose criterion for exemption of target substances in Categories 4 and 5 can be considered appropriately to be 1 mSv/year for exemption of this "existing exposure situation," because these substances become subject to both "planned exposure situations" and "existing exposure situations."

NORM-containing substances in Categories 4 and 5 are generally handled in large quantities. In addition, their activity concentrations are not uniform, or may vary with veins and shafts in the countries and areas in which they are produced. For these reasons, it is actually difficult to measure or determine their concentrations, or such measurement might incur a huge cost. It is not appropriate to define an exemption level for these substances. We consider it suitable to preliminarily identify substances whose average activity concentration could exceed a certain level and to evaluate exposure doses for actual workers and the public involving in the handling of those substances. If the exposure doses exceed 1 mSv/year, then it is appropriate to require proper control for radiation protection. In this case, the exemption levels given in the BSS [7] and RP-122 [8] should be referred to establish a certain level for determining substances to be regulated.

The use of consumer goods in Category 6 is basically equivalent to "planned exposure situations"; therefore, it can be considered that they are treated in the same manner as artificial radioactive substances. However, they have widely varying activity concentrations, are sometimes not used for radiation purposes, and are widely distributed because they have been not regulated so far. For these reasons, it is important not to apply the BSS exemption level to all consumer goods but to conduct reasonable and proper regulation. Hence, in case of consumer goods whose activity concentration and activity exceed the BSS exemption level, it is appropriate to confirm that users' exposure from each item is below 1 mSv/year (ICRP Publication 82), a maximum value of a dose constraint for the public, and to conduct rationalized regulation such as indication of inclusion of NORM and NORM information disclosure to users; those are equivalent to authorization based on their design, which is adopted in regulation of artificial radiation sources in various foreign countries.

Substances in Category 7 are those used as radiation sources, such as nuclear fuel materials and radium sources that are refined for use of their radiation, and are regulated in the same manner as artificial radiation sources.

For radon in Category 8, it is appropriate to review the action levels against radon sources after a survey on radon radiation in houses and workplaces in general.

It is not practical to provide a certain concentration and a specific activity level for intervention and exemption to NORM in the same manner as artificial radioactive substances because their activity concentrations and activity vary widely. Therefore, exposures that will cause doses within 10 µSv/year (an exemption dose criterion for "planned exposure situations") and 1 mSv/year (an exemption dose criterion for "existing exposure situations") should be reviewed. In this review, it is necessary that the exposure scenarios and exposure pathway for dose assessments be appropriately selected in an evenhanded fashion, and it is required that the dose assessment should be performed according to an adequate guidance.

From the aforementioned reasons, Categories 1, 2, and 3 will not be regulated under law, but it is considered that Categories 4, 5, and 6 should be regulated under a future law in Japan.

Scope of The University of Tokyo Global COE (GCOE) Program

Target of The University of Tokyo GCOE [9]

Mankind is having an increased effect on the environment through greenhouse gas emission; a very important and growing concern. Generally, nuclear power is seen as a method for reducing greenhouse gas emission while still satisfying our modern society's high demand for energy. We are developing a well-rounded research and education program in response to a variety of worldwide nuclear utilization subjects, such as protection of the global environment, supplying safe and stable nuclear energy, and applying radiation for healthy, productive, and prosperous lives. Our COE is the "Nuclear Education and Research Initiative."

The first systematic education on nuclear energy in the world will be performed in this GCOE, incorporating the social sciences, liberal arts, and technical subjects as they relate to nuclear utilization. Such subjects include law and legislation, communication with the public, risk management, crisis control, nuclear nonproliferation, nuclear fundamentals, and nuclear applications. Research and education will be carried out in three areas: nuclear energy, radiation application, and the social aspects of nuclear engineering, which we call nuclear energy sociology.

Nuclear Energy, Radiology, and Nuclear Energy Sociology

Our COE will create a comprehensive nuclear engineering discipline, incorporating three different aspects of nuclear engineering: nuclear energy, radiology, and nuclear energy sociology.

In the nuclear energy discipline, we focus on expanding the traditional research and educational models to include a more interdisciplinary approach. We will make use of the features of nuclear energy as the interface between science and technology and attempt to extend each individual field into this new model.

Radiology is based on the physical knowledge of various types of radiation, and interdisciplinary studies are performed that are centered on medical applications such as treatment, diagnosis, or generation of radiation. Besides this medical physics discipline, other fields are also explored such as application of electron beams and gamma rays, radiation imaging, molecule imaging, and spectrometry by accelerator. Radiation safety is mainly categorized in this area.

Nuclear energy sociology is a broad field pertaining to societal perception and interaction with nuclear energy. In the GCOE we mainly deal with nuclear energy law and legislation, nuclear nonproliferation, and harmonization of technology and society. Other fields are also treated in cooperation with people both inside and outside the university. For example, societal concern over the safety of nuclear energy is a compound problem concerning technology, law, public understanding, and ethics.

Scope of Radiation Safety Area [10]

The following three subjects represent the major directions of the radiation safety research in the GCOE.

Radiation Safety System

The radiation safety system research consists of the following four keywords: (1) radiation safety standards and criteria; (2) radioactive waste management; (3) accelerator health physics; and (4) environmental radiation/radioactivity management.

Radiation Shielding

Experimental and simulation study of neutron and photon shielding for nuclear reactors and accelerators has been one of our main activities for decades. The scope of this research covers the following three key terms: (1) radiation shielding design for nuclear reactors and accelerators; (2) shielding experiments (benchmark experiments); and (3) calculations for radiation transportation.

Radiation Measurement/Dosimetry

Radiation measurement/dosimetry study has progressed in the following two key areas: (1) dosimetry on internal/external exposure; and (2) development of new radiation detectors and measurement instruments.

References

1. Cooper JR (2007) The 'new' ICRP recommendations: implications for nuclear power. In: Abstract book of the 41st academic meeting of Japan Health Physics Society, June 2007
2. ICRP Publication 103 (2008) Recommendations of the ICRP. Annals of the ICRP, vol 37/2-4. International Commission on Radiological Protection. Elsevier, Amsterdam
3. ICRP Publication 60 (1991) 1990 Recommendations of the International Commission on Radiological Protection. Annals of the ICRP, vol 21/1-3. International Commission on Radiological Protection. Elsevier, Amsterdam
4. ICRP Publication 101 (2007) Assessing dose of the representative person for the purpose of radiation protection of the public and the optimisation of radiological protection. International Commission on Radiological Protection. Elsevier, Amsterdam
5. Kosako T, Sugiura N (2005) Development of radiation protection on TENORM. Jpn J Health Phys 40:67–78
6. http://kokai-gen.org/information/2003_menzyo.html
7. IAEA (1996) Safety Series No. 115. International Basic Safety Standards for Protection against Ionizing Radiation and for the Safety of Radiation Sources
8. European Commission (2001) Radiation protection 122. Practical use of the concepts of clearance and exemption. Part II: Application of the concepts of exemption and clearance to natural radiation sources
9. http://www.n.t.u-tokyo.ac.jp/gcoe/eng/program/objectives.html
10. http://www.n.t.u-tokyo.ac.jp/kosako/eng/modules/m0/

Network System for Radiation Emergency Medicine in Japan and the Role of Hiroshima University

Kenji Kamiya

Summary. On the basis of the lessons of the Tokai-mura nuclear criticality accident, Japan decided to develop a new system for the nation's radiation emergency medicine. A new medical system would be prepared and function depending on the severity of each patient's injury, such as primary stage (slight injury), secondary stage, or tertiary stage (serious injury). This system would create a network that would coordinate medical treatment efforts in an emergency. Tertiary radiation emergency hospitals with sufficient ability for advanced medical care and overall responsibility in a radiation emergency should be established. In 2004, the Japanese government designated Hiroshima University and the National Institute of Radiological Sciences as "regional tertiary radiation emergency hospitals" for western and eastern Japan, respectively. Construction of a radiation emergency medical care system is an urgent international issue, and the World Health Organization (WHO) and the International Atomic Energy Agency (IAEA) are pushing forward planning it in response to the nuclear terrorism threat and the Chernobyl nuclear accident. However, there are extremely few specialists, and there is almost no organization that is able to play a central role of radiation emergency medicine: regenerative medicine development. Hiroshima University has a high medical standard and does world-class research in the relevant fields, and it has already achieved a role as a WHO liaison institute. This institute will provide education in radiation emergency medicine and create an international standard.

Key words Radiation · Radiation emergency medicine · Genome damage · Regenerative medicine · Cancer · Radiation injury

---

Department of Experimental Oncology, Division of Genome Biology, Research Institute for Radiation Biology and Medicine, and Center for the Promotion of Radiation Emergency Medicine, Hiroshima University, 1-2-3 Kasumi, Minami-ku, Hiroshima 734-8553, Japan

Radiation Emergency Medicine in Japan

Outline

On the basis of the lessons of the Tokai-mura nuclear accident, the Japan Prime Minister's Cabinet Office's Nuclear Safety Commission made recommendations for a model of our nation's radiation emergency medical system. Specifically, it recommended preparation of a radiation emergency medicine system that will work depending on the severity of each patient's injury, such as primary stage (slight injury), secondary stage, or tertiary stage (serious injury). This system will create a network that will coordinate medical treatment efforts in an emergency. The recommendations also stated that tertiary radiation emergency hospitals with sufficient ability for advanced medical care and overall responsibility in a radiation emergency should be established. In 2004, the Ministry of Education, Culture, Sports, Science and Technology designated Hiroshima University and the National Institute of Radiological Sciences as "regional tertiary radiation emergency hospitals" for western and eastern Japan, respectively.

The Role of Hiroshima University

Hiroshima University has established "The Center for the Promotion of Radiation Emergency Medicine" as an organization to implement the tertiary radiation emergency hospital responsibilities and has commenced the three projects below:

1. Management of regional conferences on preparation of a system for radiation emergency medicine in cooperation with primary and secondary-stage radiation casualty medical facilities and administrations.
2. Management of meetings of radiation casualty medicine cooperating facilities to prepare a cooperative system of local hospital facilities in Hiroshima.
3. Training activities for radiation casualty medicine (e.g., radiation emergency medicine seminars).

Through these projects, we intend to work toward making an effective system of radiation emergency medicine available in the event that it is needed.

At the same time, another important aspect of the radiation emergency medicine system is to nurture the next generation of young doctors and researchers who will undertake this specialized medical treatment. At Hiroshima University, we would also like to make the most of being an educational organization and devote ourselves to training specialists in this field. Hiroshima University has a long history of achievements in atomic bomb medicine and a well-trained staff of specialists in various fields of medical treatment for radiation-induced disorders. Furthermore, the 21st Century Center of Excellence (COE) Program of Hiroshima University, called "The Radiation Casualty Medical Research Center," which was founded by the Ministry of Education, Culture, Sports, Science and Technology, has reached the last year of its 5-year program, and has succeeded in the development of the new academic field of "genome radiation medical science." This up-to-date academic program has also incorporated genome science and regenerative medicine. Promoting this science and nurturing younger scientists are two essential characteristics of Hiroshima University. Through the practice of such interesting programs, we would like to continue to nurture the next generation of specialists and promote the establishment of a continuously developing radiation emergency medicine system.

Future Direction

The use of atomic energy will dramatically increase in the future as a policy of global warming prevention. A sharp increase in radiation use by industry and medicine is expected in Asian countries in particular. It is an urgent problem to cultivate talented people involved with radiation medicine and radiation risk. Hiroshima University has distinguished itself by accepting many foreign students from Asian countries, and we have established the Asian Association of Radiation Research at this institute to facilitate the recruitment of an even larger number of talented Asian students, which is extremely important for cultivating Asian scientific leaders in medical care and industrial development. Construction of a radiation emergency medical care system is an urgent international problem, and the World Health Organization (WHO) and the International Atomic Energy Agency (IAEA) are pushing forward planning it in response to the nuclear terrorism threat and the Chernobyl nuclear accident. However, there are extremely few specialists, and there is almost no organization that is able to take on a central aspect of radiation emergency medicine: that is, regenerative medicine development. This institute will have a high medical standard and perform world-class research in the relevant fields, and it has already achieved a role as a WHO liaison institute. This institute will provide education in radiation emergency medicine and will create the international standard.

Hiroshima University 21st Century COE Program: "Radiation Casualty Medical Research Center"

Concept

The remarkable progress of the genome damage sciences, such as genome repair science and cellular response science, is making it possible to bring innovation to radiation damage research and radiation risk research. Radiation damage and risk both have genome damage in common. The time has come when we can pioneer a new academic discipline that uses genome damage research as a common platform. Because Japan is the only country to have been atomic bombed, the 21st Century COE program has led the world with the establishment of the unique science called radiation casualty medicine, which has the ability to contribute to the world with research in developing treatments for diseases caused by genome disorders. This 21st Century COE program will establish an international institute to promote a globally incomparable "Radiation Casualty Medical Research Center" by applying the results we have developed in radiation genome damage research to the treatment of acute radiation injury, radiation-induced cancers, and radiation risk.

Objectives

Our foremost aim is to cultivate global talent with the highest level research and education at a world institute for a "Radiation Casualty Medical Research Center" established by Japan, as it is the only country to have suffered atomic bombing. Therefore, we will teach a wide range of scientific fields, including genome repair and cellular response research, that are at the forefront of the life sciences, molecular oncology, radiation emergency medicine research, and an academic program of radiation risk research to provide students with interdisciplinary knowledge and methodology. As a result, the 21st Century COE will produce researchers with cutting-edge ideas and specialists who can develop new treatments and be scientific leaders in this field in Asian countries. At the same time, we will contribute to global research and risk management by establishing an academic institute for research in radiation risk and treatment.

Necessity

People receive vast benefits from radiation and the use of atomic energy in modern society, but suffer serious social and health damage by its misuse. Today, cancer onset in atomic bomb victims continues to increase even after more than 60 years have passed. The big problem that genome damage science must solve is the health problems that continue for a lifetime after receiving only one radiation exposure. In addition to the Chernobyl nuclear accident and the Tokai-mura criticality radiation exposure accident, the world faces the threat of nuclear terrorism. For these reasons, the WHO and IAEA are pushing forward the maintenance of an international radiation emergency medicine system, and Japan is expected to have a big role. Throughout Asia, along with economic development and atomic energy development, a rapid increase in the medical and industrial use of radiation is expected. However, there are definitely not enough specialists in radiation and health risk, and the cultivation of these experts is an urgent problem in Asian countries. On the other hand, progress in radiation cancer treatment and computed tomography (CT) scanning, as well as angiography diagnosis and treatment, depends on a large increase in the use of radiation.

However, the problems of low- to relatively high-dose radiation exposure, as in myocardial infarction treatment, have yet to be addressed. Based on genome damage science, advances through the understanding of the health effects are more effective to promote safe medical, energy, and industrial usage and develop new radiological diagnoses and treatments that utilize this knowledge. For this aim, it is necessary to cultivate talented people in this field. At the same time, it is also necessary to establish an academic institute for radiation risk. However, for this institute to be able to promote this kind of scientific collaboration and contribute to society and education, it is essential for us to concentrate Japan's full effort as its duty to the world as the only country that has experienced both the light and dark sides of radiation.

Research Plans

All radiation-induced diseases are caused by genome damage. The cause of death for critical acute disorders is multiple organ failure caused by apoptosis induced by genome damage. Genome mutations from repair errors cause late-onset disorders such as cancers. In our program, we will promote four research projects: (1) research on radiation damage, cellular response, and repair mechanisms; (2) research on regenerative medical treatments for acute disorders; (3) research on diagnosis and treatment based on the mechanisms of cancers and leukemias; and (4) research on comprehensive medical treatment for all radiation casualties.

In our research program, we are attempting to develop a diagnosis and prevention method for radiation diseases, new treatments for damaged genomes, and methods of tissue regeneration using pluripotent stem cells (ES cells, tissue stem cells), which can be transplanted into radiation-damaged tissues. Studies of molecular mechanisms of radiation-induced cancers/leukemia by the technology of genome science are also among our major research projects. For example, we are analyzing genes associated with leukemia and cancers and establishing a monitoring system based on information from genome alterations. From this effort, we can develop a new system of prevention and treatment of radiation-exposed patients. Our ultimate goal is the achievement of a comprehensive medical system that is capable of dealing with all types of radiation injury based on the radiation dose estimated from information from the damaged genome.

Future Direction

The fruit of this research will be to establish a new science, "Medicine for Genome Integrity," which will target all the disorders caused by genome damage. Furthermore, it will have applications in research and treatment in a wide range of medical fields such as cancer, lifestyle-related diseases, preventive medicine by gene monitoring, and even the analysis of aging mechanisms. These studies are a unique scientific contribution to the world that we are in a singular position to provide because Japan is the only country in the world with atomic bomb victims. In addition, our work can provide ideas for the safe usage of nuclear energy. Another significant role of this center is education. Through education, we will implement our research projects to support the independence of young researchers, nurture graduate students, and make our graduate school successful. At the same time, we aim to acquire advanced specialized knowledge/technology for new treatments and to nurture the research abilities of our young associates.

Non-DNA-Targeted Effects and Low-Dose Radiation Risk

Barry D. Michael

Summary. Non-DNA-targeted effects of ionising radiation are defined as effects triggered by radiative energy deposition in cellular targets other than nuclear DNA; these include radiation-induced bystander effects and processes that can be mediated via bystander mechanisms, such as genomic instability and adaptive responses. Laboratory studies show that these responses are favoured by heterogeneous irradiation conditions. Heterogeneous conditions occur at low doses and low dose rates where radiation tracks are sparsely distributed over a cell population; this situation favours bystander signalling between hit and non-hit cells. Non-DNA-targeted effects are currently considered to be candidate mechanisms for any failure of the linear no-threshold (LNT) model to extrapolate radiation risk estimates accurately down to low doses. Some non-DNA-targeted effects have the potential to increase low-dose risk above the LNT extrapolation, and others could decrease the risk.

Key words Bystander effect · Nontargeted effect, Radiation risk · Linear no-threshold hypothesis · Adaptive response · Genomic instability

Introduction

Information about the risks of cancer induction by radiation derives principally from epidemiological follow-up of the effects of the high-dose acute exposures to the atomic bombs [1]. These exposures differ radically from those at the low doses and low dose rates that are of general concern in relationship to environmental, occupational, and medical diagnostic exposures [2] because the deposition of radiation energy takes place along distinct radiation tracks, each much finer than the dimensions of a cell. With the atomic bomb exposures, all the cells of the exposed individuals were subjected almost instantaneously to hundreds or thousands of tracks, and the dose received by any one cell was similar to that received by its neighbours. This effect contrasts with typical protection-level exposures (Fig. 1) in

---

University of Oxford, Gray Cancer Institute, P.O. Box 100, Northwood, Middlesex HA6 2JR, United Kingdom

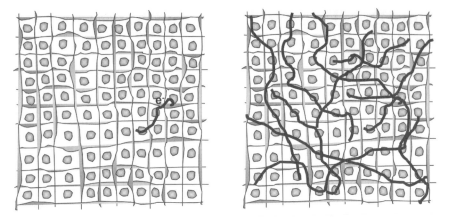

Fig. 1. Two-dimensional representation of electron tracks in tissue illustrating heterogeneous energy deposition at low doses. *Left:* 1 week of low-LET (low linear energy transfer) natural background (~20 µGy); the 4 cells that are traversed by a track receive ~1 mGy and the 96 cells that are not traversed receive 0 mGy. *Right:* 1 year of natural background (~1 mGy); most, but not all, cells are traversed at least once and receive ~1 mGy per traversal [3]

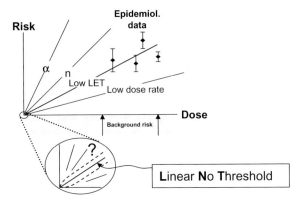

Fig. 2. Illustration of possible deviations (*dashed lines*) in the low-dose region (*inset*) from the extrapolation of high-dose epidemiological (*Epidemiol.*) data using the linear no-threshold (LNT) model. *LET*, linear energy transfer

which individual cells are on average traversed by radiation tracks at intervals ranging from months to many years [3], resulting in a highly heterogeneous distribution of dose from cell to cell. Little is known about how cells respond to isolated single tracks, and this lack therefore raises questions about whether the effects of low doses are accurately extrapolated from the high-dose data by the application of the linear no-threshold (LNT) model (Fig. 2).

Non-DNA-Targeted Effects of Radiation

There is now a considerable body of evidence showing effects of radiation that do not conform to some of the basic assumptions underlying the LNT model. The classical model of radiation effects, in which discrete cellular targets respond individually according to the amounts of unrepaired or misrepaired DNA damage, has been challenged by observations of damage-inducing and other processes that operate over distances that are comparable with or greater than the dimensions of the cell itself [4,5]. Broadly, these "non-DNA-targeted effects" can be categorized as (a) effects on the cell nucleus that result from events initiated in a target larger than, or outside, the nucleus; (b) effects that are transmitted from hit to non-hit cells ("bystander" effects); (c) delayed effects that are only expressed after a number of cell generations; and (d) cooperative responses in which interactions between hit cells influence the overall level of effect. A range of endpoints has been found to be influenced by one or more of these effects, including clonogenic survival, apoptosis, chromosome/chromatid damage, gene induction, genomic instability, adaptive responses, and delayed lethality.

Characterisation of nontargeted effects is important in defining their possible roles in radiation therapy and radiation risk and for their ultimate incorporation into mechanistic models of response. Some of the observations show specificity to high-LET radiation. A common observation of these responses is that they predominate at low doses and saturate with increasing dose (Fig. 3). With classical responses, such as cell survival of a uniformly irradiated population, all cells may show an effect at sufficiently high doses. However, with non-DNA-targeted effects, such as the bystander effect, the response saturates in a manner that indicates that only a certain fraction of the cell population responds. Several candidate mechanisms have been put forward: these include reactive oxygen species, cell signalling, and irradiated medium effects.

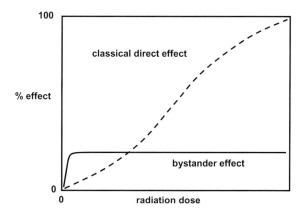

Fig. 3. Comparison of dose–effect curves of classical targeted responses and of a non-DNA-targeted response

Microbeam Studies of Non-DNA-Targeted and Low-Dose Effects

A number of laboratories have developed microbeam systems capable of targeting precise exposures of charged particles or soft X-rays to cells individually, under either manual or automatic control [6]. These devices have been used to investigate some of the foregoing phenomena by revisiting hit and non-hit cells and following responses in them and their progeny [7–9]. In addition, because of their ability to irradiate specific regions of the cell with micrometre or submicrometre accuracy, it is possible to map its responsiveness across the cell and gain information about the locations of targets and pathways involved in these transmitted effects. A recent development is to extend these microirradiation studies from purely in vitro to in vivo-like systems towards gaining an understanding of the role of nontargeted effects in the responses of organised tissues [10,11].

Discussion

Laboratory research in recent years has shown that certain low-dose responses differ both qualitatively and quantitatively from those observed at higher doses. In particular, bystander and other non-DNA-targeted effects exert a proportionately greater role with low-dose exposures. This behaviour appears to be, at least partly, a consequence of the increased heterogeneity of energy deposition that occurs with low-dose exposures, which favours signalling between hit and non-hit cells. Evaluation of the risks of exposures on the order of 1 mGy low-LET radiation depends on the extrapolation of epidemiological data from much higher doses. Although the LNT model continues to be the method of choice generally used for these extrapolations [12], any future modification in the low-dose region will rest on an improved mechanistic understanding of the biology.

References

1. Preston DL, Ron E, Tokuoka S, et al (2007) Solid cancer incidence in atomic bomb survivors: 1958–1998. Radiat Res 168:1–64
2. UNSCEAR (2000) Sources and effects of ionizing radiation. United Nations Scientific Committee on the Effects of Atomic Radiation Report to the General Assembly with scientific annexes, vol I. Sources. United Nations, New York
3. Prise KM, Folkard M, Michael BD (2003) Bystander responses induced by low LET radiation. Oncogene 22:7043–7049
4. Morgan WF (2003) Non-targeted and delayed effects of exposure to ionizing radiation: I. Radiation-induced genomic instability and bystander effects *in vitro*. Radiat Res 159: 567–580

5. Morgan WF (2003) Non-targeted and delayed effects of exposure to ionizing radiation: II. Radiation-induced genomic instability and bystander effects *in vivo*, clastogenic factors and transgenerational effects. Radiat Res 159:581–596
6. Proceedings of the 7th International Workshop (2006) Microbeam probes of cellular radiation response, Columbia University, New York, New York, March 15–17, 2006. Radiat Res 166:652–689
7. Kashino G, Prise KM, Schettino G, et al (2004) Evidence for induction of DNA double strand breaks in the bystander response to targeted soft X-rays in CHO cells. Mutat Res 556:209–215
8. Schettino G, Folkard M, Michael BD, et al (2005) Low-dose binary behavior of bystander cell killing after microbeam irradiation of a single cell with focused C(k) X-rays. Radiat Res 163:332–336
9. Hamada N, Schettino G, Kashino G, et al (2006) Histone H2AX phosphorylation in normal human cells irradiated with focused ultrasoft X-rays: evidence for chromatin movement during repair. Radiat Res 166:1–8
10. Belyakov OV, Folkard M, Mothersill C, et al (2006) Bystander-induced differentiation: a major response to targeted irradiation of a urothelial explant model. Mutat Res 597:43–49
11. Belyakov OV, Mitchell SA, Parikh D, et al (2005) Biological effects in unirradiated human tissue induced by radiation damage up to 1 mm away. Proc Natl Acad Sci U S A 102:14203–14208
12. ICRP (2005) Low-dose extrapolation of radiation-related cancer risk. ICRP Publication 99. Ann ICRP 35

Update from the Chernobyl Tissue Bank: Effect of Latency on Different Types of Thyroid Cancer Post-Chernobyl

Gerry A. Thomas

Summary. The only unequivocal radiological effect of the Chernobyl accident on human health is the increase in thyroid cancer in those exposed in childhood or early adolescence. In response to the scientific interest in studying the molecular biology of thyroid cancer post Chernobyl, the Chernobyl Tissue Bank (CTB: www.chernobyltissuebank.com) was established. The project is supported by the governments of Ukraine and Russia, and is financially supported (US $3M) by the European Commission, the National Cancer Institute of the United States, and the Sasakawa Memorial Health Foundation of Japan. The project began collecting a variety of biological samples from patients on October 1, 1988, and has supplied material to 15 research projects in Japan, the United States, and Europe. The results from these studies so far suggest that the increase in thyroid cancer is largely confined to papillary carcinoma, but follicular cancers have also now been shown to increase, suggesting that different types of thyroid cancer may have differing latencies. Molecular biological studies have indicated that there is as yet no obvious radiation signature, and that the molecular biology of the papillary cancers which have arisen may be influenced more by the age of the patient at clinical presentation than their aetiology.

Key words Molecular biology · Chernobyl · Tissue bank

Introduction

The CTB (Chernobyl Tissue Bank) is a unique venture. It is the first international cooperation that seeks to establish a collection of biological samples from patients for whom the aetiology of their disease is known—exposure to radioiodine in childhood. The project has the full support of the governments of the Russian Federation and Ukraine. The European Commission (EC), the National Cancer Institute (NCI) of the United States, and Sasakawa Memorial Health Foundation

---

Department of Histopathology, Hammersmith Hospital, Du Cane Road, London W12 0NN, on behalf of the Pathology Panel and the Scientific Project Panel of the Chernobyl Tissue Bank

of Japan (SMHF) cooperate to support the project financially. Thyroid cancers are very rare in a population of this age that has not been exposed to radioiodine. By the nature of the patients from whom the material is collected, the tumours are small. To maximise information, the CTB therefore does not supply pieces of tissue to researchers, but rather extracted nucleic acids and tissue sections. It is already clear, from the results of the Human Genome Organisation (HUGO) project, that it is likely to be the interaction of suites of genes which is responsible for both susceptibility to development of human cancer and the biological mechanism that influences tumour growth. The CTB therefore seeks also to permit multiple analyses on individual samples from the same piece of tumour and compare these with analyses on a separate area of tumour. This method will enable scientists to investigate the heterogeneity of a given tumour, a factor that may prove very important in the future design of therapeutic strategies. The CTB aims to provide material for study not only to this generation of scientists but also to the next, who may be in a position to benefit from a much more detailed analysis carried out on paraffin-embedded sections as well as the current molecular biological approaches that use frozen material. Samples of peripheral DNA from blood lymphocytes and samples of serum from each patient are also available, to permit the study of the interaction of the hormonal/immunological environment with genetics.

The project has been collecting material since October 1, 1998, and the Pathology Panel has already reviewed 2500 cases of thyroid cancer and cellular follicular adenoma from patients who were under 19 years of age at the time of the Chernobyl accident. Frozen material is available from 2083 of these cases, and DNA and RNA have already been extracted from a quarter of these cases. Collection of blood samples began in late 1999, and samples of serum and whole blood have been collected from more than 2000 patients. One important feature of the project is that it also collects biosamples from patients resident in the areas of Ukraine and Russia exposed to radioactive fallout, but who were not exposed to radioiodine, as they were born more than 9 months after the accident. These cases form an age- and residency-matched cohort of patients who develop spontaneous thyroid neoplasia; this is the ideal cohort for comparison with those who were exposed to radioiodine in 1986. The current number of cases in this valuable cohort is 138, with a further 84 coming from areas other than the exposed oblasts. The number of cases in this cohort is much lower than those exposed to radioiodine; the incidence is approximately the same as the background spontaneous rate from uncontaminated regions, of the order of 1 per million per year.

Pathology of Post-Chernobyl Thyroid Cancer

The majority of thyroid cancers diagnosed post Chernobyl in those who were children or adolescents at the time of the accident in Belarus, Ukraine, and the contaminated areas of Russia are papillary thyroid cancers (PTC). PTC is also the more common of the two main types of thyroid cancer in unexposed populations. Early reports of the pathology of post-Chernobyl thyroid cancer suggested that there was a particularly high frequency of the solid and solid follicular variants of PTC. This subtype of PTC is also seen in young children who were not exposed to radiation. An international panel of expert thyroid pathologists has reviewed all cases (aged under 19 at the time of the accident) of thyroid cancer that have occurred in the contaminated areas of Ukraine and Russia from October 1998 to date which are included in the Chernobyl Tissue Bank and all those that have occurred in Belarus from October 1998 to February 2001. Although in the majority of cases it has been easy to distinguish papillary cancers from follicular cancers, there are a few cases where a definitive diagnosis has not been possible. This type of intermediate lesion is also seen in non-radiation-exposed populations and has led to a suggested reclassification of thyroid tumours [1].

The UNSCEAR 2000 Report [2] suggested on the evidence then available that there may be a link between radiation exposure and the morphological subtype (i.e., solid/follicular variant) of PTC observed in children from the areas contaminated by the Chernobyl accident. More recent evidence raises questions as to the causal relationship between radiation exposure and the solid/follicular morphological subtype of PTC. The morphology and aggressiveness of PTC groups has been shown to be a function of latency in children exposed at different ages and was suggested to be independent of age at exposure [3]. The proportion of PTCs that are composed mainly of papillae increases with time post accident, whereas the solid/follicular variant appears to be decreasing with time post accident [4]. In addition, the percentage of small PTCs (≤ 1 cm) appears to be increasing with time [4]. This finding could be a result of more sensitive screening or that of a decrease in growth rate or aggressiveness of the tumours.

A recent study undertaken by the Pathology Panel of the CTB has defined the incidence of benign and malignant follicular lesions, as function of time since exposure (latency), in those exposed to fallout from Chernobyl as children or adolescents. The dataset, derived from cases reviewed as part of earlier research projects, comprised 1858 cases of thyroid tumour [1179 PTCs, 585 benign follicular lesions, 63 FTCs, and 31 medullary carcinomas (MTC: derived from a small subset of cells within the thyroid, the C cells, which are of a different embryological derivation than the follicular cells that are the cells of origin for both PTCs and FTCs)] from Ukraine and Russia. Eighty-one percent of the cases were from contaminated regions and 19% were from noncontaminated regions. Thyroid surgery was performed at a median age of 6.7 ± 5.6 years and at a median latency of 15 ± 4 years after exposure (75% female, 31% Russian, 69% Ukranian). All cases had been reviewed by the same pathologists and were aged either 3 months in utero or older at the time of the accident. The thyroid concentrates iodine only from 3 months of intrauterine age.

In the noncontaminated regions, the percentage and actual number of cases within each phenotype did not vary with latency analysed as four discrete quartiles (Q1–Q4, 4–19.5 years; data are available only from 1990, hence there are no cases with a latency less than 4 years) since time of exposure. However, in the contaminated regions, the percentage of benign follicular lesions rose from 32% in

Q1 to peak at 36% in Q2 and then declined over time to 32% in Q3 and 27% in Q4 ($P = 0.007$). The percentage of FTCs was lowest in Q2 (0.8%) and demonstrated a successive increase in Q3 (3.2%) and Q4 (5.8%; $P = 0.007$). The percentage of MTC and PTC did not show significant variation over time in the same population.

These data suggest that although the main increase in thyroid tumours post Chernobyl is in the papillary type, the possibility that there is a secondary rise in FTC with a longer latency, perhaps related to the progression from adenoma to carcinoma, needs further investigation. Longer-term studies are therefore required to determine the risk to the population of development of thyroid cancer post Chernobyl.

Molecular Biological Studies of Post-Chernobyl Thyroid Cancer

Earlier studies [5–7] reported that there was a higher than expected frequency of *RET* rearrangement in post-Chernobyl thyroid cancer, suggesting some *RET* rearrangements might be regarded as a marker for radiation exposure. More recent reports, however, have suggested that there is no link between radiation exposure and *RET* rearrangements. Instead, the high prevalence of one particular type of rearrangement of the *RET* gene (PTC3) in post-Chernobyl PTC may reflect the association between the solid morphological subtype with PTC3 rearrangement and the age of the patient at diagnosis, rather than the aetiology of the tumour [5,8]. There have been few statistically valid studies of *RET* rearrangement in non-Chernobyl-associated paediatric thyroid cancers [5,9], making substantiation of the association of *RET* rearrangements with age at diagnosis difficult. It is important to remember that the correlation between molecular biology and pathology is not absolute: in all the series published so far, a substantial proportion (30%–50%) of the papillary cancers do not harbour a *RET* rearrangement. A variety of different techniques have been used to assess the frequency of *RET* rearrangements and, although this may explain the variation in frequency observed among studies [10], there still remains a large proportion of PTCs for which alternative molecular pathways need to be identified. Moreover, a few studies have demonstrated *RET* rearrangements in benign tumours associated with radiation exposure [11–13]; however, other studies have failed to substantiate these findings [14], adding further uncertainty to the specific association of *RET* rearrangement with PTC. Despite the evidence that *RET* is able to transform the follicular cell in vitro, the evidence from transgenic mice suggests that other oncogenic mutations must be required for development of the tumour. The clinical relevance of *RET* rearrangements in post-Chernobyl papillary carcinoma still remains unclear. Some studies in adults have suggested that the presence of *RET* rearrangements may confer a better prognosis, but other studies suggest the opposite [15–18]. In addition, it has also been suggested that *RET* rearrangements are not found in all cells in post-Chernobyl PTCs, and that cells harbouring the rearrangement may be clustered [19]. The degree of clustering appears to be related to the latency of the tumours, with tumours of shorter latency giving a more homogeneous profile than those of longer latency [20]. This finding suggests either a polyclonal origin of these tumours or that *RET* rearrangement is a later event in thyroid papillary carcinogenesis than had previously been thought.

The BRAF oncogene has recently emerged as the most commonly mutated oncogene in PTC in adults. The frequency varied in a number of studies from 36% to 69% in adult PTC [21,22], including one study on Ukrainian tumours [8]. The frequency of BRAF mutation in post-Chernobyl cases (aged under 18 at operation) is much lower, less than 10% [23], and does not appear to be significantly different from that observed in sporadic childhood thyroid papillary carcinoma (PTC) [22,23]. This finding is perhaps not surprising as BRAF and *RET* oncogenic alterations appear to be virtually mutually exclusive in the series published thus far.

Few studies have combined analysis of both *RET* and BRAF with detailed pathology and age at operation. A recent study, conducted by members of the Pathology Panel of the CTB on the cohort of patients who were born after December 1, 1987, suggests that *RET* rearrangement is indeed associated with young age at diagnosis and the solid phenotype of PTC. The higher frequency of *RET* rearrangement seen in children may be a reflection of the pathomorphological type of tumour in the young.

Results from the study of the frequency of the BRAF mutation in the same cases suggest that indeed the molecular biology of childhood thyroid cancer is different from that of adult thyroid cancer. Only one case in the under 16 years of age group of patients was positive for BRAF rearrangement (Thomas et al., in preparation). The same analysis was repeated in 51 cases of PTC from the same Ukrainian population aged 16 to 30 years at operation. In the older group, the overall frequency of *RET* rearrangement was lower (39% vs. 54%), but the BRAF mutation was more frequent (12% vs. 2%), although significantly lower than the 58% previously reported for adult-onset PTC in the Ukrainian population [8].

These results show that there is a genuine increase in the proportion of BRAF-positive tumours with the same pathomorphology with increasing age of the patients at presentation. These results have led us to conclude that (a) *RET* rearrangement and BRAF mutation are not related to exposure to radiation, but show a strong association with age of the patient at operation; (b) *RET* rearrangement and BRAF mutation are mutually exclusive; and (c) RAS, *RET*, and BRAF oncogenes, although they all activate the MAPK pathway, are associated with tumours of different pathological phenotypes. One possible explanation is that activation via *RET* is more likely to provide a growth advantage in the child's thyroid, whereas BRAF is more likely to produce a growth advantage in the adult thyroid. These results suggest that cross talk with pathways other than MAPK may be an important factor in thyroid tumour growth at different ages.

It is, therefore, clear that all cases that are negative for BRAF in young-onset papillary cancer are not necessarily positive for *RET* rearrangement, and that there are as yet unidentified oncogenic changes in these tumours. A novel rearrangement involving inversion of chromosome 7, resulting in fusion of part of the BRAF gene with the AKAP9 gene, has also been described in three PTCs from young children in Belarus [24]. However, further studies in age-matched cases will be needed to establish whether this is a radiation-specific event.

One recent study, which will be confirmed in a larger group of PTCs requested from the CTB, investigated 25 PTCs (12 from adults and 13 from post-Chernobyl children) with known *RET* rearrangement status using 1 Mb BAC (Bacterial Artificial Chromosome) array CGH. Hierarchical cluster analysis revealed distinct groupings of tumours, one of which showed frequent genetic gains on chromosomes 19 and 21 or losses on 1, 6, 9, 13, and 20. However, the six *RET* rearrangement-negative cases from adults differed significantly from the other cases, harbouring more frequent losses of regions on chromosomes 7q and 22. Statistical analysis (maximum permutation *t* test) revealed significant differences between adult *RET* rearrangement-positive and childhood *RET* rearrangement-positive cases on chromosome 1p and between adult *RET* rearrangement-positive and *RET*-rearrangement negative cases on chromosomes 1p, 3q, 7p, 4p, 9p, 9q, 10q, 12q, 13q, and 21q. Tumour-related candidate genes within these distinctive regions are JAK1, RAB3B (1p), BCHE (3q), RBAK (7p), TXK- RHOH (4p), JAK2 (9p), DEC1, DBC1 (9q), FAX, PTEN (10q), TCF1 (12q), SLITRK1–3 (13q), and ERG (21q). Losses on chromosome 1p appear to be associated with adult PTCs whereas losses on chromosome 1q are specific for adult *RET* rearrangement-positive cases. Gain on chromosome 19 is specific for *RET* rearrangement-positive cases; losses on chromosome 19 are specific for adult *RET* rearrangement-negative cases. Deletion of chromosome 13 was found only in *RET* rearrangement-positive childhood cases. Fluorescent in situ hybridization (FISH) analysis for specific chromosomal areas has confirmed the BAC array findings [25]. Further studies are required to determine which of these genes cooperate with *RET* rearrangement to stimulate growth and which provide an alternative route to tumour growth.

BRAF gene reduplication has also been shown to be present in follicular tumours [26], suggesting that activation of this pathway is critical in thyroid follicular cell tumorigenesis. To date, there have been no studies specifically related to the molecular biology of follicular rather than papillary tumours of the thyroid following radiation. However, two applications for access to the CTB have recently been received that will address this question.

One recent publication highlights the change in proliferative activity of the thyroid during maturation. However, the authors were unable to relate the increased sensitivity of the young thyroid gland simply to proliferative rate, suggesting that a number of factors may also influence this sensitivity [27].

Thus, the evidence so far suggests that the molecular biology of post-Chernobyl childhood thyroid cancer is similar to that seen in age-matched series from non-irradiated populations. Post-Chernobyl papillary thyroid carcinomas, in common with non-radiation-associated childhood papillary carcinomas, do not harbour *RAS* [28,29] or p53 mutations [27,29] or show specific microsatellite instability [28]. However, three studies have now indicated that post-Chernobyl thyroid cancers may show gains and losses of chromosomal material when DNA is analysed on a global scale [25,29,30]. It remains to be seen whether these profiles are specific for radiation exposure or relate to the age of the patient at operation.

A number of studies have recently published transcriptomic analyses demonstrating different expression profiles between normal follicular thyroid epithelium or follicular tumours and PTCs [31–36]. Similar methods have not yet been shown to be able to differentiate between different types of PTCs, and in one recent report analysed it has been shown that the overall profile of post-Chernobyl PTCs is similar to PTCs from Belgium and France [36]. An updated analysis suggests that there are subtle differences between these two groups [37]. However, the two groups used in these studies were not age matched and the data should therefore be interpreted with caution. Further studies are now underway to link transcriptomic studies with genomic changes in an age-matched population.

Little work has been carried out regarding the effects of single nucleotide polymorphisms in peripheral DNA and post-Chernobyl thyroid carcinoma. A number of studies are underway, but their results are too preliminary to be included in this chapter. One published observation suggested that polymorphisms in the p53 gene may contribute to the risk of developing PTC after radiation exposure [38]. Further studies are clearly needed in this important area.

Conclusion

In summary, the CTB has facilitated research into the pathology and molecular biology of thyroid cancer post Chernobyl. It has highlighted the need for adequate age-matched studies to separate radiation-specific effects on tumour biology and genetic susceptibility from effects that are the result of the age of the patient at diagnosis. The research supported by the CTB has radically changed our understanding of radiation-induced thyroid cancer. The further support for the project that has now been received from the SMHF of Japan, the EC, and the NCI of the United States will allow continuation of the collection and documentation of biological material, not only from the cohort of patients exposed to radioactive iodine but also from the cohort of patients who were conceived more than 6 months after the accident and therefore not exposed to radioiodine. There are a number of large studies of the molecular biology of post-Chernobyl thyroid cancer currently underway, with pathologically verified material supplied by the Chernobyl Tissue Bank. There is no doubt that these studies will enable us to dissect out the elements that are caused by effects of age and those which are truly radiation specific.

References

1. Williams ED, Abrosimov A, Bogdanova TI, et al (2000) Two proposals regarding the terminology of thyroid tumours. Int J Surg Pathol 8:181–183
2. UNSCEAR (2000) Report. Volume 2, Annex J. United Nations, New York and Geneva

3. Williams ED, Abrosimov A, Bogdanova TI, et al (2004) Carcinoma after Chernobyl. Latent period, morphology and aggressivity. Br J Cancer 90:2219–2224
4. Bogdanova TI, Zurnadzhy LY, Greenebaum E, et al (2006) A cohort study of thyroid cancer and other thyroid diseases after the Chernobyl accident: pathology analysis of thyroid cancer cases in Ukraine detected during the first screening (1998–2000). Cancer (Phila) 107:2559–2566
5. Nikiforov YE, Rowland JM, Bove KE, et al (1997) Distinct pattern of ret oncogene rearrangements in morphological variants of radiation-induced and sporadic thyroid papillary carcinomas in children. Cancer Res 57:1690–1694
6. Fugazzola L, Pilotti S, Pinchera A, et al (1995) Oncogenic rearrangements of the RET proto-oncogene in papillary thyroid carcinomas from children exposed to the Chernobyl nuclear accident. Cancer Res 55:5617–5620
7. Klugbauer S, Lengfelder E, Demidchik EP, et al (1995) High prevalence of RET rearrangement in thyroid tumors of children from Belarus after the Chernobyl reactor accident. Oncogene 11:2459–2467
8. Powell NG, Jeremiah J, Morishita M, et al (2005) Frequency of BRAF T1794A mutation in thyroid papillary carcinoma relates to age of patient at diagnosis and not to radiation exposure. J Pathol 205:558–564
9. Fenton CL, Lukes Y, Nicholson D, et al (2000) The ret/PTC mutations are common in sporadic papillary thyroid carcinoma of children and young adults. J Clin Endocrinol Metab 85:1170–1175
10. Zhu Z, Ciampi R, Nikiforova MN, et al (2006) Prevalence of RET/PTC rearrangements in thyroid papillary carcinomas: effects of the detection methods and genetic heterogeneity. J Clin Endocrinol Metab 91:3603–3610
11. Bounacer A, Wicker R, Caillou B, et al (1997) High prevalence of activating ret proto-oncogene rearrangements, in thyroid tumors from patients who had received external radiation. Oncogene 15:1263–1273
12. Elisei R, Romei C, Vorontsova T, et al (2001) RET/PTC rearrangements in thyroid nodules: studies in irradiated and not irradiated, malignant and benign thyroid lesions in children and adults. J Clin Endocrinol Metab 86:3211–3216
13. Sadetzki S, Calderon-Margalit R, Modan B, et al (2004) Ret/PTC activation in benign and malignant thyroid tumors arising in a population exposed to low-dose external-beam irradiation in childhood. J Clin Endocrinol Metab 89:2281–2289
14. Thomas GA, Bunnell H, Cook HA, et al (1999) High prevalence of RET/PTC rearrangements in Ukrainian and Belarussian post Chernobyl thyroid papillary carcinomas: a strong correlation between RET/PTC3 and the solid/follicular variant. J Clin Endocrinol Metab 84: 4232–4238
15. Basolo F, Molinaro E, Agate L, et al (2001) RET protein expression has no prognostic impact on the long-term outcome of papillary thyroid carcinoma. Eur J Endocrinol 145:599–604
16. Bongarzone I, Vigneri P, Mariani L, et al (1998) RET/NTRK1 rearrangements in thyroid gland tumors of the papillary carcinoma family: correlation with clinicopathological features. Clin Cancer Res 4:223–228
17. Musholt TJ, Musholt PB, Khaladj N, et al (2000) Prognostic significance of RET and NTRK1 rearrangements in sporadic papillary thyroid carcinoma. Surgery (St. Louis) 128:984–993
18. Sugg SL, Ezzat S, Rosen IB, et al (1998) Distinct multiple RET/PTC gene rearrangements in multifocal papillary thyroid neoplasia. J Clin Endocrinol Metab 83:4116–4122
19. Unger K, Zitzelsberger H, Santoro M, et al (2004) Heterogeneity in the distribution of RET/PTC rearrangements within individual post-Chernobyl papillary thyroid carcinomas. J Clin Endocrinol Metab 89:4272–4279
20. Unger K, Zurnadzhy L, Walch A, et al (2006) RET rearrangements in post-Chernobyl papillary thyroid carcinomas with a short latency analysed by interphase FISH. Br J Cancer 94:1472–1477
21. Cohen Y, Xing M, Mambo E, et al (2003) BRAF mutation in papillary thyroid carcinoma. J Natl Cancer Inst 95:625–627

22. Kimura ET, Nikiforova MN, Zhu Z, et al (2003) High prevalence of BRAF mutations in thyroid cancer: genetic evidence for constitutive activation of the RET/PTC-RAS-BRAF signaling pathway in papillary thyroid carcinoma. Cancer Res 63:1454–1457
23. Ciampi R, Knauf JA, Kerler R, et al (2005) Oncogenic AKAP9-BRAF fusion is a novel mechanism of MAPK pathway activation in thyroid cancer. J Clin Invest 115:20–23
24. Ciampi R, Zhu Z, Nikiforov YE (2005) BRAF copy number gains in thyroid tumors detected by fluorescence in situ hybridization. Endocr Pathol 16:99–105
25. Unger K, Malisch E, Thomas G, et al (2007) Array-CGH demonstrates characteristic aberration signatures in human papillary thyroid carcinomas governed by RET/PTC. Oncogene (in press)
26. Saad AG, Kumar S, Ron E, et al (2006) Proliferative activity of human thyroid cells in various age groups and its correlation with the risk of thyroid cancer after radiation exposure. J Clin Endocrinol Metab 91:2672–2677
27. Suchy B, Waldmann V, Klugbauer S, et al (1998) Absence of RAS and p53 mutations in thyroid carcinomas of children after Chernobyl in contrast to adult thyroid tumours. Br J Cancer 77:952–955
28. Santoro M, Thomas GA, Vecchio G, et al (2000) Gene rearrangement and Chernobyl related thyroid cancers. Br J Cancer 82:315–322
29. Kimmel RR, Zhao LP, Nguyen D, et al (2006) Microarray comparative genomic hybridization reveals genome-wide patterns of DNA gains and losses in post-Chernobyl thyroid cancer. Radiat Res 166:519–531
30. Richter H, Braselman H, Hieber L, et al (2004) Chromosomal imbalances in post Chernobyl thyroid tumours. Thyroid 14:1061–1064
31. Barden CB, Shister KW, Zhu B, et al (2003) Classification of follicular thyroid tumors by molecular signature: results of gene profiling. Clin Cancer Res 9:1792–800
32. Chevillard S, Ugolin N, Vielh P, et al (2004) Gene expression profiling of differentiated thyroid neoplasms: diagnostic and clinical implications. Clin Cancer Res 10:6586–6597
33. Huang Y, Prasad M, Lemon WJ, et al (2001) Gene expression in papillary thyroid carcinoma reveals highly consistent profiles. Proc Natl Acad Sci U S A 98:15044–15049
34. Jarzab B, Wiench M, Fujarewicz K, et al (2005) Gene expression profile of papillary thyroid cancer: sources of variability and diagnostic implications. Cancer Res 65:1587–1597
35. Mazzanti C, Zeiger MA, Costouros NG, et al (2004) Using gene expression profiling to differentiate benign versus malignant thyroid tumors. Cancer Res 64:2898–2903
36. Detours V, Watte S, Venet D, et al (2005) Absence of a specific radiation signature in post-Chernobyl thyroid cancer. Br J Cancer 92:1545–1552
37. Detours V, Delys L. Liebert F, et al (2007) Genome wide gene expression profiling suggests distinct radiation susceptibilities in sporadic and post Chernobyl papillary thyroid cancers. Br J Cancer 97:818–825
38. Rogounovitch TI, Saenko VA, Ashizawa K, et al (2006) TP53 codon 72 polymorphism in radiation-associated human papillary thyroid cancer. Oncol Rep 15:949–956

Current Risk Estimate of Radiation-Related Cancer and Our Insight into the Future

Michiaki Kai and Nobuhiko Ban

Summary. In low doses and low dose rates, current radiation-related cancer risk is estimated based on the linear no-threshold dose–response model. This model is often used not only for radiological protection but also for risk estimation of medical exposure such as computed tomography. These uses bring about controversy. The first aspect of the current risk estimate is whether a dose below 100 mSv contributes to the increase of the probability of cancer risk and remains controversial in light of some biological evidence. The second aspect of the current risk estimate is to presume a genetically homogeneous population in which both age at exposure and attained age of cancer that influence the risk, can be considered. This chapter reviews the current risk estimate for radiological protection and considers some issues for our insight into the future.

Key words Cancer risk · Radiation-related risk · Linear no-threshold model · Dose–response models · Risk heterogeneity · *BRCA1/2*

Introduction

The latest article by Brenner and Hall published in the *New England Journal of Medicine* [1] about the health risk of widespread use of computed tomography (CT) in diagnostic radiology has commanded attention. It has been also noted that Gonzalez and Darby [2] estimated the risk from medical exposure of which the results showed 3% attributable risk of radiation-related cancer in Japan. They calculated the lifetime risk of radiation-related cancer based on the linear no-threshold (LNT) model. The organ doses from CT examinations are a few tens of mGy, which is below the level of 100 mGy at which the increase of cancer incidence is statistically detected among the atomic bomb survivors in Hiroshima and Nagasaki. The first aspect of the current risk estimate is whether a dose below 100 mSv contributes to

---

Laboratory of Environmental Health, Department of Health Sciences, Oita University of Nursing and Health Sciences, 2944-9 Megusuno, Oita 870-1201, Japan

increasing the probability of cancer risk, which remains controversial in the light of some biological evidence.

The second aspect of the current risk estimate is to presume a genetically homogeneous population, although both age at exposure and attained age of cancer that influence the risk, can be considered. Recent evidence on the specific translocations of chromosome aberrations indicates that the frequency of healthy carriers is much higher than the incidence of spontaneous leukemia. This finding will cause us to reconsider the risk heterogeneity of population in radiation-related cancer. The second aspect of the current risk estimate would impact more strongly on current radiological protection than the first aspect.

This chapter reviews the current risk estimate for radiological protection and considers some issues for our insight into the future.

The LNT Model

It is generally understood that the LNT model is a simple extrapolation from high doses and dose rates in the dose–response relationship of cancer incidence. The International Commission on Radiological Protection (ICRP), however, introduced the dose and dose rate effectiveness factor (DDREF) of 2 when the cancer and hereditary risk are estimated in low doses and dose rates [3]. Epidemiological data such as those from the atomic bomb survivors strongly indicate a linear dose response for cancer mortality and incidence. The DDREF of 2 results in one-half of the cancer risk calculated using the available data of the atomic bomb survivors in Hiroshima and Nagasaki. This risk estimation underlies both undetectability of risk below about 100 mGy and lower risks at lower dose rates that will be considered in radiological protection. Therefore, the risk estimate is uncertain even if statistical variation can be excluded, and it can be based on other dose–response relationships except the LNT model. Figure 1 shows the dose–response models of cancer probability in attained age of 70 when exposed at age of 30 years to low

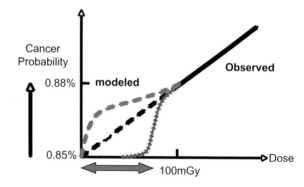

Fig. 1. Dose–response models of radiation-related cancer risk for low-dose region

doses below 100 mGy. Although unexposed people receive 0.85% of annual cancer probability, the people exposed at 100 mGy gain 0.03% increase of the risk [4]. These numerical values are so small that it is markedly difficult to validate the increase of risk resulting from radiation exposure above the spontaneous baseline cancer rate. The statistical aspect is essential to discuss whether the low-dose risk is real or a myth, because the excess cancer probability of 0.03% is less than the statistical variation of the baseline rate.

Current Risk Estimate

In its new recommendations [3], the ICRP has reestimated both cancer and hereditary risks for radiological protection (Table 1). The detrimental-adjusted nominal risk coefficients for a whole population have changed little as compared with those in the ICRP previous recommendations [5]. The hereditary risk, however, has markedly changed because risk estimation has theoretically changed. Hereditary excess risk has never been observed in humans such as in the atomic bomb survivors in Hiroshima and Nagasaki. The risk methodology in hereditary effects was changed by considering the advanced progress of genetics, although it underlies the LNT model. The resulting risk estimate of the hereditary effects has become lower.

Looking at cancer risk, there are opposing opinions to the LNT model (Fig. 1). In particular, some experts, such as the French Academy of Science, claim that the LNT model gives an overestimate and support a practical threshold of cancer risk. However, no consideration was made on uncertainty in determining the threshold. In general, it is expected that a threshold certainly gives us zero risk below the threshold dose. In contrast, the ICRP discusses the uncertainty and estimates that the upper confidence limit of the risk estimate by the threshold model is approaching to the risk estimate by the LNT model when a threshold dose is assumed to exist (Fig. 2) [6]. This uncertainty estimation tells us that no certain risk zero is possible even if a threshold certainly exists. At present, the LNT model is more reasonable for radiological protection, although many controversial issues exist.

The ICRP uses the numerical values of the current risk estimates for updating tissue weighting factors. There are some modifications in the tissue weighting factors to reflect the new information of risk estimates. In particular, the tissue

Table 1. Detrimental-adjusted nominal risk coefficients for stochastic effects at low dose rate (unit, % Sv^{-1})

Exposed	Cancer		Heritable		Total	
	1990	2007	1990	2007	1990	2007
All	6.0	5.5	1.3	0.2	7.3	5.7
Adult	4.8	4.1	0.8	0.1	5.6	4.2

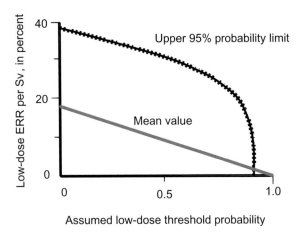

Fig. 2. Estimated excess relative risk (*ERR*) is not zero, depending on uncertainty of threshold dose when a threshold exists

weighting factor of breast cancer has increased, because the risk in women of younger age at exposure has increased in the cohort of the atomic bomb survivors. The cancer risk for radiological protection is estimated for a hypothetical population where it is computed by averaging over age groups and both sexes. The ICRP derives the cancer risk as averages across Asian and Euro-American populations. Current risk estimates can be made using either excess relative risk (ERR) models or excess absolute risk (EAR) models, when applied to populations with different baseline cancer rates. The ICRP uses different models for organs or tissues as the risk transfer models across populations. For breast and bone marrow, EAR models are used whereas the previous ICRP recommendations [5] did not use it only for these. Conversely, ERR models are only used for thyroid and skin. The combined estimates of ERR/EAR weights of 30%/70% are made for lung and 50%/50% for all others. The magnitude of weights may be judged according to epidemiological evidence. In breast, a pooled analysis of eight cohorts including the atomic bomb survivors in Hiroshima and Nagasaki provides the evidence of supporting EAR models across populations [7]. However, it is unclear why quite different models may be reasonable in estimating the risk among organs or tissues. The mechanistic process of carcinogenesis should be elucidated to choose risk transfer models for reliable risk estimation.

Susceptible Populations

Genetic susceptibility to radiation-related cancer is well known [8]. In radiological protection, the ICRP believes that high penetrance is too rare to cause significant impact on the population-based estimates of low-dose cancer risk except for susceptible individuals receiving radiotherapy [3].

Recent evidence related with carcinogenesis is increasing. It is unclear how radiation plays a role in carcinogenesis, although it is true that radiation induces mutation via DNA damage.

One interpretation of radiation contribution to leukemia is to induce two track events in the double strands of DNA, which cause chromosome translocation that might lead to preleukemic cells. In irradiated lymphocytes at 50 to 100 Gy, *BCR-ABL* translocation was observed at a low level. However, it is not likely the low frequency of these translocations could contribute to inducing chronic myelogeneous leukemia (CML) at doses of a few grays (Gy). The most prevailing translocation associated with pediatric ALL is t(21;12), which derives *TEL/AML1* fusion gene transcripts [9]. The frequency of *TEL/AML1* observed in cord blood samples is ~1% [10]. Considering the estimated extremely low probability of radiation-induced specific translocations, the role of radiation could be to raise the spontaneous mutation related to leukemia. Although this hypothesis will be biologically validated, it gives us the insight of the risk heterogeneity of a population in radiation-related leukemia. This hypothesis would influence low-dose extrapolation if radiation might contribute to carcinogenesis by disturbing stem cell kinetics.

Another source of evidence related to the second aspect is that the carriers of germline mutations of the *BRCA1* or *BRCA2* tumor suppressor gene have high radiosusceptibility for breast cancer. A relative large effect has been observed on breast cancer risk when women with the carriers of germline mutations of *BRCA1* or *BRCA2* had experienced chest X-ray examinations [11]. In particular, it has indicated higher sensitivity in the use of X-ray imaging in young *BRCA1/2* carriers.

In the atomic bomb survivors in Hiroshima and Nagasaki, the relative risk of breast cancer in younger age-at-exposure survivors is much higher than for other solid cancers. The possible reason is the existence of susceptible groups such as the carriers. It has been well known that the mutation frequencies of *BRCA1* or *BRCA2* in non-family-history cohorts range from 4% to 29% for *BRCA1* and from 0.6% to 16% for *BRCA2* [12]. Our theoretical calculation based on some evidence can provide that the high relative risk of breast cancer would be result from the existence of susceptible groups with the carriers of *BRCA1* or *BRCA2*. Further research should be highly promoted to ensure the hypothesis for radiological protection.

Conclusion

There are some controversies about current estimates of radiation-related cancer risk in low dose and dose rates using LNT models. It should be emphasized however, that the risk estimate from a low dose is so small that it may not be possible to prove or disprove the validity. A more important aspect is to presume risk homogeneity of the population in the current risk estimate. Further carcinogenesis study would give better understanding of the risk heterogeneity of a population rather than the issue of threshold existence.

References

1. Brenner DJ, Hall EJ (2007) Computed tomography-an increasing source of radiation exposure. N Engl J Med 357:2277–2284
2. Gonzalez AB, Darby S (2004) Risk of cancer from diagnostic X-rays: estimates for the UK and 14 other countries. Lancet 363:345–351
3. ICRP (2007) The Recommendations of the International Commission on Radiological Protection. Publication 103. Ann ICRP 37(2-4)
4. Pierce DA, Preston DL (2000) Radiation-related cancer risks at low doses among atomic bomb survivors. Radiat Res 154:178–186
5. ICRP (1991) 1990 Recommendations of the International Commission on Radiological Protection. Publication 60. Ann ICRP 21(1-3)
6. ICRP (2005) Low-dose extrapolation of radiation-related cancer risk. Publication 99. Ann ICRP 35(4)
7. Preston DL, Mattsson A, Holmberg E, et al (2000) Radiation effects on breast cancer risk: a pooled analysis of eight cohorts. Radiat Res 158:220–235
8. ICRP (1998) Genetic susceptibility to cancer. ICRP Publication 79. Ann ICRP 28(1-2)
9. Greaves MF, Wiemels J (2003) Origins of chromosome translocations in childhood leukemia. Nat Rev Cancer 3:639–649
10. Mori H, Colman SM, Xiao Z, et al (2002) Chromosome translocations and covert leukemic clones are generated during normal fetal development. Proc Natl Acad Sci U S A 99: 8242–8247
11. Andrieu N, Easton DF, Chang-Claude J, et al (2006) Effect of chest X-rays on the risk of breast cancer among *BRCA1/2* mutation carriers in the International *BRCA1/2* Carrier Cohort Study. A report from the EMBRACE, GENEPSO, GEO-HEBON, and IBCCS Collaborators' Group. J Clin Oncol 24:3361–3366
12. Fackenthal JD, Olopade OI (2007) Breast cancer risk associated with *BRCA1* and *BRCA2* in diverse populations. Nat Rev Cancer 7:937–948

Atomic Bomb Disease Medicine

Introduction of Atomic Bomb Disease Medical Research in Global COE Program

Kunihiro Tsukasaki[1], Masahiro Nakashima[2], and Naoki Matsuda[3]

Summary. Leukemia was the first radiation-induced malignancy observed among atomic bomb survivors. Radiation Effects Research Foundation researchers and others revealed that solid cancers began to increase in incidence with dose response after 1960 until now, along with the aging of the population, following the decline of leukemia incidence. In our previous Center of Excellence (COE) program, frequencies of multiple primary cancers and some hematological malignancies were found to have increased among atomic bomb survivors in relationship to exposure–distance response. Following these results, we have begun to establish a prospective banking system consisting of information about atomic bomb survivors on their exposure status, medical examination/care, including cancer diagnosis/treatment and tissue/blood specimens. Cancerous and surrounding tissues obtained from atomic bomb survivors are now being collected after informed consent during surgical operations at major collaborative hospitals in Nagasaki City. Blood specimens will be similarly collected during health examinations. All specimens and medical records will be stored in a deep freezer and in the computer database, respectively, at our institute. Questionnaires given to participating atomic bomb survivors about their lifestyle and disease history, including cancers, will be collected by interview and linked with acute symptoms resulting from atomic bomb exposures, which were recorded in our database. This databank will prove a valuable source for elucidating clinical and molecular pathophysiology of cancers still persisting after more than 60 years among atomic bomb survivors.

Key words Atomic bomb survivors · Databank, Late-onset carcinogenesis · Radiation health-risk control · Regenerative medicine

---

[1]Department of Molecular Medicine and Hematology, Nagasaki University Graduate School of Biomedical Sciences, 1-12-4 Sakamoto, Nagasaki 852-8523, Japan
[2]Tissue and Histopathology Section, Atomic Bomb Disease Institute, Nagasaki University School of Biomedical Sciences, Nagasaki, Japan
[3]Department of Radiation Biology and Protection, Nagasaki University Graduate School of Biomedical Sciences, Nagasaki, Japan

Introduction

Our multidisciplinary center of excellence (COE) program for the Global Strategic Center for Radiation Health Risk Control focuses on three major core fields: Atomic Bomb Disease Medical Research, International Radiation Health Science Research, and Radiation Basic Life Science Research. We are focusing on atomic bomb disease medical research, which is medical care for the effects of radiation, particularly still-persistent cancer risks in approximately 50000 aging Nagasaki atomic bomb survivors. Leukemia was the first radiation-induced malignancy observed among atomic bomb survivors. Radiation Effects Research Foundation (RERF) researchers and others revealed that solid cancers began to increase in incidence with dose response after 1960 until now, along with the aging of the population, following the decline of leukemia incidence [1]. In our previous COE program, frequencies of multiple primary cancers (MPC) and some hematological malignancies were found to have increased among atomic bomb survivors in relationship to exposure–distance response [2,3]. These findings suggest that late health effects of the atomic bomb are still persisting after more than 60 years. Following these results, we have begun to establish a prospective banking system consisting of information about atomic bomb survivors from Nagasaki on their exposure status, medical examination/care, including cancer diagnosis/treatment and tissue/blood specimens.

Achievements in the Previous COE

In our previous COE program, we retrospectively surveyed for MPC and myelodysplastic syndrome (MDS), a syndrome of so-called preleukemia among atomic bomb survivors in Nagasaki [2,3]. Development of MPC has been increasing in recent decades, possibly because of aging and improvement in the treatment of the primary cancer. We found that the incidence of MPC and MDS increased in relationship to exposure–distance response. Multiple myeloma is a malignancy of plasma cells secreting immunoglobulin and is frequent in the aged population. We prospectively surveyed for monoclonal gammopathy of undetermined significance (MGUS), so-called premyeloma, by screening for monoclonal gammopathy in serum at annual health examinations [3]. The incidence of premyeloma was about 2% in atomic bomb survivors, and the incidence increased with age. A significant inverse relationship between MGUS prevalence rate and exposure distance was seen only in the group who had been exposed while under 20 years of age [3]. Further detailed analyses are necessary to confirm these results.

Hypothetically, the radiation-damaged hematological stem cell could persist and acquire malignant characteristics during a long period of over 50 years. A study in 1995 of chromosomal abnormalities caused by radiation injury among healthy atomic bomb survivors has shown that lymphocyte and myeloid progenitor cells are carrying identical and distinct chromosomal abnormalities [4,5]. Recently, we encountered a characteristic proximally exposed survivor with a late hematological effect. This 79-year-old woman, who developed acute myeloid leukemia (AML), had complex and distinct cytogenetic abnormalities in leukemic cells, in nonleukemic bone marrow myeloid cells, and in peripheral blood T cells during remission of the disease. These data suggest that radiation may affect the development of malignancies six decades after exposure to the atomic bomb, especially in proximally exposed atomic bomb survivors. Therefore, in this global COE program, the mechanism of late effects of the atomic bomb is being further analyzed.

High-dose radiation exposure is a serious problem in the era of nuclear power generation. For the treatment of tissue damage caused by exposure, regenerative medicine is among the promising options. We are collaborating with the hematopoietic stem cell transplantation team and blood service team at our university hospital to continue clinical research on therapeutic angiogenesis. Implantation of autologous bone marrow mononuclear cells, including endothelial progenitor cells, into ischemic limbs increases collateral vessel formation in patients with arteriosclerosis [6]. Furthermore, ischemic symptoms were relieved for more than 6 months. We are now trying to purify stem cells from bone marrow using FACS-vantage (Becton Dickinson, Franklin Lakes, USA), by collecting side population cells after staining with Hoechist dye, for a source of regeneration medicine.

Establishment of a Databank in the Global COE

The risk of cancer persists and will reach a peak in 10 to 20 years in approximately 50 000 aging Nagasaki atomic bomb survivors, especially in proximally exposed survivors. Therefore, translational research is warranted to develop risk-adopted comprehensive methods for cancer diagnosis/treatment for atomic bomb survivors through the introduction of new molecular diagnosis and molecular-targeting therapy. For this purpose, in this global COE program, we are now establishing a databank consisting of information on atomic bomb survivors concerning their exposure status, medical examination/care, including cancer diagnosis/treatment and tissue/blood specimens (see Fig. 1). This project follows the regulations on human genome research by the Japanese government and was approved by the institutional review committee on the human genome at Nagasaki University in March 2008. Cancerous and surrounding tissues obtained from atomic bomb survivors have been collected after informed consent during surgical operations at major collaborative hospitals in Nagasaki City. Blood specimens will be collected similarly during health examinations. All specimens and medical records will be stored in a deep freezer and in the computer database, respectively, at our institute. Blood specimens will be processed into and stored as serum and mononuclear cells. Furthermore, B cells from peripheral blood will be immortalized and expanded with Epstein–Barr virus for banking. Questionnaires given to participating atomic bomb survivors about their lifestyle and disease history, including cancers, will be collected by interview and linked with acute symptoms resulting from atomic bomb

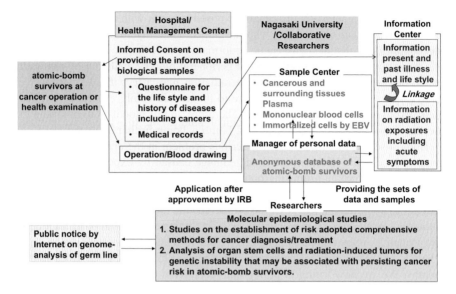

Fig. 1. Establishment of the databank consisting of information on radiation exposures, medical records, and biological samples from atomic bomb survivors. IRB, Institutional Review Board, EBV, Epstein–Barr virus

exposures, and recorded in our database. This provision will be especially meaningful for proximally exposed atomic bomb survivors who have been and who continue to be at high risk for multiple cancers.

The bank will provide a database for clinical and molecular epidemiological studies on late-onset carcinogenesis among atomic bomb survivors (see Fig. 1). To this end, the following research will be considered: (1) studies on the establishment of risk-adopted comprehensive methods for cancer diagnosis/treatment based on clinical and molecular pathophysiology of cancers among atomic bomb survivors, and (2) analysis of organ stem cells from proximally exposed survivors and radiation-induced tumors for genetic instability that may be associated with persisting cancer risk in atomic bomb survivors.

Future Direction

Research using this databank, consisting of information on radiation exposures, medical records and biological specimens from atomic bomb survivors, will generate implications for health risk assessment/management of low-dose radiation and developmental studies for education on "Radiation health risk control." This databank will be available to collaborative efforts in molecular epidemiological studies, to both clinical and basic research in atomic bomb diseases.

Project Members

Establishment of the databank consisting of information on radiation exposures, medical records and biological samples from atomic bomb survivors: M. Nakashima, K. Tsukasaki, M. Iwanaga, N. Matsuda, M. Mine, and K. Yokota (Nagasaki University).

Clinical and molecular epidemiological studies on the late-onset carcinogenesis among atomic bomb survivors: M. Nakashima, K. Tsukasaki, Y. Miyazaki, M. Iwanaga, S. Ulzibat, N. Matsuda, M. Mine, and K. Yokota (Nagasaki University).

Studies on the establishment of risk-adopted comprehensive methods for cancer diagnosis/treatment based on clinical and molecular pathophysiology of cancers among atomic bomb survivors: K. Tsukasaki, Y. Miyazaki, M. Nakashima, and K. Nagai (Nagasaki University).

Health risk assessment/management of low-dose radiation, and developmental studies for education on "Radiation Health Risk Control": N. Matsuda, M. Yoshida, H. Takao, M. Miura, N. Morita, T. Nakayama, and K. Shitijo (Nagasaki University); M. Akahoshi and A. Suyama (RERF).

Analysis of stem cell abnormalities of tumors in atomic bomb survivors: Y. Miyazaki, S. Ulzibat, K. Tsukasaki, T. Nakayama, K. Nagai, and K. Suzuki (Nagasaki University).

Studies on the genome abnormalities in lymphocytes of atomic bomb survivors at near distance: K. Tsukasaki, S. Ulzibat, K. Yoshiura, and K. Nagai (Nagasaki University).

Studies on the establishment of medical support using physio-mental evaluations of atomic bomb survivors, including those living abroad: H. Nakane, H. Kinoshita, M. Iwanaga, K. Tsukasaki, and A. Ohtsuru (Nagasaki University).

Studies on the development of regenerative medicine for the treatment of high dose radiation exposure: K. Nagai, Y. Miyazaki, N. Matsuda, M. Miura, N. Morita, and K. Shichijo (Nagasaki University).

References

1. Preston DL, Ron E, Tokuoka S, et al (2007) Solid cancer incidence in atomic bomb survivors: 1958–1998. Radiat Res 168:1–64
2. Nakashima M, Kondo H, Miura S, et al (2008) Incidence of multiple primary cancers in Nagasaki atomic bomb survivors: associated with radiation exposure. Cancer Sci 99:87–92
3. Tsukasaki K, Iwanaga M, Tomonaga M (2007) Late hematological effects in the atomic bomb survivors. In: Shibata Y, Namba H, Suzuki K, et al (eds) Radiation risk perspectives. Elsevier, Amsterdam, pp 67–72
4. Amenomori T, Honda T, Otake M, et al (1988) Growth and differentiation of circulating hemopoietic stem cells with atomic bomb irradiation-induced chromosome abnormalities. Exp Hematol 16:849–854

5. Kusunoki Y, Kodama Y, Hirai Y, et al (1995) Cytogenetic and immunologic identification of clonal expansion of stem cells into T and B lymphocytes in one atomic-bomb survivor. Blood 86:2106–2112
6. Nagai K, Matsumaru I, Fukushima T, et al (2007) Therapeutic angiogenesis by autologous transplantation of bone marrow cells for peripheral artery disease. In: Shibata Y, Namba H, Suzuki K, et al (eds) Radiation risk perspectives. Elsevier, Amsterdam, pp 67–72

The Offspring of Atomic Bomb Survivors: Cancer and Non-Cancer Mortality and Cancer Incidence

Akihiko Suyama[1], Shizue Izumi[2], Kojiro Koyama[3], Ritsu Sakata[4], Nobuo Nishi[4], Midori Soda[1], Eric J. Grant[4], Yukiko Shimizu[4], Kyoji Furukawa[5], Harry M. Cullings[5], Fumiyoshi Kasagi[4], and Kazunori Kodama[6]

Summary. The Radiation Effects Research Foundation (RERF) has conducted several studies of the potential impact of genetic effects on the mortality and cancer incidence among about 41 000 offspring born to atomic bomb survivors. The purpose of this research is to determine the degree to which parental radiation exposure affects mortality and cancer incidence in their offspring. Cause-specific risk analyses were performed with respect to parental gonadal doses. This chapter summarizes the findings to date, including the conclusion that there is no evidence of a significant association between parental gonadal doses and F_1 mortality or cancer incidence. This report is a summary of previously published results based on the long-term follow-up of the children of the atomic bomb survivors.

Key words F_1 cohort study, Mortality, Cancer incidence, Cancer mortality

Introduction

Various studies using different experimental methods have been conducted for several decades to find radiation-induced genetic effects. However, the results, particularly in mammals, have been inconsistent and controversial. A number of studies (Table 1) have been conducted at the Atomic Bomb Casualty Commission/ Radiation Effects Research Foundation (ABCC/RERF) to investigate whether genetic effects can be found in this human cohort [1]. For example, a study was conducted on abnormal pregnancy outcomes between 1948 and 1954. A total of 77 000 pregnancies were investigated. However, no statistically significant genetic

---

[1]Department of Epidemiology, Radiation Effects Research Foundation, 1-8-6 Nakagawa, Nagasaki 850-0013, Japan
[2]Faculty of Engineering, Oita University, Oita, Japan
[3]Division of Urology, Sanyo Hospital, Fukuyama, Japan
[4]Department of Epidemiology, Radiation Effects Research Foundation, Hiroshima, Japan
[5]Department of Statistics, Radiation Effects Research Foundation, Hiroshima, Japan
[6]Radiation Effects Research Foundation, Hiroshima, Japan

Table 1. Atomic Bomb Casualty Commission (ABCC)/Radiation Effects Research Foundation (RERF) genetic studies: past studies

Study	Period	No. of subjects	Genetic effect
Stillbirth, deformity, infant mortality	1948–1954	~77 000	Absent
Sex ratio	1948–1966	~140 000	Absent
Chromosomal aberration	1967–1985	~16 000	Absent
Protein analysis	1977–1984	~24 000	Absent

Source: Nakamura N (2006) *J Radiat Res* 47:B67–B73 [1]

effects caused by atomic bomb radiation were observed in any category examined, including stillbirths, deformities, and infant mortality [2]. The sex ratio was investigated in 140 000 offspring of survivors between 1948 and 1966, but no apparent effects were observed [2]. A study on chromosomal aberrations was performed between 1967 and 1985 that examined 16 000 offspring. In that study, sex chromosomal abnormalities, such as XYY, XXY, XXX, and mosaicism or inversion of the Y chromosome, were investigated. Furthermore, autosomal structural rearrangements, such as reciprocal translocations, inversions, and also chromosome trisomy were investigated. However, there were no significant differences or increases [2]. Between 1975 and 1984, 23 000 offspring were examined for protein variants using two techniques, starch-gel electrophoresis and enzyme activity measurements, to determine whether variants had been produced as a result of mutations in their parental germ cells. However, no indication of radiation effect was seen in that study [3]. Despite the data already mentioned, because of the primitive state of our knowledge of the genetic risks accruing in humans exposed to ionizing radiation and the fact that the children of atomic bomb survivors are currently entering their most cancer-prone years, an inquiry into the effects of parental exposure on the mortality and cancer incidence of their offspring remains an important and timely undertaking. This report is a summary of previously published results based on the long-term follow-up of the children of the atomic bomb survivors.

Subjects and Methods

F_1 Follow-Up Cohort

The original cohort was a selection of offspring born between 1946 and 1958, which was enlarged by including additional offspring born to parents located 0–1999 m from the hypocenter between 1959 and 1984. The original cohort consisted of three groups: offspring born to one or both parents located 0–1999 m away; offspring with one or both parents located 2500 m away but with neither parent located at 0–2499 m; and offspring born to parents not in either city (NIC) at the time of the bombings. The offspring were selected on the basis of city, sex, year of birth, and parental exposure to atomic bomb radiation. Family and biological relationships were established from birth records, parental interviews, and maternal pregnancy data. The cohort did not include offspring born to atomic bomb survivors who had moved away from the cities after the bombings. The study sample included 59 657 subjects with one or both parents in Hiroshima or Nagasaki on August 6 or August 9, 1945, when the atomic bombs were dropped.

Dose Distributions of F_1 Parents

The atomic bomb dosimetry system was established based on physical characteristics of the atomic bombs dropped on Hiroshima and Nagasaki as well as nuclear physical theoretical models based on data concerning how much radiation was released, how it was transmitted through the air, and how it was attenuated when it passed through buildings and human body tissues. The model was validated by actual measurements of exposed samples (such as wall and roof tiles). Individual radiation dose has been estimated based on information on a person's location and shielding status at the time of the bombings. After the initial T65D radiation dosimetry system, DS86 was established[*1], and since 2005, DS02 has been used [4].

For parental dose, the paternal testicle dose or maternal ovary dose was used. The paternal and maternal exposure dose distributions are shown in Table 2. Most parental doses were relatively low, with the proportion of those whose parental exposure dose was greater than 500 mGy being about 5%.

Confirmation of "Cancer and Non-Cancer Mortality" and Cancer Incidence

Study of the F_1 cohort has been facilitated by access to the official family registration records, called 'Koseki' in Japanese. By checking 'Koseki' records every 2 to

Table 2. Parental dose (DS02) distributions of F_1 cohort

Parental dose (mGy)	Paternal dose (%)	Maternal dose (%)
NIC	48.5	31.6
0–5	20.0	28.9
5–500	12.9	19.0
500–10 000	2.0	3.0
>1 000	1.9	1.8
Unknown	3.9	5.2
No information	10.8	10.5

NIC, not in city at the time of bombings

[*1] A dose category was defined as 'Unknown' for survivors who were close enough to the hypocenters to have received doses in excess of 10 mGy but for whom doses cannot be computed because of the complexity or lack of information regarding their shielding conditions.

3 years, virtually complete ascertainment of the vital status of cohort members is achieved, regardless of the location of their Japanese residence.

ABCC, in collaboration with local medical associations, started tumor registries in Hiroshima and Nagasaki in 1957 and 1958, respectively. Those tumor registries also provide linkage with our RERF study cohorts providing monitoring of incident cancer cases in all cohorts, including the F_1 cohort.

Statistical Methods

For the mortality and cancer incidence analyses, subjects were excluded if the national family registry indicated foreign nationality or if they had unknown status, the radiation dose was unknown or zero (NIC) for both parents, neither parent had exposure information, or subjects did not survive for at least 1 year. Finally, the total number of subjects for these analyses was about 41 000.

We analyzed cancer and non-cancer mortality and cancer incidence, both before and after 20 years of age. Cox regression models were used to compute hazard ratios and 95% confidence intervals (CIs) for paternal and maternal radiation dose (using either groups or continuous values) with adjustments made for city, sex, year of birth, parental age at childbirth, and age at entry on the baseline hazard rates. For non-cancer mortality before 20 years of age, baseline rates were also adjusted for birth weight. Confounding variables for baseline rates were chosen on the basis of their biological relevance.

Results

Cancer and non-cancer mortality rates during the period of 1946–1999 and cancer incidence during the period of 1958–1997 were assessed in relationship to individual paternal and maternal gonadal doses (Table 3). We found no evidence of significantly increased cancer and non-cancer mortality (Table 4) or cancer incidence rates associated with parental radiation exposures [5,6].

Table 3. Hazard ratios per 100 mGy for cancer mortality and incidence

Age in years	Cancer mortality		Cancer incidence	
	Maternal exposure	Paternal exposure	Maternal exposure	Paternal exposure
Ages 1–19	1.38	0.04	1.02	1.03
	(0.4–2.9)	(0–1.4)	(0.9–1.1)	(0.8–1.1)
Ages 20+	0.92	0.64	1.01	0.96
	(0.6–1.4)	(0.3–1.2)	(0.98–1.04)	(0.92–1.00)

Confidence intervals in parentheses
Source: Izumi et al. *Int J Cancer* 2003;107:292–297 [5]; *Br J Cancer* 2003;89:1709–1713 [6]

Table 4. Hazard ratios per 100 mGy for non-cancer mortality

Age in years	Maternal exposure	Paternal exposure
Ages 1–19	0.77 (0.6–1.0)	1.16 (0.9–1.5)
Ages 20+	1.15 (0.8–1.6)	1.01 (0.7–1.4)

Confidence intervals in parentheses
Source: Izumi et al. *Int J Cancer* 2003;107:292–297 [5]

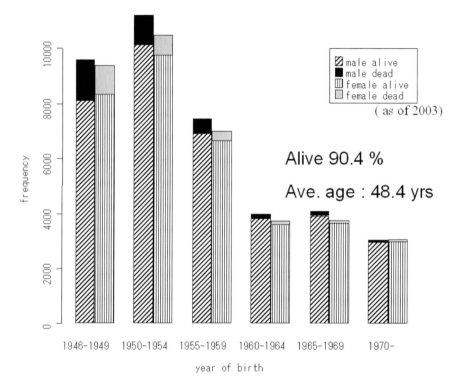

Fig. 1. Number of subjects at year of birth

Discussion

The epidemiological cohort study results with respect to F_1 cancer and non-cancer mortality and cancer incidence reported in 2003 [5,6] and summarized here are consistent with earlier results from ABCC/RERF [7–9]. The results suggest that parental exposure to atomic bomb radiation has not led to an increased cancer or non-cancer mortality or cancer incidence among the subsequently conceived offspring from parents exposed in Hiroshima and Nagasaki. This conclusion applies to deaths and cancer incidence of offspring occurring both before and after 20 years of age, even though the major causes of death tend to change with increasing age. The survival rate for the F_1 generation as of 2003 was about 90%, and the average age of F_1 cohort members (48 years) is still young (Fig. 1). As the number of deaths from cancer is very small to date, statistical power to detect small differences or to reach conclusive results is still lacking. Therefore, additional follow-up of cancer and non-cancer mortality and cancer incidence is needed.

Conclusion

After more than 50 years of follow-up, no evidence was found that parental pre-conception exposure to the atomic bombs altered cancer and non-cancer mortality or cancer incidence rates in children or young adults who were offspring born to parents exposed in Hiroshima and Nagasaki. These results may provide useful information relevant to current public concerns about the health of offspring whose parents were exposed to ionizing radiation before conception.

Acknowledgments. The Radiation Effects Research Foundation (RERF), Hiroshima and Nagasaki, Japan, is a private, non-profit foundation funded by the Japanese Ministry of Health, Labour and Welfare (MHLW) and the U.S. Department of Energy (DOE), the latter in part through the National Academy of Sciences. This publication was conducted under RERF Research Protocol 4-75.

References

1. Nakamura N (2006) Genetic effects of radiation in atomic-bomb survivors and their children: past, present and future. J Radiat Res 47:B67–B73
2. Neel JV, Schull WJ (eds) (1991) The children of atomic bomb survivors. National Academy Press, Washington, DC
3. Neel JV, Satoh C, Goriki K, et al (1988) Search for mutations altering protein charge and/or function in children of atomic bomb survivors: final report. Am J Hum Genet 42:663–676
4. Young RW, Kerr GD (eds) (2005) Reassessment of the atomic bomb radiation dosimetry for Hiroshima and Nagasaki: dosimetry system 2002. Radiation Effects Research Foundation, Hiroshima
5. Izumi S, Suyama A, Koyama K (2003) Radiation-related mortality among offspring of atomic bomb survivors: a half-century of follow-up. Int J Cancer 107:292–297
6. Izumi S, Koyama K, Soda M, et al (2003) Cancer incidence in children and young adults did not increase relative to parental exposure to atomic bombs. Br J Cancer 89:1709–1713
7. Kato H, Schull WJ, Neel JV (1966) A cohort-type study of survival in the children of parents exposed to atomic bombings. Am J Hum Genet 16:214–230
8. Neel JV, Kato H, Shull WJ (1974) Mortality in the children of atomic bomb survivors and controls. Genetics 76:311–326
9. Yoshimoto Y, Shull WJ, Kato H, et al (1991) Mortality among the offspring (F_1) of atomic bomb survivors, 1946–1985. J Radiat Res 32:327–351

Ischemic Heart Disease Among Atomic Bomb Survivors: Possible Mechanism(s) Linking Ischemic Heart Disease and Radiation Exposure

Masazumi Akahoshi

Summary. It has been demonstrated that exposure to atomic bomb radiation appears to be associated with an increased risk of ischemic heart disease (IHD). In addition, atomic bomb radiation dose is associated with many of the IHD risk factors such as high blood pressure, hypertension, high cholesterol level, inflammatory markers, and aortic arch calcification. Because visceral fat accumulation or metabolic syndrome clusters many of the IHD risk factors such as obesity, insulin resistance, dyslipidemia, glucose intolerance, hypertension, and inflammatory markers, and predicts IHD, results observed in atomic bomb survivors led us to hypothesize that visceral fat accumulation or metabolic syndrome may explain the association between atomic bomb radiation and IHD. Therefore, to examine this possibility, we used fatty liver, which is a surrogate marker of visceral fat accumulation or metabolic syndrome, and examined whether fatty liver: (1) clusters the IHD risk factors; (2) is related to radiation dose; and (3) predicts IHD in atomic bomb survivors. We defined that fatty liver: (1) is associated with obesity ($P < 0.001$), hypertension ($P < 0.001$), hypercholesterolemia ($P < 0.001$), low-HDL cholesterol ($P < 0.001$), hypertriglyceridemia ($P < 0.001$), and diabetes mellitus ($P < 0.001$); (2) is associated with atomic bomb radiation ($P = 0.02$); and (3) predicts IHD ($P = 0.04$). These results suggest that visceral fat accumulation or metabolic syndrome might be involved in the basic mechanism(s) explaining the association between atomic bomb radiation and IHD.

Key words Radiation exposure · Ischemic heart disease · Risk factor clustering · Visceral fat accumulation · Metabolic syndrome · Fatty liver

---

Department of Clinical Studies, Radiation Effects Research Foundation, 1-8-6 Nakagawa, Nagasaki 850-0013, Japan

Introduction

It has been well recognized that atomic bomb radiation exposure increases the risk of malignant neoplasms, even 60 years after the bombing [1,2]. In addition, an association between atomic bomb radiation and ischemic heart disease (IHD) has been reported in previous studies [3,4]. Examination of mortality in the Life Span Study cohort of atomic bomb survivors revealed that mortality from heart disease increased with radiation dose, although the relative risk for non-cancer disease was smaller than that for all solid cancers. An incidence study of the Adult Health Study cohort also revealed that myocardial infarction newly detected during 1968–1998 among Adult Health Study participants who were less than 40 years old at the time of the bombing increased significantly with radiation dose [4].

Other evidence supporting the association between atomic bomb radiation and IHD has been reported. Aortic arch calcification detected by plain chest radiography was significantly associated with radiation exposure in multiple logistic analysis after controlling for age, smoking, systolic blood pressure (SBP), body mass index (BMI), hemoglobin A1c, and white blood cell counts [5]. In a cataract study, retinal arteriosclerosis was associated with radiation dose after adjusting for age, sex, city, and smoking [6].

Radiation effects on conventional IHD risk factors have been reported in atomic bomb survivors. Growth-curve analysis showed that SBP and diastolic blood pressure trends among the younger exposed subjects [7], and cholesterol trends among all exposed subjects, shifted upward [8], although the basic mechanism(s) to explain how radiation exposure worsens the conventional IHD risk factors have not been elucidated. Effects of atomic bomb radiation on glucose metabolism have not been studied using sophisticated methods. However, recent unpublished data demonstrated that prevalence of diabetes mellitus (DM) was significantly higher among high-dose survivors who were exposed at younger than 20 years of age [8].

Recently, it has been reported that inflammation is closely related to the atherosclerotic process [9]. In atomic bomb survivors, it has been reported that C-reactive protein, interleukin 6, tumor necrosis factor-α, interferon-γ, and erythrocyte sedimentation rate increase with radiation dose [10,11]. Those results suggest that atomic bomb radiation has caused an increase in inflammatory activity, and this may partially explain the association between atomic bomb radiation and IHD.

Thus, studies of atomic bomb radiation and IHD risk factors revealed that atomic bomb survivors cluster many IHD risk factors such as DM, hypertension, abnormal lipid profiles, and inflammation, giving us the idea that visceral fat accumulation or metabolic syndrome may contribute to explaining the association between atomic bomb radiation and IHD. It has been reported that visceral fat accumulation plays a central role for this syndrome [12] and is closely related to fatty liver [13].

Therefore, to examine the possibility that visceral fat accumulation or metabolic syndrome may explain the association between atomic bomb radiation and IHD, we used fatty liver, which is a surrogate marker of visceral fat accumulation or metabolic syndrome, and examined whether fatty liver: (1) clusters the IHD risk factors; (2) is related to radiation dose; and (3) predicts the future development of IHD in atomic bomb survivors.

Subjects and Methods

A total of 2083 atomic bomb survivors (810 men and 1273 women) in Nagasaki underwent physical examinations [height (m), weight (kg), and blood pressure (mmHg)], fasting blood collection for biochemical measurements [cholesterol (mg/dl), high density lipoprotein (HDL) cholesterol (mg/dl), triglycerides (mg/dl), blood glucose (mg/dl), and uric acid (mg/dl)], and inquiries about smoking and drinking habits from November 1990 through October 1992. In addition, a radiologist conducted abdominal ultrasonographic examinations to make the diagnosis of fatty liver without reference to histories of liver disease, clinical findings, and/or biochemical examinations. We defined obesity, hypertension, hypercholesterolemia, low-HDL cholesterol, hypertriglyceridemia, impaired glucose tolerance, and hyperuricemia using the following criteria. Obesity was defined as a BMI (kg/m^2) of 26.0 kg/m^2 or more, hypertension as a mean blood pressure of 107 mmHg or more, hypercholesterolemia as a cholesterol level of 220 mg/dl or more, low-HDL cholesterol as an HDL cholesterol level below 40 mg/dl, hypertriglyceridemia as a triglycerides level of 150 mg/dl or more, and hyperuricemia as a uric acid level of 7.0 mg/dl or more. Participants with a fasting blood glucose of 110 mg/dl or more and those undergoing medical treatment for DM or impaired glucose tolerance were defined as having impaired glucose tolerance. The 2024 subjects who were free from IHD and/or cerebrovascular disease (CVD) at basic examination from November 1990 through October 1992 were followed until December 2000 to identify newly developed IHD and/or CVD cases during the follow-up period. IHD includes myocardial infarction and angina pectoris. Myocardial infarction was confirmed by the presence of one or more of the following conditions: typical electrocardiographic evidence of myocardial infarction compared with previous electrocardiographic findings; chest pain with typical electrocardiographic changes; elevation of myocardial enzymes; and coronary arteriographic (CAG) findings. Angina pectoris was confirmed by the presence of one or more of the following conditions: a positive result in an exercise electrocardiogram; chest pain with typical electrocardiographic changes; effectiveness of medical treatment for the disorder; and CAG findings. CVD was defined as rapid onset of a new neurological deficit in the absence of underlying potentially important nonvascular causes and lasting at least 24 h. Brain computed tomography

(CT) images and other diagnostic tests were also used to determine CVD. In this way, we detected 49 incident IHD cases and 84 incident CVD cases. DS86 was the radiation dosimetry used to estimate the association between fatty liver and radiation dose. The relationships between fatty liver and IHD risk factors and between fatty liver and radiation dose were evaluated by logistic analyses. The Cox proportional hazard regression model was used to estimate the relative risk and 95% confidence interval for fatty liver and each IHD risk factor for incident IHD.

Results

Odds ratios of fatty liver for IHD risk factors adjusted for age, smoking, and drinking are shown in Table 1. Fatty liver was significantly related to hypercholesterolemia and hypertriglyceridemia, a relationship suggestive for hypertension and low-HDL cholesterol in men; in women, fatty liver was significantly related to all the IHD risk factors.

Radiation dose had an effect on prevalence of fatty liver, low-HDL cholesterol, and hypertriglyceridemia, whereas it had no effects on obesity, hypertension, hypercholesterolemia, and impaired glucose tolerance (Table 2).

Univariate analysis showed that among IHD risk factors examined, impaired glucose tolerance, hyperuricemia, and fatty liver were predictive variables for IHD risk (Table 3). In multivariate analysis including age, sex, smoking, drinking, impaired glucose tolerance, hyperuricemia, and fatty liver, hyperuricemia and fatty liver predicted IHD development.

Table 1. Age-, smoking-, and drinking-adjusted odds ratios of fatty liver for coronary risk factors

Coronary risk factor	Sex	Odds ratio of fatty liver	Confidence interval, 95%
Hypertension	Male	1.923*	0.961–3.846
	Female	2.075***	1.238–3.472
Hypercholesterolemia	Male	4.132***	2.096–8.130
	Female	2.336***	1.447–3.774
Low-HDL cholesterol	Male	1.938*	0.965–3.891
	Female	3.115***	1.808–5.348
Hypertriglyceridemia	Male	2.857***	1.447–5.650
	Female	4.098***	2.519–6.667
Impaired glucose tolerance	Male	1.435	0.631–3.268
	Female	3.571***	2.012–6.329

*Relationship is suggested ($0.05 \leq P < 0.1$)
**Significance of $P < 0.05$
***Significance of $P < 0.01$
Source: Modified from *Hypertension Research* 2001;24(4):337–343 [14]

Table 2. Age-, smoking-, and drinking-adjusted odds ratio of radiation dose

Dependent variable	Explanatory variables	
		Radiation dose (Gy)
Fatty liver	Male: 28	1.32 (1.05–1.64), $P = 0.0201$
	Female: 57	
Obesity	Male: 61	0.89 (0.74–1.06), $P = 0.2060$
	Female: 163	
Hypertension	Male: 119	1.03 (0.88–1.19), $P = 0.7407$
	Female: 177	
Hypercholesterolemia	Male: 106	1.08 (0.95–1.23), $P = 0.2361$
	Female: 390	
Low HDL-cholesterol	Male: 127	1.24 (1.06–1.44), $P = 0.0062$
	Female: 107	
Hypertriglyceridemia	Male: 136	1.19 (1.03–1.36), $P = 0.0162$
	Female: 184	
Impaired glucose tolerance	Male: 94	0.87 (0.70–1.05), $P = 0.1579$
	Female: 84	

Values are odds ratio, 95% confidence interval in parentheses, and P value
Source: Modified from *Hypertension Research* 2003;26(12):965–970 [15]

Table 3. Relative risk of classic risk factors and fatty liver for ischemic heart disease development

	Univariate analysis	Multivariate analysis
Obesity	1.21 (0.56–2.58), $P = 0.63$	
Hypertension	1.34 (0.71–2.51), $P = 0.36$	
Hypercholesterolemia	1.38 (0.77–2.46), $P = 0.27$	
Low-HDL cholesterol	0.96 (0.46–1.99), $P = 0.91$	
Hypertriglyceridemia	0.91 (0.47–1.79), $P = 0.79$	
Impaired glucose tolerance	2.00 (1.02–3.91), $P = 0.04$	1.59 (0.76–3.34), $P = 0.22$
Hyperuricemia	2.59 (1.26–5.34), $P < 0.01$	2.30 (1.08–4.89), $P = 0.03$
Fatty liver	2.54 (1.06–6.05), $P = 0.04$	2.53 (1.06–6.06), $P = 0.04$

Values are odds ratio, 95% confidence interval in parentheses, and P value
Multiple Cox regression analysis was conducted using variables of impaired glucose tolerance, hyperuricemia, and fatty liver in addition to age, sex, smoking, and drinking
Source: Modified from *Hypertension Research* 2007;30(9):823–829 [16]

Discussion

Fatty liver was associated with hypertension, hypercholesterolemia, low-HDL cholesterol, hypertriglyceridemia, and impaired glucose tolerance after controlling for age, sex, and smoking and drinking habits in atomic bomb survivors [14]. Fatty liver was also associated with radiation dose after controlling for age, sex, and smoking and drinking habits [15]. Fatty liver predicted the future development of

IHD independently from conventional IHD risk factors in atomic bomb survivors [16]. The results suggest that visceral fat accumulation or metabolic syndrome might be involved in the basic mechanism(s) explaining the association between atomic bomb radiation and IHD. Future studies of radiation effects on adipogenesis and insulin resistance are necessary to evaluate this possibility further.

Acknowledgments. The Radiation Effects Research Foundation (RERF), Hiroshima and Nagasaki, Japan is a private, non-profit foundation funded by the Japanese Ministry of Health, Labour and Welfare (MHLW) and the U.S. Department of Energy (DOE), the latter through the National Academy of Sciences. This publication was supported by RERF Research Protocol RP 2-75.

References

1. Imaizumi M, Usa T, Tominaga T, et al (2006) Radiation dose-response relationships for thyroid nodules and autoimmune thyroid diseases in Hiroshima and Nagasaki atomic bomb survivors 55–58 years after radiation exposure. JAMA 295:1011–1022
2. Pierce DA, Preston DL (2000) Radiation-related cancer risks at low doses among atomic bomb survivors. Radiat Res 154:178–186
3. Preston DL, Shimizu Y, Pierce DA, et al (2003) Studies of mortality of atomic bomb survivors. Report 13: Solid cancer and noncancer disease mortality: 1950–1997. Radiat Res 160:381–407
4. Yamada M, Wong FL, Fujiwara S, et al (2004) Noncancer disease incidence in atomic bomb survivors, 1958–1998. Radiat Res 161:622–632.
5. Yamada M, Naito K, Kasagi F, et al (2005) Prevalence of atherosclerosis in relation to atomic bomb radiation exposure: an RERF Adult Health Study. Int J Radiat Biol 81:821–826
6. Minamoto A, Taniguchi H, Yoshitani N, et al (2004) Cataract in atomic bomb survivors. Int J Radiat Biol 80:339–345
7. Sasaki H, Wong FL, Yamada M, et al (2002) The effects of aging and radiation exposure on blood pressure levels of atomic bomb survivors. J Clin Epidemiol 55:974–981
8. Wong FL, Yamada M, Sasaki H, et al (1999) Effects of radiation on the longitudinal trends of total serum cholesterol levels in the atomic bomb survivors. Radiat Res 151:736–746
9. Ross R (1999) Atherosclerosis: an inflammatory disease. N Engl J Med 340(2):115–126
10. Hayashi T, Kusunoki Y, Hakoda M, et al (2003) Radiation dose-dependent increases in inflammatory response markers in A-bomb survivors. Int J Radiat Biol 79:129–136
11. Hayashi T, Morishita Y, Kubo Y, et al (2005) Long-term effects of radiation dose on inflammatory markers in atomic bomb survivors. Am J Med 118:83–86
12. Sattar N, Gaw A, Scherbakova O, et al (2003) Metabolic syndrome with and without C-reactive protein as a predictor of coronary heart disease and diabetes in the West of Scotland Coronary Prevention Study. Circulation 108:414–419
13. Hayashi T, Boyko EJ, Leonetti DL, et al (2003) Visceral adiposity and the prevalence of hypertension in Japanese Americans. Circulation 108:1718–1723
14. Akahoshi M, Amasaki Y, Soda M, et al (2001) Correlation between fatty liver and coronary risk factors: a population study of elderly men and women in Nagasaki, Japan. Hypertens Res 24:337–343
15. Akahoshi M, Amasaki Y, Soda M, et al (2003) Effects of radiation on fatty liver and metabolic coronary risk factors among atomic bomb survivors in Nagasaki. Hypertens Res 26:965–970
16. Baba T, Amasaki Y, Soda M, et al (2007) Fatty liver and uric acid levels predict incident coronary heart disease but not stroke among atomic bomb survivors in Nagasaki. Hypertens Res 30:823–829

Leukemia, Lymphoma, and Multiple Myeloma Incidence in the LSS Cohort: 1950–2001

Wan-Ling Hsu[1], Midori Soda[2], Nobuo Nishi[3], Dale Preston[4], Sachiyo Funamoto[1], Masao Tomonaga[5], Masako Iwanaga[5], Akihiko Suyama[2], and Fumiyoshi Kasagi[3]

Summary. Leukemia was one of the first late health effects of radiation exposure observed among the atomic bomb survivors, initially appearing in the late 1940s. Several Atomic Bomb Casualty Commission/Radiation Effects Research Foundation studies have reported a highly significant radiation-associated excess risk for leukemia, although the evidence for increased risks of lymphoma and myeloma are less clear in the Life Span Study (LSS) cohort. As this cohort ages, the number of incident leukemia and lymphoma cases continues to increase. The current analyses update the incidence risk estimates with a particular focus on how the radiation-associated excess risk varies with age at exposure, gender, and attained age or time since exposure. Consideration is also given to characterization of curvature in the leukemia dose response.

Key words Leukemia incidence · Atomic bomb survivor · Radiation · Temporal pattern

Introduction

A marked radiation-related increase in leukemia incidence was apparent within 5 years of the bombings of Hiroshima and Nagasaki. The excess risk appeared to reach a peak in the mid-1950s and is generally believed to have declined since that time [1]. The most recent detailed report on the risks of radiation-induced leukemia and lymphoma in the Life Span Study (LSS) cohort of atomic bomb survivors considered the nature of the risks for the period from 1950 to 1987 [2]. This study

---

[1]Department of Statistics, Radiation Effects Research Foundation, 5-2 Hijiyama Park, Minami-ku, Hiroshima 732-0815, Japan
[2]Department of Epidemiology, Radiation Effects Research Foundation, Nagasaki, Japan
[3]Department of Epidemiology, Radiation Effects Research Foundation, Hiroshima, Japan
[4]Hirosoft International, Eureka, CA, USA
[5]Department of Molecular Medicine and Hematology, Atomic-Bomb Disease Institute, Nagasaki University Graduate School of Biomedical Sciences, Nagasaki, Japan

aims to extend the follow-up through the end of 2001 using cases from the Hiroshima and Nagasaki Tumor Registries, validated by available information from the Leukemia Registry (1950–1987) through the end of 2001. One goal of the current study is to investigate whether simpler statistical models can describe the radiation at least as well as those used in the earlier analyses. In this chapter, we provide a short description of the new risk models used in the new analyses and briefly outline the nature of the excess relative risk (ERR) model for all leukemias as a group. Additional details on the leukemia excess risk and the risks for other lymphohematopoietic malignancies will be presented elsewhere.

Material and Methods

The LSS consists of a cohort of Japanese residents in Hiroshima or Nagasaki born before August 1945 and whose members were alive on October 1, 1950. The cohort currently includes 93 741 people (atomic bomb survivors) who were within 10 km of the hypocenters at the time of the bombings and 26 580 people who were not near the cities at the time of the bombings. Cases of leukemia, lymphoma, and multiple myeloma were identified from the Leukemia and Tumor Registries. Details on the registries are given in Mabuchi et al. [3] and Preston et al. [2]. By the end of 2001, there were 488 cases of leukemia, 542 of lymphoma, and 179 of multiple myeloma. Cases were eligible for analysis if they were a first-primary cancer diagnosed after October 1, 1950, among cohort members (including those who were not in the city at the time of the bombings), with dose estimates. There were 360 eligible leukemia cases, 434 lymphomas, and 134 multiple myelomas among 113 000 people, with 3 610 000 person-years of follow up (after allowing for migration).

Radiation effects on the leukemia, lymphoma, and multiple myeloma incidence rates were investigated using Poisson regression models. Both ERR and excess absolute rate (EAR) models were considered. The general forms of the models used in the study were these:

$$\text{ERR:} \quad \text{Total Risk} = B(c,s,b,a)[1 + \text{ERR}(d,s,e,a)]$$

$$\text{EAR:} \quad \text{Total Risk} = B(c,s,b,a) + \text{EAR}(d,s,e,a)$$

where c = city, s = gender, b = birth year, a = attained age, d = radiation dose, e = age at bombing, and B(c, s, b, a) is the background risk for the people with zero radiation exposure. Radiation dose was estimated using Dosimetry System 2002 (DS02) weighted bone marrow dose. Various dose–response functions, such as linear, linear-quadratic, and threshold models, were examined. The risks were estimated using the AMFIT module of the Epicure risk modeling software.

In the previous LSS leukemia report (1994), radiation effects were described using EAR models in which the risk varied with time since exposure and gender within age at exposure groups. As we examined the current data, it was found that models in which the excess risk (ERR or EAR) varied smoothly with attained age and age at exposure and a simple multiplicative gender effect described the data at least as well as the more complicated models used previously. Those relatively simpler models were the focus of these analyses.

The conduct of the LSS was approved by the Human Investigation Committee of Radiation Effects Research Foundation (RERF). The use of death certificates of the LSS subjects was approved by the Ministry of Internal Affairs and Communications. The respective committees of Hiroshima City Cancer Registry, Hiroshima Prefecture Tissue Registry, and Nagasaki Prefecture Cancer Registry approved the use of cancer registry data for the present study.

Results

For leukemia of all types, the logarithm of the background rates could be fit quite well using a linear-quadratic function of the log of attained age; that is, background rate is a power function of age in which the power increases with log age (Fig. 1) with a simple main effect of gender (men having higher risks than women) and birth cohort (with higher age-specific rates for later birth cohorts).

The linear-quadratic dose response with upward curvature fitted significantly better ($P = 0.002$) than a simple linear model. The temporal pattern and gender variation in the excess risk could be described equally well using either ERR or EAR models in which the excess risk decreases with increasing attained age and,

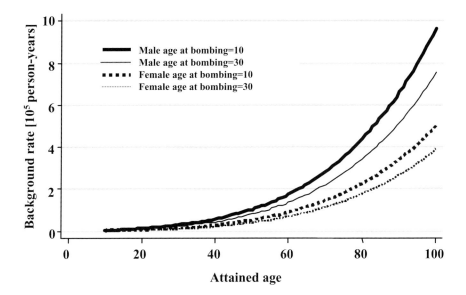

Fig. 1. Fitted background rate for leukemia of all types (ages in years)

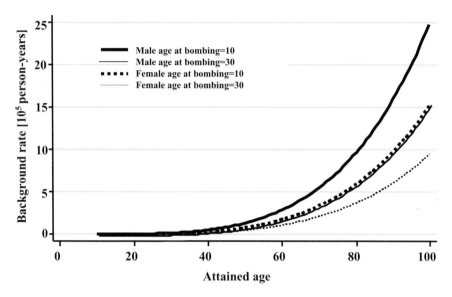

Fig. 2. Fitted background rate for lymphoma (ages in years)

for a given attained age, increases with increasing age at exposure. There was no indication of a statistically significant gender difference in the ERR model ($P > 0.5$), but in the EAR model excess rates for women were significantly lower than those for men ($P = 0.03$). Although the highest excess rates (or excess relative risks) were seen at the youngest attained ages, for a given attained age, the EAR increased by about 60% per decade increase in age at exposure. City was not a significant risk modifier ($P > 0.05$).

For lymphoma, the increase in the background rate was roughly proportional to the fourth power of attained age (Fig. 2), with significant age-specific background ($P < 0.001$) and gender effects ($P < 0.001$). There was a significant linear dose response in men ($P < 0.001$) but not in women. The background rate of multiple myeloma increased proportionally to the sixth power of attained age. There was a significant trend with age-specific rates that increased by 2.2% for each year increase in the year of birth ($P < 0.001$). The rate did not appear to differ by city ($P > 0.1$) or by sex ($P > 0.1$). As reported in the previous study, there was no indication of a significant dose response for multiple myeloma.

Conclusion

We have briefly outlined some of the main features of our new analyses of radiation effects on the risk of leukemia and other lymphohematopoietic malignancies in atomic bomb survivors for the period from 1950 through 2001. The results, which are based on almost twice as many cases as the previous incidence analyses of these outcomes, indicate that excess risks for leukemia can be described by simpler ERR or EAR models than were used in the earlier report. As in the earlier report, although a significant dose response was seen for leukemia, the situation for lymphoma is complicated in that there is no indication of a dose response for women but some evidence for a radiation effect in men. There is no indication of a significant increase in the risk of multiple myeloma. The results of the new analyses will be presented in detail in forthcoming publications.

Acknowledgments. The Radiation Effects Research Foundation (RERF), Hiroshima and Nagasaki, Japan is a private, non-profit foundation funded by the Japanese Ministry of Health, Labour and Welfare (MHLW) and the U.S. Department of Energy (DOE), the latter in part through the National Academy of Sciences. This publication was supported by RERF Research Protocol 29-60.

References

1. Ichimaru M, Ishimaru T, Mikami M, et al (1981) Incidence of leukemia in a fixed cohort of atomic-bomb survivors and controls, Hiroshima and Nagasaki, October 1950-December 1978. TR13-81, Radiation Effects Research Foundation
2. Preston DL, Kusumi S, Tomonaga M, et al (1994) Cancer incidence in atomic-bomb survivors. Part III: Leukemia, lymphoma and multiple myeloma, 1950–1987. Radiat Res 137:S68–S97
3. Mabuchi K, Soda M, Ron E, et al (1994) Cancer incidence in atomic-bomb survivors. Part I: Use of tumor registries in Hiroshima and Nagasaki for incidence studies. Radiat Res 137: S1–S16

Follow-Up Study of 78 Healthy Exposed Atomic Bomb Survivors for 35 Years in Hiroshima, with Special Reference to Multiple Cancers

Nanao Kamada

Summary. From 1968 to 1972, a survey was carried out to find persons who had miraculously survived being exposed to the atomic bomb within 500 m from the hypocenter by Hiroshima University and Hiroshima City. After the confirmation of these 78 survivors, Hiroshima University started a project called "Comprehensive Study on Heavily Exposed Survivors" in 1972. Exposed radiation doses estimated by chromosome aberrations of the peripheral blood lymphocytes ranged from 1 to 5.1 seiverts (Sv). Of the 78 survivors, 58 had died in the past 35 years. Biannual health examination revealed 29 survivors with cancers, including 5 double and 1 triple cancer. The incidence of multiple cancers increased with their age. The survivors who were exposed to the atomic bomb at an early age are reaching the cancer prediction age. Therefore, the tendency for multiple cancers among the survivors will continue to increase.

Key words Atomic bomb survivors · Double or triple cancers · Radiation dose

Introduction

The health consequences of radiation exposure to the people are a very important matter. The Radiation Effects Research Foundation (RERF) has investigated for a long time the late effects of atomic bomb radiation from an epidemiological point of view, using a cohort group [1,2]. As a result, high frequencies of leukemia and solid tumors among the exposed people in Hiroshima and Nagasaki have been established.

Recently, a number of survivors, especially heavily exposed persons, have developed double or triple cancers [3]. This chapter provides the present state of multiple cancers among heavily exposed survivors during the past 35 years of follow-up.

Hiroshima Atomic Bomb Survivors Relief Foundation (HABREF), 3-50-1 Kurakake, Asakita-ku, Hiroshima 739-1743, Japan

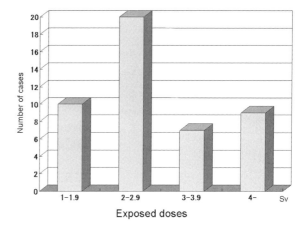

Fig. 1. Estimated radiation doses of the heavily exposed survivors group

Material and Methods

Patients and Exposed Doses

Seventy-eight atomic bomb survivors were examined for their health condition for 35 years at Hiroshima University Clinic. They had been exposed within 500 m from the hypocenter in heavily shielded conditions. Their exposure doses were estimated by chromosome aberration rates of the peripheral blood lymphocytes [4]. Exposed radiation doses ranged from 1 to 5.1 Sv (Fig. 1). The mean exposed dose was 2.9 Sv.

Confirmation of Diagnosis

Medical charts and medical films, as well as pathological tissue slides, were used for confirmation of the diagnosis for multiple cancers.

Results

Percentage of Survival and Cause of Death. Of the 78 survivors, 58 have died in the past 35 years. The cumulative survival curve showed a gradual decrease of survivors (Fig. 2). The cause of death was mainly cancers (40%) and cerebro-cardiovascular diseases (33%) (Table 1).

Numbers and Types of Cancer. Among the 78 survivors, 36 cancers were observed: 7 stomach cancer, 5 colon cancer, 4 each of breast cancer and

Fig. 2. Cumulative survival curve of the 78 survivors

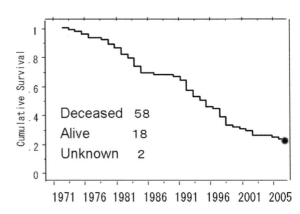

Table 1. Cause of death

Cancer (including 3 double cancers)	23 (40%)
Cerebro-cardiovascular disease	19 (33%)
Renal failure	4 (7%)
Interstitial pneumonia	3 (5%)
Pneumonia	3 (5%)
Accident (1 suicide)	2 (3%)
Others	4 (7%)
Total	58 (100%)

Table 2. Number of persons with multiple cancers among 78 survivors

Single cancer	23
Double cancers	5
Triple cancers	1
Combination of multiple cancers	
Stomach and liver	
Stomach and colon	
Meningioma and colon	
Colon and lung	
Multiple myeloma and breast	
Thyroid, colon, and meningioma	

meningioma, 3 each of liver cancer and leukemia, 2 lung cancer and ovarian cancer, and 6 other, such as prostate and skin cancers.

Number of Multiple Cancers and Their Combination. Among the 29 survivors with cancer, 5 had double cancers and 1 had triple cancers. The combination of multiple cancers were stomach and liver, stomach and colon, meningioma and colon, colon and lung, and multiple myeloma and breast. Triple cancers were found in a survivor who had thyroid cancer at age 57, colon cancer at age 66, and meningioma at age 69 (Table 2). The incidence of multiple cancers increased with their age (Fig. 3).

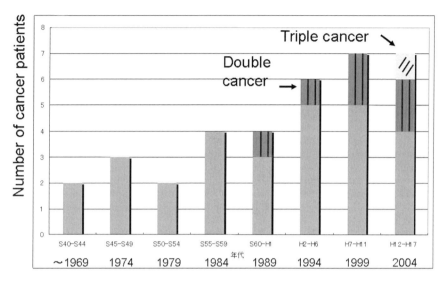

Fig. 3. Chronological incidence of multiple cancers

Discussion

Why the survivors develop multiple cancers of different organs has not yet been completely explained. Several factors are considered, such as aging of the survivors, tissue stem cells damaged by radiation, or the hormone environment. Recently, a report was published in *Science* stating that the origin of stomach cancer is from bone marrow-derived cells, not from stomach tissue stem cells, and providing a new theory on the origin of cancer [5]. When we consider the situation in the atomic bomb survivors, it has been reported that a number of cytogenetically abnormal cells exist in the bone marrow, some of which are forming abnormal clones [6]. Furthermore, it was found that some of the abnormal stem cells are circulating in the peripheral blood of the survivors [7]. Therefore, multiple cancers among the atomic bomb survivors may be reflecting the presence of bone marrow cells with radiation-induced damage.

It is well known that the *ras* gene mutation takes place at an early stage of tumorigenesis. An N- or K-*ras* point mutation was found in bone marrow cells from healthy atomic bomb survivors, and those who had the mutation developed leukemia or solid cancer 4 to 9 years after the examination [4]. These *ras* gene mutations in their tissues may have contributed to multiple cancer development among the exposed survivors.

References

1. Preston DL, Ron E, Tokuoka S, et al (2007) Solid cancer incidence in atomic bomb survivors: 1958–1998. Radiat Res 168:1–64
2. Yamada M, Wong FL, Fujiwara S, et al (2004) Noncancer disease incidence in atomic bomb survivors, 1958–1998. Radiat Res 161:622–632
3. Nakashima M, Kondo H, Miura S, et al (2008) Incidence of multiple primary cancer in Nagasaki atomic bomb survivors: association with radiation exposure. Cancer Sci 99:87–92
4. Kamada N (1999) Biological dosimetry of atomic bomb survivors exposed within 500 meters from the hypocenter and the health consequences. J Radiat Res 40:S155–S164
5. Houghton J, Stoicov C, Nomura S, et al (2004) Gastric cancer originating from bone marrow-derived cells. Science 306:1568–1571
6. Kamada N, Tanaka K (1983) Cytogenetic studies of hematological disorders in atomic bomb survivors. In: Ishihara T, Sasaki M (eds) Radiation-induced chromosome damage in man. Liss, New York, pp 455–474
7. Amenomori T, Honda T, Otake M, et al (1988) Growth and differentiation of circulating hemopoietic stem cells with atomic bomb irradiation-induced chromosome abnormalities. Exp Hematol 16:849–854

International Radiation Health Sciences

Research Activities and Projects Within a Framework of International Radiation Health Sciences Research

Noboru Takamura[1], Akira Ohtsuru[2], Hiroki Ozawa[3], and Shunichi Yamashita[4]

Summary. In our Global Center of Excellence (COE) program, one of the main tasks is to develop international radiation health research based on the worldwide consortium that we established within the framework of our 21st Century COE program, "International Consortium for Medical Care of Hibakusha and Radiation Life Sciences." Through the promotion of comprehensive medical support and academic joint research on those exposed to low-dose radiation after the accident at the Chernobyl nuclear power plant, the project for radiation risk evaluation regarding internal exposure and physiological effect elucidation is scheduled to be completed. It is expected that large-scale analysis of single nucleotide polymorphisms will succeed in identifying radiosensitive or disease-sensitive gene groups. Also, a joint project to strengthen the medical infrastructure around the Semipalatinsk Nuclear Testing Site and to promote academic joint research will continue. Furthermore, to evaluate the mental effects caused by radiation exposure in the population, including atomic bomb survivors, and to develop basic and clinical strategies for future unexpected radiation emergencies, we promote a number of research projects, in collaboration with the World Health Organization and other institutions. Our final goal through the implementation of these projects is to establish a human resource center that can explore human health risks from radiation on a global scale, to develop measures for overcoming the negative legacies of radiation, and to establish a scientific center for contributing to the safety and security of human beings.

Key words Chernobyl nuclear power plant · Semipalatinsk Nuclear Testing Site · Atomic bomb survivors · Mental effects · Radiation emergency

---

[1]Department of Public Health, Nagasaki University Graduate School of Biomedical Sciences, 1-12-4 Sakamoto, Nagasaki 852-8523, Japan
[2]Takashi Nagai Memorial International Hibakusha Medical Center, Nagasaki University Graduate School of Biomedical Sciences, Nagasaki, Japan
[3]Department of Neuropsychiatry, Nagasaki University Graduate School of Biomedical Sciences, Nagasaki, Japan
[4]Department of Molecular Medicine, Nagasaki University Graduate School of Biomedical Sciences, Nagasaki, Japan

The Global Center of Excellence (COE) Program "Global Strategic Center for Radiation Health Risk Control" and International Radiation Health Sciences Research

Our global COE program, the Global Strategic Center for Radiation Health Risk Control, has been initiated based on the consortium with relevant institutions in the former USSR, the United States, and Europe, which was constructed within the framework of the previous 21st Century COE program. Based on this consortium, we will focus on the control of radiation health risk through the cooperation of international organizations such as the World Health Organization (WHO), International Atomic Energy Agency (IAEA), and International Association for Research on Cancer (IARC); overseas institutions that have been participating in our consortium; and Japanese research institutions such as the National Institute of Radiological Research, the Radiation Effects Research Foundation, and Hiroshima University. In addition to the continuation of collaborations with these institutions, we will expand our consortium to Asian countries that are developing nuclear facilities, including nuclear power plants. Through the implementation of such cooperation, we will train personnel in various fields and contribute to society through the evaluation and control of radiation health risk.

Research Activities Around the Chernobyl Nuclear Power Plant and the Semipalatinsk Nuclear Testing Site

A dramatic increase of thyroid cancer has been observed since the accident at the Chernobyl nuclear power plant. According to a report of the WHO and the United Nations (UN) Chernobyl forum, about 4800 people who were less than 18 years old at the time of the accident have been diagnosed with thyroid cancer (Table 1) [1,2]. We need to continue molecular epidemiological studies to clarify the mechanism of carcinogenesis resulting from radiation exposure and to supply scientific evidence pertinent to the establishment of guidelines for radiation safety. In cooperation with the European Union, the National Cancer Institute, WHO, Sasakawa Memorial Health Foundation, and the governments of Ukraine and the Russian

Table 1. Number of cases of thyroid cancer diagnosed between 1986 and 2002 by country and age at exposure

Age at exposure (years)	Number of cases			
	Belarus	Russia	Ukraine	Total
0–14	1711	349	1762	3822
15–17	299	134	582	1015
Total	2010	483	2344	4837

Federation, we established the Chernobyl Tissue Bank, which is the first international cooperative venture that seeks to establish a collection of biological samples from tumors and normal tissues from patients who were exposed to radioiodine in childhood [3,4].

Furthermore, it has been clarified that the target age of thyroid cancer is shifting from children to young adults who were 0 to 5 years old at the time of the accident. Careful follow-up of this particular group, as well as of patients who underwent thyroidectomy, is definitely needed. We established an e-health system including telepathology and a tele-education system in cooperation with WHO, the Ministry of Health of Belarus, and Sasakawa Memorial Health Foundation to facilitate the diagnosis of thyroid diseases and to strengthen the infrastructure of medical education in this area [5]. In the Global COE program, we will continue the establishment of an e-health system in the former USSR, in cooperation with the Japanese embassies in these countries as well as with each relevant institution (Fig. 1).

Since the Chernobyl Sasakawa project, we have evaluated the trend of internal body burden of ^{137}Cs as determined by whole-body counter in the general population, in cooperation with the medical facilities of Russia, Ukraine, and Belarus, and we showed that 99.9% of the population now receives less than 1 mSv internal radiation exposure annually [6]. In addition to follow-up of internal body burden of residents in contaminated areas, development of a monitoring system of radiation

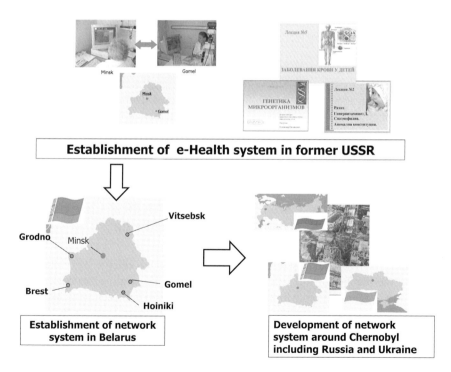

Fig. 1. Framework of an e-health system in the former USSR

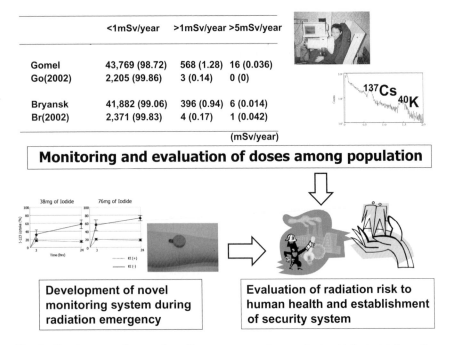

Fig. 2. Development of a novel small sensor system for monitoring biological information, including radiation doses

exposure doses for nuclear workers, as well as for the general population, is essential. For this purpose, we are developing a novel small sensor system that can monitor biological information including radiation doses. Through the development of such a monitoring system, we will evaluate the radiation risk to human health and establish a security system for use during radiation emergencies (Fig. 2).

Establishment of an International and Domestic Radiation Emergency Medical Care Network and a Medical Care System for Atomic Bomb Survivors Residing Worldwide

An international network system for coping with a radiation emergency is important because the number of medical specialists in the world qualified to deal with a radiation emergency is quite limited. Nagasaki University has been participating in the worldwide network system called REMPAN (Radiation Emergency Medical Preparedness and Assistance Network), which is organized by WHO Headquarters, as a collaborating center [7]. In cooperation with other collaborating centers and liaison institutions in the world, we will contribute to medical assistance during radiation emergencies.

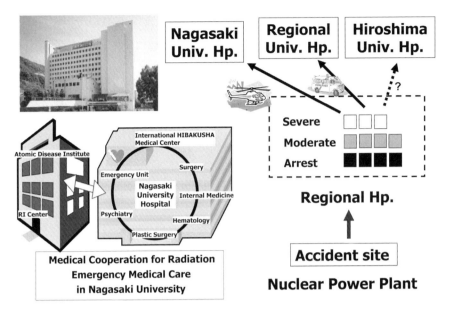

Fig. 3. Establishment of "Nagasaki Radiation Emergency Medical Care Network." Univ., university; Hp., hospital

Also, we have established the Nagasaki Radiation Emergency Medical Care Network in Japan, in cooperation with Hiroshima University and the National Institute of Radiological Sciences, for risk and crisis management of radiation accidents or nuclear terrorism in Kyushu area, Japan (Fig. 3). Within the framework of this network system, we have annually held special lectures and practical training courses to develop and maintain our ability to manage radiation-exposed patients. Also, we have published guidelines for radiation emergencies, including iodine prophylaxis, in Japanese.

Clinically, development of novel therapies for acute radiation syndrome is definitely needed. In particular, treatment of radiation burns is one of the most important issues. We have promoted stem cell research for future regenerative therapy of acute radiation injury, in cooperation with the Department of Plastic Surgery of Nagasaki University. These clinical studies will be also promoted within the framework of our global COE program.

There are atomic bomb survivors currently residing in Korea, the United States, and South American countries. In cooperation with Nagasaki Prefecture and Nagasaki City, we have performed medical screening and counseling in each country. Furthermore, in cooperation with the Korean Red Cross, we have begun an evaluation of the mental health of Korean atomic bomb survivors (Fig. 4). We hope that these studies will provide insight into mental health disorders, such as post-traumatic stress disorder, occurring after environmental disasters, including radiation exposure.

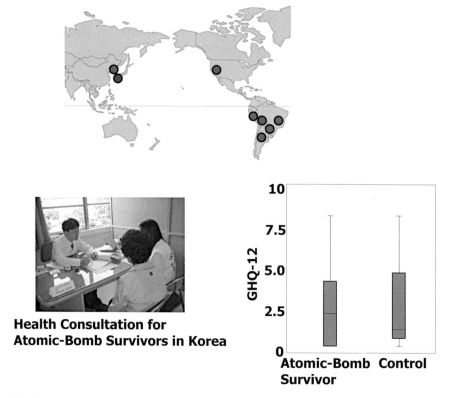

Fig. 4. Areas where atomic bomb survivors are currently residing in the world (*upper*), medical counseling for atomic bomb survivors in Korea (*lower left*), and preliminary results of mental health disorders among Korean atomic bomb survivors (*lower right*)

Development of International Collaborations with Asian Countries

Currently, nuclear power plants are important sources of electric power for many countries. For example, in Japan, there are 55 nuclear power plants currently operating, 1 is being built, and 1 is in the planning stage. Currently, almost 35% of electricity is supplied by nuclear power plants in this country. Therefore, science-based radiation risk communication with the general population, as well as specialists, has become an important issue.

Worldwide, 439 nuclear power plants are operating, and most of them are located in Western countries or Japan (Table 2). However, many of the plants currently being built or planned are located in Asian countries, including China and Korea. In India, where the economy has developed dramatically and the population has increased in recent years, there are 11 plants in the building or planning stages.

Table 2. Operating conditions of nuclear power plants in the world

Country	Operating	Power(MN)	Building	Planning
Total	**439**	**370 721**	**28**	**62**
America	104	99 209	1	
France	59	63 363	1	
Japan	55	47 593	1	1
Russia	31	21 743	4	1
UK	23	11 852		
Korea	20	16 810		8
Canada	18	12 599		2
Germany	17	20 339		
India	16	3 557	7	4
Ukraine	15	13 107		2
Sweden	10	8 910		
China	10	7 572	5	5
Spain	8	7 446		
Belgium	7	5 824		
Taiwan	6	4 884	2	
Czech	6	3 368		
Slovakia	6	2 442		
Switzerland	5	3 220		
Bulgaria	4	2 722		2
Finland	4	2 676	1	1
Hungary	4	1 755		
Brazil	2	1 901		1
South Africa	2	1 842		1
Romania	2	1 355		2
Mexico	2	1 310		
Argentina	2	935	1	
Pakistan	2	425	1	
Lithuania	1	1 185		
Slovenia	1	656		
Holland	1	449		
Armenia	1	376		
Iran	0	0	1	2
North Korea	0	0	4	
Turkey	0	0		3

We have already initiated collaborative studies with Barathiar University, which is located in the Tamil-Nadu region in India, involving the screening of the population residing near the Kudankulam nuclear power plant, which has been constructed with the technical cooperation of the Russian Federation [8–10]. Furthermore, we are going to promote collaborative study relating to the high natural background radiation area along the seacoast near the power plant resulting from the presence of monazite, which includes thorium-232 (Fig. 5). Through the continuous evaluation of the health risks of the population residing near the nuclear power plant and

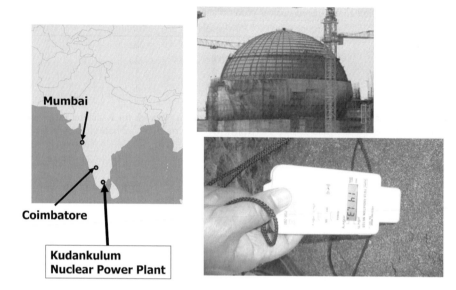

Fig. 5. Locations of Mumbai, Coimbatore, and Kudankulam Nuclear Power Plant (*left*), a power plant under construction in Kudankulam (*upper right*), and the area of high natural background radiation along the seacoast near the power plant (*lower right*)

in the high natural background radiation area, we would like to promote collaborative studies between Japan and India and possibly to develop a novel consortium among Asian countries.

Conclusion

Based on these international and domestic field studies of radiation medicine, we would like to train specialists for radiation risk control. Furthermore, we would like to establish a short-term training course and fellowship for radiation risk control and management, in cooperation with international organizations, such as WHO. Within the framework of this global COE program, our ultimate goal is to produce specialists who can formulate guidelines and standards based on scientific evidence in the field of radiation medicine.

References

1. Yamashita S, Shibata Y (eds) (1997) Chernobyl: a decade. Elsevier, Amsterdam
2. Cardis E, Howe G, Ron E, et al (2006) Cancer consequences of the Chernobyl accident: 20 years on. J Radiol Prot 26:127–140

3. Thomas GA, Williams ED, Becker DV, et al (2001) Creation of a tumour bank for post Chernobyl thyroid cancer. Clin Endocrinol 55:423
4. Thomas GA, Williams ED, Becker DV, et al (2000) Chernobyl tumor bank. Thyroid 10:1126–1127
5. Takamura N, Nakashima M, Ito M, et al (2001) A new century of international telemedicine for radiation-exposed victims in the world. J Clin Endocrinol Metab 86:4000
6. Morita N, Takamura N, Ashizawa K, et al (2005) Measurement of the whole-body ^{137}Cs in residents around the Chernobyl nuclear power plant. Radiat Prot Dosim 113:326–329
7. Souchkevitch G (1997) The World Health Organization Network for Radiation Emergency Medical Preparedness and Assistance (REMPAN). Environ Health Perspect 105:1589–1593
8. Brahmanandhan GM, Selvasekarapandian S, Malathi J, et al (2008) Population dose from indoor gamma exposure in the dwellings around Kudankulam Nuclear Power Plant. Radiat Prot Dosim 129:481–485
9. Malathi J, Selvasekarapandian S, Brahmanandhan GM, et al (2008) Gamma dose measurement in dwellings of Agastheeswaram Taluk of Kanyakumari district, lying 30 km radius from Kudankulam nuclear power plant site. Environ Monit Assess 137:163–168
10. Malathi J, Selvasekarapandian S, Brahmanandhan GM, et al (2005) Study of radionuclide distribution around Kudankulam nuclear power plant site (Agastheeswaram taluk of Kanyakumari district, India). Radiat Prot Dosim 113:415–420

Age and Prognosis: Do Adjuvant Therapies Influence the Real Prognosis?

Robert C.F. Leonard[1], Mariko Morishita[1], and Gerry A. Thomas[2]

Summary. The optimal management of older women with breast cancer remains an unanswered question. Clinical trial data on the use of chemotherapy are lacking, even in overview analyses. There are emerging data from laboratory studies that show that the biology of breast cancer may also be related to age of onset, even within the same pathology grade category. This finding means we must conduct carefully devised clinical research studies that also include a preplanned element of pathology investigation to decide which elderly patients may benefit from adjuvant chemotherapy.

Key words Adjuvant chemotherapy · Breast cancer · Molecular markers

Introduction

Breast cancer is, in common with most cancers, a disease associated with advancing age. In general, it is perceived that the biology of the disease is influenced by age in that proportionately more young patients present with aggressive, often oestrogen receptor (ER)-negative disease, whereas older postmenopausal women present with proportionately less aggressive, ER-positive disease. There is also the associated paradox that the mortality of older women from the disease remains higher than that of younger women, that is, that age, as such, is an adverse prognostic factor for breast cancer-specific survival. This paradox may be explained by factors such as access to appropriate surgical care, inadequate staging, and underusage of complex and often toxic supportive drug and radiation therapies, which are known to be important in improving the outcomes of the treatment of early-stage disease.

In addition to the way in which a patient is treated, a number of other factors associated with the clinical presentation and biology of disease have been found to

---

[1]Department of Oncology, Imperial College School of Medicine, Hammersmith Hospital, Du Cane Road, London, W12 ONN United Kingdom
[2]Department of Histopathology, Imperial College School of Medicine, Hammersmith Hospital, London, United Kingdom

relate to the prognosis of patients with breast cancer. Among these are tumour size, node status, and oestrogen receptor (ER) status [1]. ER represents a critical growth and survival pathway in most breast tumours; agents that block the ER signalling pathway (endocrine therapies) have been shown to be extremely effective in the treatment of breast cancer. Endocrine therapy has therefore been the most widely used adjuvant therapy for "early-stage" breast cancer. Initially, this was achieved by surgical ovarian ablation, but it is now attained by the use of drugs, ovarian suppression agents such as goserelin, and specific ER antagonists such as tamoxifen, or, more recently, agents that block the enzymes responsible for the synthesis of oestrogens, the aromatase inhibitors anastrozole, letrozole, and exemestane. The benefit of these drugs for patients with ER-negative disease is virtually nil, but women with ER-positive disease show a greater than 40% reduction in the odds of recurrence and a 22% reduction in the odds of death when given these drugs after "curative" surgery [2]. Endocrine agents have therefore considerably changed the approach to targeted treatment during the past two decades. The likelihood of a patient presenting with an ER-positive tumour is also affected by age. Eppenberger-Castori et al. [3] studied an American collection of 800 samples and a European collection of 3000 samples of breast cancers to "explore the hypothesis that ageing not only increases breast cancer incidence but also alters breast cancer biology." The study concluded that breast cancer is indeed significantly affected by patient age; in particular, that breast tumours arising in older patients have slower growth rates and are more likely to be ER positive. However, there may be no absolute association between ER status and proliferation rate, and there may be other effects that age at clinical presentation has on the biology of the tumour.

A significant contributor to the increase in survival of breast cancer has also been the appropriate use of cytotoxic chemotherapy following, or preceding, surgery. The odds reduction in death from modern, complex, and intensive combination chemotherapy given for several months after surgery is significant in both ER-positive and ER-negative disease and is similar in magnitude to the endocrine effect (although the latter is limited in its effect to ER-positive disease). In contrast to endocrine therapy, the side effects of chemotherapy can be dangerous as well as debilitating, and it cannot be used without serious attention to the patient's comorbid factors. It is also observed that the impact of chemotherapy-associated survival benefit tends to be greater in young, premenopausal women and falls progressively in the older-age cohorts of postmenopausal women.

This realization has resulted in clinicians now wanting to determine whether we have been too cautious in treating older patients with chemotherapy and to demonstrate, in randomised phase III trials of chemotherapy, whether by careful evaluation of an older cohort of women over the age of 70 at diagnosis, chemotherapy can be shown to provide an acceptable and effective addition to standard surgery and radiotherapy. This concern is the subject of a new clinical trial (ACTION): further information on the trial can be found on www.angloceltic.org.uk.

The study reported here was carried out to provide information on the effects of age, biology, and treatment on outcome from a representative population of patients in the UK, and to provide clinical data for linkage with further biological studies being carried out within our group.

Subjects and Methods

Patient data for the study were obtained from the Cantoris database (South West Wales Network) and from study of the patients' notes. This database collected clinical information on breast cancer patients treated in the Cancer Centre in Swansea from 1996 to 2002. The study was approved by the Local Research Ethics Committee in Swansea. A total of 918 breast cancer patients undergoing surgery during 1996–2000 were reviewed, and their outcome relative to prognosis defined by the Nottingham Prognostic Index (NPI) was determined. Patients were assigned to one of three groups based on their NPI score: expected good prognosis (G, NPI ≤ 3.4), moderate prognosis (M, NPI 3.41–5.4), or poor prognosis (P, NPI > 5.4). Age groups are divided as 35–44 ($n = 93$), 45–54 ($n = 277$), 55–64 ($n = 251$), 65–74 ($n = 196$), and over 75 years of age ($n = 101$). ER status was available in the majority of cases, but should be interpreted with caution as the methods used to assess ER status varied over time.

Results

Prognostic groups related to the age of the patient at diagnosis are given in Table 1. Median follow-up time was 5.5 years. Most patients had received adjuvant hormonal therapy in all age groups (94.6%–96.4%) regardless of ER status. Neoadjuvant and/or adjuvant chemotherapy was used most frequently in the youngest group and decreased with the age of the patient (see Table 1). Chemotherapy regimens

Table 1. Age distribution of patients with varying Nottingham prognostic index (NPI) and age in relationship to neo/adjuvant chemotherapy treatment

Age group (years)	NPI category			Percent receiving neo/adjuvant chemotherapy
	Good	Moderate	Poor	
34–44	31%	50%	19%	81%
45–54	36%	49%	15%	66%
55–64	51%	30%	19%	34%
65–74	38%	46%	16%	16%
>75	32%	48%	20%	1%

consisted of CMF (cyclophosphamide, methotrexate, fluorouracil) (84%), anthracycline based (11%), and others (5%). Percentages of death from breast cancer were similarly seen in each age group: 22%, 17%, 16%, 20%, and 21%, respectively. Most of the deaths from breast cancer (>60%) were seen in poor prognostic groups (NPI > 5.4) in older age groups (>55 years old); 15% of breast cancer deaths occurred in the younger age group (35–44 years old). Neo/adjuvant chemotherapies were used in most cases in the younger age group (>80% in 35- to 44-year-old patients), which may contributed to lower mortality (17%) in the high-risk group (NPI > 5.4) in those young patients; however, 33% of patients in the moderate-risk group (NPI 3.41–5.4) died. Many cases, 66% in 45- to 54-year-old and 34% in 55- to 64-year-old groups, received neo/adjuvant chemotherapy; however, the actual mortality was not significantly different with those of older groups (>65 years old), the majority of whom did not have adjuvant chemotherapy (only 16% in the 65–74 and 1% in the over 75 years old group). However, elderly patients among the high-risk group (NPI > 5.4) may have had benefit from adjuvant chemotherapy if it had been provided.

Discussion

A recurrent problem in analysis of the results reported here was the lack of information for cases in the oldest age group, particularly regarding node status, NPI, and tumour size. Nodes were less likely to be sampled in the oldest age groups, probably to reduce the side effects of more radical surgery in the elderly patient. There was a clear inverse association with ER status and age, and histological grade and disease, in this study, as noted by other authors [4]. All breast cancers of histological grade 1 are ER positive, whereas only 60% of those of histological grade 3 are positive, suggesting that the relationship between ER and age may be related to the finding that older patients present with tumours of a lower histological grade than younger patients. Grade, included in the NPI, is considered to be a major contributor to prognosis similar to lymph node status, and tumour size is given rather less weight in the algorithm. It is, therefore, interesting that the NPI score increased with age, suggesting that older patients may present with larger tumours and, as size relates to the chance of invasion, with more advanced disease. This difference may be a result of sociological factors (less likely to seek advice from their general practitioner, less aware of self-screening procedures, etc.) rather than a true reflection of altered biology of the disease. However, the variability of these key clinical prognostic factors should be taken into account when interpreting studies on the biology of the tumour related to age. Our recent results, using BAC array CGH (Unger et al., in preparation), suggest that there are indeed biological differences associated with age when analysis is restricted only to grade 3, node-negative cancers, and that distinct biological subgroups exist within an individual clinical category. The relationship between these findings and prognosis is currently under investigation by our group.

Conclusion

This study is the first to bring together local data to find trends in breast cancer biology. It is the springboard for much further study and investigation into the differences in biology between pre- and postmenopausal tumours. Nevertheless, the results of this study have indicated clear differences in tumour biology. There is a striking difference in ER status between older and younger patients, and this is very closely linked with tumour grade. Although low grade and ER expression are associated with older age, their 'benign' effect in older patients may be overridden by the two other dominant factors in the Nottingham Prognostic Index (NPI), namely tumour size and nodal involvement. Thus NPI risk worsens and survival is compromised in older patients. Even though there may be sociological reasons for the latter, it is clear that more widely used chemotherapy in the older patient with a high NPI score may be beneficial. This realization has encouraged us to proceed with a clinical trial of chemotherapy versus no chemotherapy in women over the age of 70. This clinical trial, called ACTION, commenced in autumn 2007, and further details may be found on www.angloceltic.org.uk. A number of biological investigations are underway on the cases identified in this study and will be related to clinical outcome. In addition, biological specimens are being requested from patients enrolled in the ACTION clinical trial to determine whether biological profiles will help clinicians select elderly patients for the likelihood of response to chemotherapy, thereby reducing the proportion of patients who are unlikely to benefit from toxic chemotherapy regimes and who may indeed suffer treatment-related side effects unnecessarily.

References

1. Lønning PE (2007) Breast cancer prognostication and prediction: are we making progress? Ann Oncol 18(suppl 8):viii3–viii7
2. Hawkins RA, White G, Bundred NJ, et al (1987) Prognostic significance of oestrogen and progesterone receptor activities in breast cancer. Br J Surg 74:1009–1013
3. Eppenberger-Castori S, Moore DH Jr, Thor AD, et al (2002) Age-associated biomarker profiles of human breast cancer. Int J Biochem Cell Biol 34:1318–1330
4. Extermann M, Balducci L, Lyman GH (2000) What threshold for adjuvant therapy in older breast cancer patients? J Clin Oncol 18:1709–1717

Mortality of the Chernobyl Emergency Workers: Analysis of Dose Response by Cohort Studies Covering Follow-Up Period of 1992–2006

Victor K. Ivanov, Sergey Yu Chekin, Valery V. Kashcheyev, Marat A. Maksioutov, and Anatoly F. Tsyb

Summary. This chapter discusses the dynamics in mortality rates and radiation risks of death among the Chernobyl emergency workers who arrived to the Chernobyl zone in 1986 and 1987, for the follow-up period from 1992 to 2006. The total size of the cohort was 47 820 persons, and the mean external radiation dose was 128 mGy. A statistically significant radiation risk of death was found for death from all causes [excess relative risk per 1 Gy (ERR/Gy), 0.42; 95% confidence interval (CI), 0.14–0.72], death from solid malignant neoplasms (ERR/Gy, 0.74; 95% CI, 0.03–1.76), and death from diseases of the circulatory system (ERR/Gy, 1.01; 95% CI, 0.51–1.57).

Key words Mortality · Chernobyl emergency workers · Analysis of dose response · Cohort studies · 1992–2006

Introduction

This work is a continuation of the analysis of mortality rates and radiation risks among the Chernobyl emergency workers undertaken by the authors [1] describing the cohort of emergency workers from six regions (comprising 40 oblasts and republics) in the European part of Russia from 1991 to 1998, and considering four groups of death causes: from malignant neoplasms [codes of the International Classification of Diseases (ICD)-9, 140–239], cardiovascular diseases (codes ICD-9, 390–459), injuries and poisoning (codes ICD-9, 800–999) and other causes. For all death cause groups, the standardized mortality rate was lower or equal to unity (for cardiovascular diseases). A statistically significant mortality rate was found for all malignant neoplasms [excess relative risk per 1 Gy (ERR/Gy), 2.11; 95% confidence interval (CI), 1.31–2.92)] and cardiovascular diseases (ERR/Gy, 0.54; 95% CI, 0.18–0.91).

Medical Radiological Research Center of Russian Academy of Medical Sciences, 4 Korolyov Str., Obninsk, Kaluga Region, 249036 Russia

Radiation risks of non-cancer diseases including blood circulation system and cerebrovascular diseases were also estimated for the same cohort of emergency workers from 1986 to 1998 [2,3]. Moreover, mention should be made of the important findings concerning radiation risks of cancer and non-cancer diseases among nuclear workers published in recent years [4–7].

As of today, the Russian National Medical and Dosimetric Registry (RNMDR) contains data permitting us to extend the analysis of the cohort up to 2006 inclusive and to single out a subcohort of the emergency workers who entered the Chernobyl zone in the period 1986–1987. The point is that the emergency workers who arrived at the Chernobyl zone from 1986 to 1987, in keeping with the Russian Federation law currently in force, are entitled to extended and specialized health care. Identifying them as a separate cohort allows distortions in radiation risk estimates to be avoided.

Materials and Methods

Cohort Description

Based on the medical and dosimetric data of the RNMDR (as of the end of 2007), a retrospective cohort of emergency workers was formed for the study. The selection criteria included the following: the subjects were males living in six regions of Russia (North-West, North-Caucasus, Volgo-Vyatsky, Povolzhsky, Central Chernozem, and Urals), registered in the RNMDR before January 1, 1992, and having a known whole-body dose from external gamma radiation and results of at least one health examination during the time period from January 1, 1992 to December 31, 2006. These men were emergency workers who arrived at the Chernobyl zone from 1986 to 1987. The total number of emergency workers meeting these criteria was 47 820 persons.

Distribution of emergency workers in the cohort as a function of age at the time of entry showed that the largest group was in the age range of 35–39 years ($n = 19\,592$) and the smallest group was 45 years and older ($n = 1\,952$). The mean dose received by emergency workers in different age groups showed that the highest mean dose (145 mGy) was found in the youngest age group (18–29 years). In the age groups of 35–39, 40–44, and 45 years and older, the emergency workers had the same mean dose (132 mGy), and the mean dose is the lowest (110 mGy) in the age group of 30–34 years. The mean dose in all cohort members of emergency workers who entered to the 30-km zone in 1986–1987 was 128 mGy.

Distribution of emergency workers as a function of dose group showed that the number of emergency workers in the dose groups of 50–150 mGy and more than 150 mGy was approximately the same: 21 086 and 19 171 persons, respectively, while the dose group of 0–50 mGy, as the internal control, includes 7 924 persons. Also, the mean dose received by emergency workers in the dose groups showed that mean dose was 21.8 mGy for the dose group of 0–50, 94.3 mGy for the dose group of 50–150, and 208.8 mGy for the dose group of more than 150 mGy. Furthermore, the distribution of the crude mortality rate (CMR) per 1 000 persons from all causes by regional centers showed that the distribution was not uniform, which suggests a possible difference in the spontaneous/background death rates from all causes in the regional centers under study—the factor to be taken into account in our study.

Registration of Death Causes in RNMDR

Death data for the follow-up cohort are among the best, ascertained characteristics in the RNMDR system. Each case is reported in primary medical documents, and on their basis the RNMDR Record of Death Causes (RDC) is completed. Medical workers filling out these documents identify, with coding, the primary cause of death and submit information to the vital statistics bureau. For outpatient hospitals, the procedures of registration and coding for cause of death are set forth by the ICD-10, as well as recommendations, guidelines, and orders of the Ministry of Health Care of the Russian Federation.

To exclude incorrect interpretation and errors during data copying and to ascertain death causes and conditions leading to death, requests are sent to the regional centers for the following documents: copies of death certificates, abstracts of medical records, histopathological and autopsy reports, forensic records, conclusions of experts, conclusions of a surgeon, general practitioner, or oncologist, and death certificate from the vital statistics bureau. All obtained documents are entered into the RNMDR mortality subregistry and used for data verification and control. Then, the Records of Death Causes are checked for completeness using primary medical documents and availability of copies of medical death certificates, autopsy reports, and other necessary documents, and following the comparative analysis of different information sources, the accuracy of data copied out from primary documents to the RDC and correctness of the death cause are ascertained.

Statistical Methods

The time an individual is at risk to die from any disease of the class under consideration (or a specific disease under study) is estimated as the difference of dates *T1* and *T0*, where *T0* is January 1, 1992, when the follow-up was begun, and *T1* is the date of the latest health examination or the date of death. To study the radiation dose response of the mortality rates, the cohort method was used. The personalized data on emergency workers were grouped in 5 strata by age at the time of arrival to the Chernobyl zone (18–29, 30–34, 35–39, 40–44, 45 years and older), 6 strata by the RNMDR regional center they belong to (North-West, North-Caucasus,

Volgo-Vyatsky, Povolzhsky, Central Chernozem, and Urals), and 15 strata by calendar year covering the follow-up period of 1992–2006. The stratification by age was performed to level off the effect of age differences, while the stratification by regional center and calendar year was required to allow for differences in the background mortality rates in the above regions in 1992–2006.

The ERR was estimated equal to the estimate of parameter β in the regression model:

$$\lambda(D)_{ijk} = \lambda 0_{ijk}(1+\beta D) \qquad (1)$$

where $\lambda(D)_{ijk}$ is the mortality rate as a function of age at time of exposure, regional center, calendar year, and external radiation dose, $\lambda 0_{ijk}$ is the background (for zero dose) mortality rate as a function of age at time of exposure, regional center, and calendar year, and D is the individual external radiation dose in Gy. The likelihood ratio statistic for testing the significance (P) of the parameter β in the model (1) and the maximum likelihood estimate for the parameter β and respective 95% CI were calculated using the Epicure software [8].

In addition, a nonparametric assessment of relative risks (RR) was made using the internal control group of emergency workers with doses from 0 to 50 mGy and the exposed groups of 50 to 150 mGy and more than 150 mGy:

$$\lambda(D)_{ijk} = \lambda 0_{ijk} \cdot RR_n \qquad (2)$$

where RR_n is the relative risk for the nth exposed group ($n = 1$ for the exposed group at 50–150 mGy, $n = 2$ for emergency workers with dose above 150 mGy, and $n = 0$ and $RR_0 = 1$ for the exposed group at 0–50 mGy). The maximum-likelihood estimates for the relative risks RR_0 and RR_1 and respective 95% confidence interval in the model (2) were also calculated using the Epicure software [8].

Results

The registered number of deaths from all death causes in the RNMDR for the described cohort of emergency workers (47 820 persons) from the start of follow-up (January 1, 1992) to the end of follow-up (December 31, 2006) inclusive, was 10 896 cases, which is 22.8% of the cohort size. The distribution of deaths in the emergency workers cohort by disease classes and their percentage of the total number of deaths are shown in Table 1. The largest number of deaths registered was from circulation system diseases (4 306 cases). In addition, there were many deaths from injuries and poisoning (2 782 cases), and it is also worth pointing out the malignant solid neoplasms (1 393 cases). The mortality from these three causes comprised 77.8% of the total number of deaths.

Table 1. Observed number of cases and estimated radiation risk for cause of death in emergency workers by main disease classes

Main disease class	ICD-10	Observed number of cases (%)	Excess relative risk per 1 Gy (95% CI)	P value
All		10 896 (100)	0.42 (0.14, 0.72)	0.003
Infectious and parasitic diseases	A, B	272 (2.5)	0.86 (−0.83, 3.57)	0.37
Malignant neoplasms (solid)	C00–C80	1 393 (12.8)	0.74 (0.03, 1.76)	0.06
Diseases of circulatory system	I	4 306 (39.5)	1.01 (0.51, 1.57)	<0.001
Diseases of respiratory system	J	623 (5.7)	−0.80 (−1.52, 0.18)	0.10
Diseases of digestive system	K	729 (6.7)	0.35 (−0.65, 1.68)	>0.5
Injuries and poisoning	S, T	2 782 (25.5)	−0.09 (−0.57, 0.46)	>0.5
Others		791 (7.3)		

ICD, International Classification of Diseases; CI, confidence interval

Table 2. Observed number of cases and estimated radiation risk for cause of death in emergency workers by selected diseases

Selected disease	ICD-10	Observed number of cases (%)	Excess relative risk per 1 Gy (95% CI)	P value
Malignant neoplasms of stomach	C16	181 (1.7)	1.08 (−0.86, 4.43)	0.33
Malignant neoplasms of lungs and bronchi	C34	485 (4.5)	0.53 (−0.65, 2.16)	0.42
Acute myocardial infarction	I21	233 (2.1)	1.59 (−0.47, 5.15)	0.15
Other forms of IHD	I24	225 (2.1)	−0.27 (−1.63, 1.90)	>0.5
Chronic IHD	I25	1763 (16.2)	0.62 (−0.08, 1.45)	0.09
Cardiomyopathy	I42	339 (3.1)	−0.43 (−1.43, 1.00)	>0.5
Cardiac insufficiency	I50	237 (2.2)	1.29 (−0.54, 4.30)	0.20
Cerebrovascular diseases	I60–I69	695 (6.4)	1.67 (0.35, 3.47)	0.009

IHD, ischemic heart disease; ICD, International Classification of Diseases; CI, confidence interval

Table 2 shows the types of solid neoplasms and blood circulation system diseases that occurred most frequently among emergency workers. The most frequent cause of death in the studied disease classes was chronic ischemic heart disease (IHD) (1763 cases), and for solid cancers the main cause was neoplasms of lungs and bronchi (485 cases).

Figure 1 shows the dynamics of the standardized mortality ratio (SMR) for all death in our cohort. The external controls were official age-specific mortality rates for males in Russia adopted by the World Health Organization. During the follow-up period from 1992 to 1996, the SMR was below the control, and its value ranged from 0.73 to 0.89. Since 1997, the value of SMR increased but did not exceed unity with statistical significance. The maximum value of SMR was reported for 1998 (1.07; 95% CI, 0.99–1.15; $P = 0.08$). Figure 2 shows the dynamics of the SMR for blood circulation system diseases (Fig. 2A) and cancers (Fig. 2B).

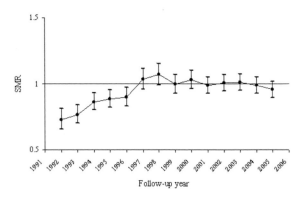

Fig. 1. Dynamics of the standardized mortality ratio (*SMR*) for all causes of death

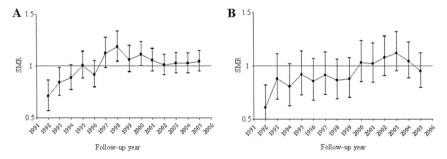

Fig. 2. Dynamics of the standardized mortality ratio (*SMR*) for blood circulation system diseases (**A**) and cancers (**B**) as cause of death

Concerning possible dependence of mortality in emergency workers on external radiation dose, Table 1 also shows estimates of ERR/Gy of death in emergency workers for main disease classes, as derived by model (1). A statistically significant risk as a function of the external radiation dose was obtained for several classes: for deaths from all causes (ERR/Gy, 0.42; 95% CI, 0.14–0.72), for deaths from solid malignant neoplasms (ERR/Gy, 0.74; 95% CI, 0.03–1.76), and for deaths from blood circulation system diseases (ERR/Gy, 1.01; 95% CI, 0.51–1.57). For other death causes, the risk was not statistically significant.

Table 2 includes the estimates of ERR/Gy of death from selected diseases among emergency workers. A statistically significant risk as a function of external radiation dose was obtained for deaths from cerebrovascular diseases (ERR/Gy, 1.67; 95% CI, −0.35 to 3.47). For other causes of death, the dose response was found not to be statistically significant. Nevertheless, a pronounced positive trend can be seen for chronic IHD (ERR/Gy, 0.62; 95% CI, −0.08 to 1.45).

Figure 3 shows the estimates of RR for solid cancers (Fig. 3A), blood circulation system diseases (Fig. 3B), and all causes (Fig. 3C) calculated by model (2) for the dose groups of 50–150 mGy and more than 150 mGy, with the dose group of

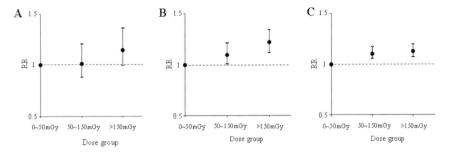

Fig. 3. Estimated relative risk (*RR*) for solid cancers (**A**), blood circulation system diseases (**B**), and all causes (**C**) by each dose group (0–50 mGy, 50–150 mGy, and more than 150 mGy). The dose group of 0–50 mGy is used as a control for calculating RR. Vertical lines show each 95% confidence interval. **A** RRs for mean dose 94.3 mGy and 210 mGy are 1.01 and 1.14, respectively. **B** RRs for mean dose 92.8 mGy and 210 mGy are 1.10 and 1.22, respectively. **C** RRs for mean dose 94.3 mGy and 210 mGy are 1.10 and 1.13, respectively

0–50 mGy used as a control. The risk for solid cancers in the dose group of 50–150 mGy seemed to be same in the control group (RR, 1.01; 95% CI, 0.87–1.19), while the risk in the dose group of more than 150 mGy was found to be increased as compared with the control group (RR, 1.14; 95% CI, 0.98–1.34), although statistical significance was not evident. The risk for blood circulation system diseases in the dose group of 50–150 mGy was significantly higher than in the control group (RR, 1.10; 95% CI, 1.01–1.21), and the risk in the dose group of more than 150 mGy was significantly higher than in the control group (RR, 1.22; 95% CI, 1.12–1.34). For all causes, the risk in the dose group of 50–150 mGy was significantly higher than in the control (RR, 1.11; 95% CI, 1.05–1.17); furthermore, the risk in the dose group of more than 150 mGy was significantly higher than in the control group (RR, 1.13; 95% CI, 1.07–1.20).

Discussion and Conclusion

The present study provided a basis for the following conclusions. (1) A statistically significant dose response for mortality rates among emergency workers who entered the 30-km zone in 1986–1987 was revealed in all disease classes (ERR/Gy, 0.42), malignant neoplasms (solid) (ERR/Gy, 0.74), and diseases of the blood circulation system (ERR/Gy, 1.01). (2) The obtained data with allowance for confidence intervals were in good agreement with the estimates of radiation risks in the Japanese cohort of Hiroshima and Nagasaki [9–11]. (3) Epidemiological studies of the cohort of emergency workers still need to be continued to refine the key characteristics of the dose–time matrix of risk, such as age at exposure, attained age, and time since exposure.

References

1. Ivanov VK, Gorski AI, Maksioutov MA, et al (2001) Mortality among the Chernobyl emergency workers: estimation of radiation risks (preliminary analysis). Health Phys 81: 514–521
2. Ivanov VK, Maksioutov MA, Chekin SY, et al (2000) Radiation-epidemiological analysis of incidence of non-cancer diseases among the Chernobyl liquidators. Health Phys 78: 495–501
3. Ivanov VK, Maksioutov MA, Chekin SY, et al (2006) The risk of radiation-induced cerebrovascular disease in Chernobyl emergency workers. Health Phys 90:199–207
4. Howe GR, Zablotska LB, Fix JJ, et al (2004) Analysis of the mortality experience amongst U.S. nuclear power industry workers after chronic low-dose exposure to ionizing radiation. Radiat Res 162:517–526
5. Cardis E, Vrijheid M, Blettner M, et al (2005) Risk of cancer after low doses of ionising radiation: retrospective cohort study in 15 countries. BMJ 89:1–7
6. Ivanov V, Ilyin L, Gorski A, et al (2004) Radiation and epidemiological analysis for solid cancer incidence among nuclear workers who participated in recovery operations following the accident at the Chernobyl NPP. J Radiat Res 45:41–44
7. Ivanov VK, Tsyb AF, Rastopchin EM, et al (2001) Cancer incidence among nuclear workers in Russia based on data from the Institute of Physics and Power Engineering: a preliminary analysis. Radiat Res 155:801–808
8. Preston DL, Lubin JH, Pierce DA, McConney ME (1993) EPICURE. Hirosoft International Corporation, Seattle
9. Pierce DA, Shimizu Y, Preston DL, et al (1996) Studies of the mortality of atomic bomb survivors. Report 12, Part I. Cancer: 1950–1990. Radiat Res 146:1–27
10. Pierce DA, Mendelsohn ML (1999) A model for radiation-related cancer suggested by atomic bomb survivor data. Radiat Res 52:642–654
11. Shimizu Y, Pierce DA, Preston DL, et al (1999) Studies of the mortality of atomic bomb survivors. Report 12, Part II. Noncancer mortality: 1950–1990. Radiat Res 152:374–389

Twenty Years After Chernobyl: Implications for Radiation Health Risk Control

Yoshisada Shibata

Summary. We surveyed the major health outcomes observed in the general population exposed to the Chernobyl accident. In contrast to the predictions made by Western scientists soon after the accident, the health effects noted up to now in the general population around Chernobyl are markedly contrasted with those ascertained in atomic bomb survivors of Hiroshima and Nagasaki, indicating that dose and dose rate of radiation resulting from the accident were probably much lower than those of the atomic bomb radiation. A remarkable increase in childhood thyroid cancer was noted in Belarus, Russia, and Ukraine. The incidence of thyroid cancer in Belarus suggested that people exposed to the Chernobyl accident in their childhood would still be at high risk of thyroid diseases, including cancer. Thyroid cancer in children (aged 0–14 years at diagnosis) began to significantly increase about 4 years after the accident, reached a peak around 10 years after the accident, then began to regress to the level recorded before the accident, whereas that in adolescents (aged 15–19 years at diagnosis) showed a time trend similar to that in children with about a 5-year lag, and in young adults (20–24 years at diagnosis) the incidence was seemingly still increasing. If the former USSR government had disclosed the accident immediately after the occurrence and had taken appropriate measures, the aforementioned victims would have been markedly fewer in number. The most common health outcome of the Chernobyl accident observed so far in the general population is mental health issues, as in the case of the Three Mile Island accident. One of the key points we should learn from the Chernobyl accident is the importance of radiation health risk control.

Key words Chernobyl · Thyroid cancer · Non-cancer thyroid disease · Leukemia · Mental health · Radiation health risk control

---

Atomic Bomb Disease Institute, Nagasaki University Graduate School of Biomedical Sciences, 1-12-4 Sakamoto, Nagasaki 852-8523, Japan

Introduction

An earthquake, later named the Niigata Prefecture Chuetsu Offshore Earthquake, with a magnitude of 6.8, jolted Niigata and northern Nagano prefectures at 10:13 A.M. on July 16, 2007, killing 7 people, injuring at least 790, and damaging hundreds of buildings. Although the Kashiwazaki-Kariwa nuclear power plant in Niigata Prefecture suffered damage, including a small fire at a power transformer, the safety of the plant's nuclear reactors was never jeopardized. The leak of radioactive substances was less than 10^{-6} of the dose of radiation to which an ordinary person is naturally exposed per year.

However, sensational images of black smoke billowing from a fire in one of the nuclear power plant's transformers were repeatedly broadcast to symbolize damage caused by the earthquake. Although the fire and radioactive leaks were unrelated, the combined reporting of the two incidents may have inferred a link. Foreign news media reported that the earthquake had caused deaths and injuries at the nuclear power plant, making it look as if people had been injured and killed in a nuclear accident. Indeed, Italian Serie A Club Catania canceled its scheduled tour of Japan because of fears over the leak of radioactive materials at the nuclear power plant. Some foreign news media even linked the incidence to the 1986 Chernobyl nuclear accident in the former USSR, and reported that residents living near the plant could not sleep for concerns over possible radioactive leaks.

The present study surveys the findings on the health effects of the Chernobyl accident and discusses the lessons of the accident from the point of view of radiation health risk control.

Chernobyl Accident

The accident occurred at 1:23 A.M. on April 26, 1986, at the No. 4 Unit of the Chernobyl nuclear power plant, resulting in the release into the atmosphere of radionuclides of about 8 EBq, including ^{131}I (1.2–1.7 EBq) and ^{133}I (2.5 EBq) [1]. Evacuation from Pripyat, where staff members of the Chernobyl nuclear power plant and their families were living, started at 2 P.M. on April 27, more than 36 h after the accident, and ended at 7 P.M. on the same day. Evacuation from the 30-km zone (areas within a radius of 30 km from the nuclear power plant) started much later, that is, on May 2, and ended on May 6 when the release of radionuclides from the reactor into the atmosphere ceased.

Surface deposition of ^{137}Cs greater than 185 kBq/m^2 was recorded in 15 500 km^2 of Belarus, 8 100 km^2 of Russian Federation, and 4 600 km^2 of Ukraine [1]. Table 1 summarizes the average accumulated doses to the affected population [2]. We note that approximately 1 000 emergency workers and on-site personnel received the highest doses of 2–20 Gy during the first days of the accident.

Table 1. Summary of average accumulated doses to affected population from Chernobyl fallout

Population category	Number	Average dose (mSv)
Liquidators (1986–1989)	600 000	~100
Evacuees from highly contaminated zone (1986)	116 000	33
Residents of "strict-control" zone (1986–2005)	270 000	>50
Residents of other "contaminated" areas (1986–2005)	5 000 000	10–20

Source: Chernobyl Forum [2]

Dose Estimation

Estimation of radiation dose received by individuals of the general population exposed to the Chernobyl accident is quite difficult because the major contribution was internal exposure to radio-contaminated food and drink ingested by complex routes. Furthermore, in contrast to radiation exposure by an atomic bomb exploded at a certain distance above the ground, which is essentially external exposure, verification of the estimated dose is almost impossible. Nonetheless, great efforts have been made in dose estimation so as to precisely as possible enable quantitative estimation of radiation risks by the accident.

Somatic Effects of the Chernobyl Accident

When the Chernobyl accident was officially disclosed by the former USSR government, most people of the world projected the experiences of the atomic bomb survivors of Hiroshima and Nagasaki on the future outcomes in the general population exposed to the accident. In atomic bomb survivors, leukemia began to emerge 2–3 years after the bombing, reaching the peak of incidence 6–7 years after the bombing, then began to decrease steadily, and was followed by an increase in thyroid cancer, breast and lung cancers, and in stomach cancer about 10 years, 20 years, and 30 years after the bombing, respectively [3]. What was observed regarding the health effects of the accident among the general population around Chernobyl in the past 20 years?

Thyroid Diseases

The somatic outcomes observed in the past 20 years among the general population around Chernobyl contrast with those observed among atomic bomb survivors. In the general population exposed to the accident, no significant increase in leukemia has been noticed, whereas a marked increase in childhood thyroid cancer has been noted.

Table 2. Number of cases of thyroid cancer diagnosed during 1986–2002 by country and age at exposure

Age at exposure (years)	Belarus	Country Russia	Ukraine	Total
0–14	1711	349	1762	3822
15–17	299	134	582	1015
Total	2010	483	2344	4837

Source: Bennett et al. [6]

In 1992, Belarusian scientists first reported in the journal *Nature* a significant increase in childhood cancer [4], but its association with radiation exposure was questioned, attributing to other factors such as deep screening after the accident [5]. Although the incidence of childhood thyroid cancer is extremely low, for example, 1 or 2 per million per year, many cases subsequently began to be reported also from Ukraine and Russia. In people of the three countries aged 17 years or less at the time of the accident, 4 837 were diagnosed with thyroid cancer in 1986–2002 [6] (Table 2).

In 2000, two articles [7,8] reported the time trend of childhood thyroid cancer incidence since the accident in Ukraine and Belarus, suggesting an association with the accident; however, the results were not decisive. The study, which by paying attention to the relatively short (8 days) half-life of ^{131}I compared the prevalence of thyroid diseases between children born before and after the accident, reported 31 cancer cases (7 males and 24 females) in 9 720 children born January 1, 1983 to April 26, 1986, whereas no cases were found in 9 472 children born January 1, 1987 to December 31, 1989 [9]; the subjects were all living in the districts of Rechitskii, Loevskii, Gomelskii, and Hoynikskii, and Gomel city in Gomel region of Belarus. These areas are within a radius of 150 km from the Chernobyl nuclear power plant, and health screening was carried out under the same protocol at all schools, except for Gomel city, where the screening was conducted at seven schools with an enrollment of more than 1 000 that were selected by a stratified random sampling procedure.

Two population-based case-control studies, aiming at reliable estimation of individual thyroid dose resulting from the Chernobyl accident and of childhood thyroid cancer risk, were recently reported by Cardis et al. [10] and Kopeckey et al. [11]. Cardis et al. [10] studied 276 cases living in areas of Belarus and Russia affected by the accident, who were aged less than 15 years at the time of the accident and diagnosed with thyroid cancer through 1998, and 1300 controls matched to cases by gender, year of birth, and the region where they were living at the time of the accident. The analysis based on several logistic models demonstrated a significant ($P < 0.001$) association between thyroid cancer risk and dose, and the odds ratio (OR) per 1 Gy varied from 5.5 [95% confidence interval (CI) = 3.1–9.5] to 8.4 (95% CI = 4.1–17.3), according to the models. Subjects studied by Kopeckey et al. [11] were 66 cases living in Bryansk region of Russia, aged 0–19 years at the time of the accident and diagnosed with thyroid cancer through 1998, and 132 controls matched to cases by gender, year of birth, and the region of residence and type of settlement (urban, town, rural) at the time of the accident. The excess relative risk per 1 Gy (ERR/Gy) was estimated as 48.7 (95% CI = 4.8–1151).

Two large-scale cohort studies on thyroid cancer and other thyroid diseases were launched by the United States in Belarus and Ukraine in 1996 and 1998, respectively, as binational research projects [12]. Subjects were those who were living in highly contaminated areas and were aged 18 years or less at the time of the Chernobyl accident, and who underwent measurement of the radioactivity of their thyroid glands in 1986. A total of 38 543 and 32 385 people were selected in Belarus and Ukraine, respectively, as candidates for follow-up and contact. However, the number of people contacted was 16 213 (42.1%) in Belarus and 19 612 (60.6%) in Ukraine, and among them, 11 918 (73.5%) and 13 243 (67.5%) participated in the first cycle of biennial health examinations in Belarus and Ukraine, respectively.

The first report of this USA–Ukraine cohort study was published in 2006, indicating excess relative risk per gray (ERR/Gy) of 5.25 (95% CI = 1.70–27.5) on the basis of 45 cancer cases diagnosed in 13 127 cohort members who participated in the first cycle of health examinations in the period 1998–2000 [13].

Figure 1 [14] supports our prediction that thyroid cancer risk in children born in 1987 or later would regress to the level recorded before the Chernobyl accident,

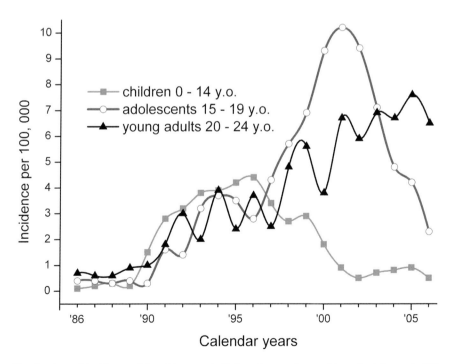

Fig. 1. Annual incidence of thyroid cancer in Belarus by age (years old, *y.o.*) at diagnosis [14]

because those children would not be exposed to radioiodine [9]. Because children born by the end of 1986 reached the age of 15 years or older in 2002, the incidence of childhood thyroid cancer thenceforth is practically zero, while the incidence of thyroid cancer is increasing, along with the growth of exposed children, in adolescents (aged 15 years or over and under 19 years) and in adults (aged 19 years or over); we note that the incidence of thyroid cancer in adolescents reached a peak in 2001 and steadily decreased thereafter (Fig. 1).

Data showing an association of non-cancer thyroid diseases with the accident are still few. The aforementioned health screening comparing the prevalence of thyroid diseases between children born before and after the accident indicated a significant difference between the two groups in the prevalence of thyroid nodules after adjustment for sex and age (OR = 3.0; 95% CI = 1.6–6.0). In 12 504 members of the USA–Ukraine cohort study, who participated in the first cycle of the screening (1998–2000) and were found to have a history of thyroid diseases, thyroid follicular adenoma was diagnosed in 23, and ERR/Gy was estimated as 2.07 (95% CI = 0.28–10.31) [15].

Leukemia

Findings on leukemia reaching consensus by experts to date are as follows [6]:

1. There has been no strong evidence supporting or denying the association between exposure in utero and an increase in leukemia.
2. Existing evidence does not support the conclusion that rates of leukemia have increased as a result of childhood radiation exposure from the Chernobyl accident.
3. Although there is a report showing an association between radiation exposure and an increase in leukemia, further detailed studies are necessary to confirm this finding.
4. There has been no definite evidence for an increase in leukemia among adults living in contaminated areas.

Solid Cancers Other Than Thyroid Cancer

No solid cancers other than thyroid cancer suggesting effects of the Chernobyl accident have been reported yet. However, the studies of the atomic bomb survivors indicated the necessity to carefully monitor the health status in people who participated in liquidation work in 1986–1987 and those living in highly contaminated areas.

Non-Cancer Diseases Other Than Thyroid

Findings on non-cancer diseases other than thyroid reaching consensus by expertise to the present are as follows [6]:

1. Ophthalmologic studies of children and liquidators suggested an association between radiation exposure by the Chernobyl accident and posterior subcapsular cataracts.

2. There is a large study on Chernobyl emergency workers that has shown a significant excess relative risk per sievert (Sv) for death from cardiovascular disease in the exposed individuals, but this has been found only in the Russian cohort, and there are some differences between incidence and mortality data. This result needs further evaluation and new studies designed to overcome the effects of bias and confounding factors.

3. Although effects on levels of immune cells and function have been reported in a number of studies, there is a significant variation in the results of different Chernobyl studies, and some results are at variance with data from the atomic bomb survivors. The possible confounding factors, such as heavy metals and the effect of radioiodine on the thyroid, also complicate the issue. To date, at doses of less than several tens of mSv, no clinical effects have been clearly related to abnormal immune function.

4. Given the range of absorbed doses received by the vast majority of parents before or during conception, the Chernobyl epidemiological studies are consistent with evidence in previous scientific literature. They do not indicate a radiation-related increase in malformations or infant mortality as a direct result of radiation exposure.

Mental Health Effects of the Chernobyl Accident

Radiation is not detectable by us without special apparatus, and the somatic effects of radiation exposure, which are mostly stochastic, are usually difficult to realize for the general public; thus people, except those who received medical exposure at their own risk, have a strong tendency to worry about their future health once they know that they have been exposed to radiation even though the dose they had received was negligible.

Although the amount of ^{131}I discharged by the accident at Three Mile Island of the United States in 1979 was less than 1 millionth of that discharged by the Chernobyl accident, the accident seriously affected the mental health of the general population [16].

Residents in the Chernobyl 30-km zone who were evacuated soon after the accident were promised they could expect an early homecoming, but this expectation has not yet been realized. Most of these people faced difficulty in adapting themselves to life in strange places, in addition to the concern about late effects of radiation exposure, and not a few of them showed neurotic disorders. Because the collapse of the former USSR has resulted in dramatic changes of the socioeconomic environment, not a few of the people who were not exposed to the Chernobyl accident have had to endure a hard life as well.

To evaluate the psychosomatic effects of the Chernobyl accident on people who were evacuated from the Chernobyl 30-km zone, we compared two groups of women living in the same district of Kiev, Ukraine, who were aged 15–45 years at the time of the accident: 1558 women who evacuated to Kiev from the Chernobyl 30-km zone (group 1) and 1931 women who had been living in Kiev since before the accident (group 2). All the subjects participated in regular health examinations at the Scientific Center for Radiation Medicine, Kiev, Ukraine, and were also administered, in 2003 (group 1) and 2004 (group 2), Goldberg's 12-item version of the General Health Questionnaire (GHQ-12), and anxiety and depression scales. For each question of GHQ-12, we assigned a score of 0 or 1 to the first two and the last two answers, respectively, defined the GHQ-12 score as the sum of the 12 scores, and classified the subjects into high-score and low-score groups depending on whether their GHQ-12 score exceeded 3. The study demonstrated that the frequency of a high GHQ-12 score was significantly higher ($P < 0.05$) in group 1 (18.7%, or 292/1558) than in group 2 (8.2%, or 159/1931) after adjustment for age and prevalence of diseases, suggesting probable effects of evacuation on mental health in people exposed to the Chernobyl accident.

Radiation Health Risk Control

Whenever serious accidents with probable late effects have occurred, the newspaper reports future outcomes that are predicted by specialists, but the prediction rarely proves right. The Chernobyl accident is also such a case. We read the following reports in a newspaper issued a few days after the accident, "A nuclear physicist of West Germany told that lung cancer deaths in the future 10 years will reach 10,000 in areas within a radius of 500 km from the nuclear power plant." (*Asahi*, April 30, 1986)

The 20-year observation of health status in the general population around Chernobyl suggests if the accident were disclosed to people immediately after the accident by informing them that children would be most vulnerable, and asked them not to take local milk and to stay inside their house as much as possible, the incidence of thyroid cancer would have been much less. Unfortunately, the measures taken first by the former USSR government for the general population consisted of evacuation from Pripyat to Kiev, which removal started more than 36 h after the outbreak of the accident; people were not told the reason for evacuation but were told that they could come back soon to their homes. Evacuation from other areas within the 30-km zone started later, beginning May 2, 1986 and completing May 6, 1986. These people have not been able to go back to their homes since that evacuation, and mental health disorders and accompanying somatic disorders are now of great concern in the general population surrounding Chernobyl.

One of the major lessons from Chernobyl is the importance of radiation health risk control. We note that it is not the safety, but the risk, which we can measure; a thing is safe if its risks are judged to be acceptable, and most expressions of risk are compound measures describing both the probability of harm and its severity [17]. Radiation health risk control is a synthesis of the following: (1) risk identification, (2) qualitative risk assessment, (3) quantitative risk assessment, (4) risk management, and (5) risk communication. Among these, risk communication is worthy of a brief comment. Radiation exposure and its outcomes are usually difficult to realize for the general public; they "understand" the effects of radiation through information reported by mass media. However, reports by the mass media are usually sensational and sometimes are far from reality.

Conclusion

In conclusion:

1. The Chernobyl accident and the atomic bombing markedly contrast with respect to radiation exposure and health effects so far observed.
2. Such a contrast indicates that the dose and dose rate of radiation resulting from the Chernobyl accident were probably much lower than those of atomic bomb radiation.
3. People exposed to the Chernobyl accident in their childhood will be at high risk of thyroid diseases, including cancer.
4. If the former USSR government had disclosed the accident immediately after the occurrence and had taken appropriate measures, the number of these victims would have been much smaller.
5. The most common health outcome of the Chernobyl accident observed so far in the general population is mental health issues, as in the case of the Three Mile Island accident.
6. A long-term follow-up of people exposed to the Chernobyl accident, especially of those exposed in their childhood, should contribute to radiation health risk control.
7. Risk communication is one of the key issues for radiation health risk control.
8. Specialists should help people acquire media literacy.

References

1. Dreicer M, Aarkrog A, Alexakhin R, et al (1996) Consequences of the Chernobyl accident for the natural and human environments. In: One decade after Chernobyl: summing up the consequences of the accident. Proceedings of an International Conference, Vienna, April 8–12, 1996. International Atomic Energy Agency, Vienna, pp 319–361

2. The Chernobyl Forum (2006) 2003–2005: Chernobyl's legacy: health, environmental and socio-economic impacts and recommendations to the governments of Belarus, the Russian Federation and Ukraine. International Atomic Energy Agency, Vienna
3. Shimizu Y, Kato H, Schull WJ (1988) Life span study report 11, Part 2: cancer mortality in the years 1950–1985 based on the recently revised doses (DS86). Tech Rep RERF TR 5-88
4. Kazakov VS, Demidchik EP, Astakova LN (1992) Thyroid cancer after Chernobyl. Nature (Lond) 359:21
5. Ron E, Lubin J, Schneider AB (1992) Thyroid cancer incidence. Nature (Lond) 360:113
6. Bennett B, Repacholi M, Carr Z (eds) (2006) Health effects of the Chernobyl accident and special health care programmes. World Health Organization, Geneva
7. Heidenreich WF, Bogdanova TI, Jacob P, et al (2000) Age and time patterns in thyroid cancer after the Chernobyl accidents in the Ukraine. Radiat Res 154:731–732
8. Jacob P, Kenigsberg Y, Goulko G, et al (2000) Thyroid cancer risk in Belarus after the Chernobyl accident: comparison with external exposures. Radiat Environ Biophys 39:25–31
9. Shibata Y, Yamashita S, Masyakin VB, et al (2001) 15 years after Chernobyl: new evidence of thyroid cancer. Lancet 358:1965–1966
10. Cardis E, Kesminiene A, Ivanov V, et al (2005) Risk of thyroid cancer after exposure to ^{131}I in childhood. J Natl Cancer Inst 97:724–732
11. Kopeckey KJ, Stepanenko V, Rivkind N, et al (2006) Childhood thyroid cancer, radiation dose from Chernobyl, and dose uncertainties in Bryansk Oblast, Russia: a population-based case-control study. Radiat Res 166:367–374
12. Stezhko VA, Buglova EE, Danilova LI, et al; Chornobyl Thyroid Diseases Study Group of Belarus; Chornobyl Thyroid Diseases Study Group of Ukraine; Chornobyl Thyroid Diseases Study Group of the USA (2004) A cohort study of thyroid cancer and other thyroid diseases after the Chornobyl accident: objectives, design and methods. Radiat Res 161:481–492
13. Tronko MD, Howe GR, Bogdanova TI, et al (2006) A cohort study of thyroid cancer and other thyroid diseases after the Chernobyl accident: thyroid cancer in Ukraine detected during first screening. J Natl Cancer Inst 98:897–903
14. Demidchik YE, Saenko VA, Yamashita S (2007) Childhood thyroid cancer in Belarus, Russia, and Ukraine after Chernobyl and at present. Arq Bras Endocrinol Metabol 51:748–762
15. Zablotska LB, Bogdanova TI, Ron E, et al (2008) A cohort study of thyroid cancer and other thyroid diseases after the Chornobyl accident: dose-response analysis of thyroid follicular adenomas detected during the first screening in Ukraine (1998–2000). Am J Epidemiol 167:305–312
16. Fabrikant JI (1983) The effects of the accident at Three Mile Island on the mental health and behavioral responses of the general population and nuclear workers. Health Phys 45:579–586
17. Lowrance WW (1976) Of acceptable risk. Kaufman, Los Altos

Fallout Exposure of the Population and Thyroid Nodular Diseases

Zhaxybay Sh. Zhumadilov and Assem M. Orymbaeva

Summary. The ecological disasters that face Kazakhstan make environmental and health research a very large priority for the people of Kazakhstan. It is well known now that the Polygon region in east Kazakhstan was the site of nuclear weapons testing under the former Soviet Union, and 40 years of testing have scarred both the population and the environment. Childhood radiation exposure is a known risk factor for subsequent thyroid cancer and thyroid nodular diseases. In 1998, for the first time, scientists of Kazakhstan and the United States used ultrasound and fine-needle aspiration biopsy to screen the thyroid glands of 3000 selected residents of six exposed and two nonexposed villages in the Semipalatinsk region. An international group with expertise in fallout-related dose reconstruction developed highly sophisticated algorithms for estimating individual radiation dose from external and internal sources as a function of bomb characteristics and movement of the fallout cloud, residential history, age at time of exposure, time spent outdoors, shielding provided by buildings, and dietary history obtained by questionnaire-guided interview and from archival data. This study revealed that there is an apparently strong association between fallout exposure and thyroid nodule prevalence, which is a marker for thyroid cancer risk. Different treatment modalities have been developed and implemented to improve treatment outcomes of patients with thyroid nodular diseases.

Key words Fallout exposure · Thyroid screening · Radiation-associated thyroid tumors

Introduction

Kazakhstan, a country rich in mineral wealth, is actively carrying out reforms with a view to integrating its economy into a well-developed worldwide economy. Destiny has placed Kazakhstan at the heart of the Eurasian continent. Economic

---

Department of Scientific & Clinical Affairs, Semey State Medical Academy, 103 Abaya Str., Semey 071400, Kazakhstan

growth, industrialization, and the grave consequences of nuclear weapons testing are causing heavy environmental and health problems. Economic growth that will benefit present and future generations and establishment of both healthy economics and a healthy environment are of great public concern in Kazakhstan. The ecological disasters that face Kazakhstan mean that environmental and health research is a very large priority for its people. Many of the environmental problems can benefit from the application of state-of-the-art research techniques that have recently been developed or can be developed in the course of working on these challenging problems.

Kazakhstan is poised to become one of the most important 21st-century laboratories for studying and solving the large-scale environmental problems, including pollution, nuclear waste, nuclear weapons testing, and elevated natural background radiation, that face it and the rest of the world. It is well known now that the Polygon region in east Kazakhstan was the site of nuclear weapons testing under the former Soviet Union, and 40 years of testing have scarred the population and the environment [1,2]. Based on reconstructed estimates of external radiation exposure in both countries, radiation doses to local population were 10 to 100 times higher around the Semipalatinsk Nuclear Test Site (SNTS) than among populations downwind of the Nevada Test Site (NTS) [3–5]. The incidence of cancer, lung diseases, congenital birth defects, and tuberculosis in East Kazakhstan is disproportionately high. For example, the incidence of breast cancer in East Kazakhstan is 1.5 fold higher in comparison with the average rate of breast cancer in Kazakhstan and 2.5 fold higher than that in South Kazakhstan. Many patients are admitted to regional hospitals with advanced stages of breast cancer, colon cancer, and skin cancer, and this fact dictates the necessity of improvement of the primary health care system in Kazakhstan.

Childhood radiation exposure is a known risk factor for subsequent thyroid cancer and thyroid nodular diseases [6–8]. In 1998, for the first time, scientists of Kazakhstan and the United States used ultrasound and fine-needle aspiration biopsy to screen the thyroid glands of 3000 selected residents of six exposed and two nonexposed villages in the Semipalatinsk region. The study was conducted within the framework of the U. S. Civilian Research and Development Foundation (International Award No. KN2-434). The co-principal investigators were Charles Land, Ph.D. [National Cancer Institute (NCI), Bethesda, MD, USA] and Zhaxybay Zhumadilov, M.D., Ph.D., D.M.Sc. [Semey State Medical Academy (SSMA), Semey, Kazakhstan].

Subjects and Methods

Subjects

Four thousand inhabitants of the east Kazakhstan region adjacent to the SNTS were screened for thyroid nodular diseases during two thyroid studies from 1998 to 2007.

We conducted analysis of screening results of 4000 study participants (3000 from the joint NCI/SSMA study and 1000 from the subsequent SSMA study), which included ultrasound examination of thyroid gland, cytopathology, fine-needle aspiration biopsy, detection of thyroid hormone levels and antibodies, and height and weight measurements.

Statistical Analysis

Historical behavioral and consumption rate data were collected from residents of Kazakhstan exposed to nuclear weapons testing fallout using a focus group data collection strategy (NCI/SSMA study in 2007). Experts of SSMA conducted implementation of novel screening algorithm and treatment modalities for patients with thyroid nodular diseases, especially from exposed villages as well as patient follow-up examinations and evaluation of late treatment outcomes.

Results

The NCI/SSMA study in 1998 identified 920 cases of nodular thyroid gland among 3000 screened inhabitants (at least 1 nodule 3 mm or greater in maximum diameter), in whom 29 papillary cancers were diagnosed by cytopathology. The study population was 60% female and 40% male, with a mean age of 56.2 years at the time of examination. The two major ethnic groups, with different diets and lifestyles, were Kazakhs (66%) and Europeans, including Russians, Ukrainians, and Germans (34%). Biopsy and cytopathology of 635 nodules from 491 subjects found 30 malignant thyroid papillary tumors in 27 participants (3 males and 24 females) The prevalence of thyroid nodules was significantly higher among females compared to males (39% and 18%, respectively) and increased by 3.5% per year from age 40 to age 70 at examination.

Prevalence of benign nodules and malignant tumors was positively related to exposure (Table 1). Among presumably exposed subjects, the relative risk for all nodules was 1.8 (95% confidence interval, 1.5–2.1). For papillary thyroid carcinoma, the increased relative risk was not significant, a result that is not surprising given the small number of cases. Determination of malignancy was not always possible; there were 86 cases of "deferred diagnosis" (13.3% of all biopsy cases), which may have included undetected cancers.

Another 53 subjects (2 males and 51 females) had undergone thyroid surgery before our screening program in 1998. An international group with expertise in fallout-related dose reconstruction developed highly sophisticated algorithms for estimating individual radiation dose from external and internal sources as a function of bomb characteristics and the movement of the fallout cloud, residential history, age at time of exposure, time spent outdoors, shielding provided by buildings, and

Table 1. Prevalence and relative risks (RRs) by cohort status of thyroid nodules, papillary carcinoma, and follicular neoplasms

Thyroid disease	Number of cases	Prevalence (%)	RR (95% CI)
All nodules			
Exposed	700	35.2	
Nonexposed	220	21.8	1.8 (1.5–2.1)
Papillary carcinoma			
Exposed	20	1.0	
Nonexposed	7	0.7	1.2 (0.6–5.6)
Follicular neoplasm			
Exposed	5	0.3	
Nonexposed	5	0.5	0.5 (0.1–1.8)

CI, confidence interval

dietary history obtained by questionnaire-guided interview and from archival data. This study revealed that there is an apparently strong association between fallout exposure and thyroid nodule prevalence, which is a marker for thyroid cancer risk. Information obtained from the focus groups are being used to derive the settlement-, ethnicity-, age-, and gender-specific (where appropriate) probability density distributions on individual consumption rates of milk and dairy products, duration of breast feeding, time spent indoors, fraction of population living in wooden and adobe homes, and other important parameters of the dosimetry model.

The study results allowed us to develop some new approaches to treatment of patients with thyroid nodular diseases and thyroid cancer. It was also very important to develop a set of clinical guidelines for use by primary care physicians in the evaluation and management of patients with thyroid nodules or thyroid cancer. Various treatment modalities can be used to improve treatment outcomes in patients with radiogenic thyroid nodular diseases. In recent times, the real nature, definitions, and descriptions of clinical, immunohistological, cytopathological, and genetic aspects of a variety of thyroid neoplasms have been defined. Modern medical equipment and scientific techniques can help us to identify particular specific types of thyroid nodules during thyroid screening. We have found a prevalence of atrophic variants of thyroid gland among inhabitants from heavily exposed villages, as well as chronic lymphocytic thyroiditis, and thyroid cancer among exposed population (Table 2).

In accordance with our experience and clinical requirements, thyroid nodules are subclassified according to the volume of the thyroid lesions for five groups: (1) micro-nodule: up to 0.5 cm^3; (2) small nodule: 0.6–2.5 cm^3; (3) middle-sized nodule: 2.6–5.0 cm^3; (4) big nodule: 5.1–8.0 cm^3; and (5) gigantic nodule: $\geq 8.1 \text{ cm}^3$. Among the nonexposed population, we have revealed the prevalence of thyroid cysts, chronic lymphocytic thyroiditis, and adenomas [9,10]. We did not find any significant differences in size, consistency, quantity, symmetry, or nodularity of thyroid nodules among exposed and nonexposed population, which can be possibly considered for thyroid radiation dosimetry. From our own experience and study

Table 2. Cytological characteristics of thyroid nodules in subjects from exposed and control settlements

Cytology	Sarzhal	Dolon	Kokpekti	Kainar	Karaul
Atrophic variant	7.1%	29.0%	0	0	0
Cyst	1.2%	1.4%	11.5%	4.2%	3.0%
Colloid nodule	19.2%	12.1%	5.3%	6.4%	27.3%
Adenoma	0	0	12.3%	6.4%	0
Adenoma with cystic and necrotic degeneration	13.4%	5.8%	0	25.5%	12.1%
Chronic thyroiditis	16.3%	18.9%	10.6%	6.4%	9.0%
Cancer	1.8%	2.9%	0	0	0

results, we believe that it would be interesting and possibly more informative for thyroid dosimetry studies to consider the incidence of thyroid nodules and their specific morphological types. We need more detailed research to apply these findings for dose–response relationship study. Some new approaches for diagnosis and treatment of thyroid nodular diseases were obtained from our joint collaborative research studies [5,9,10].

It is quite common in rural areas that patients really need noninvasive, inexpensive, effective, and rapid treatment modalities. In the past decade, several studies have evaluated and proposed percutaneous intranodular ethanol injection therapy (PIEIT) and percutaneous ultrasound-guided intranodular polidocanol injection therapy (PIPIT), as well as percutaneous intranodular injection therapy by "Paoscle" (PIITP), as treatments for thyroid nodular diseases [9,10]. It helps to avoid an invasive surgical operation as well as the development of some postoperative complications. We have implemented in our clinic various treatment modalities for percutaneous intranodular sclerotherapy of thyroid nodules and treated more than 350 patients. The study group included patients with thyroid nodular diseases (mainly "pretoxic" and "compensated" nodules). We have long-term results of using PIITP in a group of patients from the Semipalatinsk region of Kazakhstan with benign thyroid nodular diseases, as well as PIEIT, and we also implemented percutaneous intranodular injection therapy by using Ethoxisclerol (Polidocanol). This method was attempted to improve the results of treatment for patients having contraindications or refusing standard treatment modalities, and to study the indications, contraindications, effectiveness, and late outcomes of these methods.

Complex analysis of treatment outcomes of patients with thyroid nodular diseases revealed, in general, good treatment results for all implemented treatment modalities. At the same time, some treatment modalities should be used by an experienced specialist to identify an exact indication and contraindication for a particular treatment method. It is common for all treatment modalities that reduction of a nodule began 1 month after the treatment started and reached a maximum 6 or 12 months later. Then, the subsequent process of reduction proceeded very slowly. Analysis of the results of treatment revealed that the nodule volume reduction rate in cases of thyroid adenomas and colloid nodules was less intensive than that of adenomas with necrotic and cystic degeneration. There was a more intensive tendency in the reduction rate for thyroid adenomas with necrotic and cystic degeneration compared to thyroid adenomas and thyroid colloid nodules, but it was not statistically significant. On the basis of our experience we concluded that the nodule volume reduction rate for adenomas with necrotic and cystic degeneration is higher than that for adenomas and colloid nodules, and it was quite typical for all treatment modalities. In the case of malignant thyroid tumors we recommended and performed thyroid surgery. The suggested method is indicated in cases of benign nodular thyroid diseases (cysts, adenomas, adenomas with necrotic and cystic degeneration, colloid nodules, polynodular goiter). We did not observe any long-term complications or thyroid test abnormalities after treatment. It should be noted that after using ethanol some patients experienced temporary intensive pain. Instead of ethanol we using polidocanol more frequently, because it does not cause any pain after precise percutaneous intranodular injection. We did not find any complications after using polidocanol. The tendency to normalization of the blood serum thyroglobulin level and antibodies to thyroglobulin was documented. Analysis of treatment results has revealed that this approach is effective, inexpensive, safe, well tolerated, and can be used on an outpatient basis. In ecologically unfavorable regions, for treatment of exposed patients with benign thyroid nodular diseases, implementation into clinical practice of noninvasive and more effective treatment modalities should be recommended.

Discussion

It is well known that in ecologically unfavorable regions the incidence of thyroid nodular diseases and thyroid cancer is very high. Thyroid cancer is a rare disease in comparison with other malignant tumors. Childhood radiation exposure is a known risk factor for subsequent thyroid cancer and thyroid nodular diseases. The nuclear reactor disaster in Chernobyl resulted in the high incidence of thyroid nodular diseases and thyroid cancer among the exposed population [6]. In our study we characterized thyroid disease prevalence in terms of radiation dose from fallout in a well-defined population exposed at young ages to both internal and external sources of radiation. Prevalence of benign nodules has been shown to be associated with radiation dose from X-rays and γ-rays [3–5]. It was documented in our thyroid studies that modern medical equipment and scientific technique can help us to identify particular specific types of thyroid nodules during thyroid screening. A modern screening algorithm should be implemented in regions adjacent to SNTS. For treatment of exposed patients with benign thyroid nodular diseases, we can recommend noninvasive treatment approaches.

Acknowledgments. The authors wish to thank all team members from NCI, SSMA, and KRIRME (Kazakh Research Institute for Radiation Medicine and Ecology) who participated and aided in the field study carried out in August 1998. We are grateful to specialists from Hiroshima University, Japan, who participated in our subsequent thyroid studies.

References

1. Nugent RW, Zhumadilov ZS, Gusev BI, et al (2000) Health effects of radiation associated with nuclear weapons testing at the Semipalatinsk Test Site, 1st edn. Nakamoto Sogo Printing, Hiroshima, Japan
2. Zhumadilov Z, Gusev B, Takada J, et al (2000) Thyroid abnormalities trend over time in northeastern regions of Kazakhstan, adjacent to the Semipalatinsk Nuclear Test Site: a case review of pathological findings for 7271 patients. J Radiat Res 41:55–59
3. Simon SL, Bouville A (2002) Radiation doses to local populations near nuclear weapons test sites worldwide. Health Phys 82:706–725
4. Simon SL, Bouville A, Land CE (2006) Fallout from nuclear weapons tests and cancer risks. Am Sci 94:48–57
5. Land C, Zhumadilov Z, Simon S, et al (2003) Thyroid disease prevalence and fallout exposure in the Semipalatinsk region of Kazakhstan. Science Health Care 2:28–31
6. Ito M, Yamashita S, Ashizava K, et al (1995) Childhood thyroid diseases around Chernobyl evaluated by ultrasound examination and fine needle aspiration cytology. Thyroid 5: 365–368
7. Martino E, Murtas M, Loviselli A, et al (1992) Percutaneous intranodular ethanol injection for treatment of autonomously functioning thyroid nodules. Surgery (St. Louis) 112: 1161–1165
8. Gharib H (1997) Management of thyroid nodules: another look. Thyroid Today 20:1–11
9. Zhumadilov Z, Hoshi M, Takeichi N, et al (2003) Approaches to treatment of patients with thyroid nodular diseases in the Semipalatinsk region of Kazakhstan. Hiroshima J Med Sci 52:81–89
10. Zhumadilov Z (2006) Thyroid nodules in the population living around Semipalatinsk Nuclear Test Site: possible implications for dose–response relationships study. J Radiat Res 47: A183–A187

Radiation Basic Life Sciences, Part 1

Higher-Order Chromatin Structure and Nontargeted Effects

Keiji Suzuki, Motohiro Yamauchi, Yasuyoshi Oka, and Shunichi Yamashita

Summary. Ionizing radiation causes deleterious effects in cells that have directly absorbed its energy as well as in those which are not exposed to radiation directly. The latter are often referred to as radiation-induced nontargeted effects. Radiation-induced genomic instability is one of those effects, and it is manifested as the expression of various delayed effects, such as delayed cell death, delayed chromosomal instability, and delayed mutagenesis. Because this instability accumulates genetic changes in the genome, it has been hypothesized to be a driving force to accelerate multistep carcinogenesis. Exposure to ionizing radiation causes double-strand breaks in DNA, which result in deletion of the genome through illegitimate rejoining of the broken ends. Recently, we found that large deletions could be transmitted in the progeny of cells surviving ionizing radiation. As large deletions disrupt higher-order chromatin structure and chromatin codes, they possibly comprise potentially unstable chromatin regions, whose disintegration causes delayed manifestation of radiation-induced genomic instability. Our present study defines the molecular nature of DNA damage memory, which is associated with nontargeted effects.

Key words Radiation · Genome instability · Chromatin · Nontargeted effect

Introduction

Ionizing radiation has now been recognized to induce adverse consequences in cells that do not receive the direct deposition of radiation energy. These so-called non-targeted effects are manifested in cells receiving bystander signals produced by directly irradiated cells, or the descendants of cells surviving direct irradiation [1–3]. The latter effect, known as radiation-induced genomic instability, has been extensively studied, and several laboratories have reported the induction of delayed reproductive death or delayed lethal mutation, delayed chromosomal instability, and

Department of Molecular Medicine, Atomic Bomb Disease Institute, Nagasaki University Graduate School of Biomedical Sciences, 1-12-4 Sakamoto, Nagasaki 852-8523, Japan

delayed mutagenesis in many types of mammalian cells. Because delayed phenotypes are not induced uniformly among the progeny of surviving cells, and because the frequency of genomic instability is significantly higher than that of typical gene mutations, it is not likely that it arises from gene mutation directly caused by radiation. Furthermore, because radiation-induced genomic instability persists over many generations of cell division, it is suggested that there is a mechanism by which exposed cells transmit the memory of DNA damage through their progeny. A number of studies have suggested that oxidative stress is involved in persistence of radiation-induced genomic instability [3,4]. However, our recent results provide an alternative mechanism: that ionizing radiation-induced destabilization of higher-order chromatin structure, transmitted down many generations through the progeny as DNA damage memory, is associated with radiation-induced genomic instability [4]. A possible mechanism of how the higher-order chromatin structure disrupted by radiation exposure is involved in nontargeted effects is discussed.

Materials and Methods

Normal human cells immortalized by transfecting SV40 DNA were cultured in minimum essential medium (MEM) supplemented with 10% fetal bovine serum (Trace Bioscience, Australia). Exponentially growing cells were irradiated with X-rays from an X-ray generator at 150 kVp and 5 mA with a 0.1-mm copper filter (Softex M-150WE; Softex, Osaka, Japan). The dose rate was 0.44 Gy/min. Dose rates were determined with an ionization chamber. After X-irradiation, 6-thioguanine (6-TG)-resistant clones were isolated. Deletion of the exons of the HPRT gene was determined by multiplex polymerase chain reaction (PCR). Deletion sizes over megabases were analyzed by PCR amplification using sequence tagged site (STS) primers. Delayed chromosomal instability was determined by Giemsa staining and by X-chromosome-specific whole chromosome painting (WCP)-fluorescence in situ hybridization (FISH). DNA double-strand breaks were visualized by the foci of phosphorylated ATM protein, which were examined under the fluorescence microscope. Digital images were captured by a charge-coupled device (CCD) camera, and the images were analyzed by Leica FW4000 software.

Results and Discussion

Previous studies demonstrated that genomic instability was induced by DNA-damaging agents [5,6]. In particular, those that induce DNA double-strand breaks cause delayed effects, indicating that DNA is a critical target for radiation-induced genomic instability. It is well known that DNA double-strand breaks are repaired through various pathways, including two major pathways, nonhomologous end-joining (NHEJ) and homologous recombination (HR). Although most DNA damage is repaired correctly, it is obvious that the repair process by itself results in disruption of the genome structure. For example, using the I-*Sce*I endonuclease expression system, it has been shown that nonhomologous end-joining or microhomology-directed repair generally result in small deletions or insertions at the break points, whereas homologous recombination results in loss of heterozygosity or chromosomal translocations [7]. Therefore, we have hypothesized that interchromosomal deletion disrupts the higher-order chromatin structure, which results in perturbation of chromatin organization within the nuclei [4].

Abnormal chromatin structures are transmissible as DNA damage memory for many generations after irradiation, which may be involved in delayed manifestation of radiation-induced genomic instability. To prove this hypothesis, the stability of X chromosomes, which have large deletions at the *HPRT* locus, was examined [8]. SV40-immortalized normal human fibroblast cells were irradiated with 3 Gy X-rays, and the independently arising *HPRT* mutants were isolated. Multiplex-PCR analysis revealed that 52% of clones lost entire exons of the *HPRT* gene. Deletion size in the total deletion mutants was examined by PCR using STS primers, and the size was expanded from 0.44 to 3.6 Mb. WCP-FISH analysis revealed that total deletion mutants frequently induce chromosome aberrations including translocations, dicentrics, and fragments. Interestingly, more than 95% of delayed induced translocations and dicentrics were observed in the q-arm of the X chromosome, where the *HPRT* gene is assigned. The results indicated that X chromosomes with large deletions showed a higher probability to induce delayed chromosomal instability, and thus radiation-induced gross genome rearrangement could be transmitted through the progeny of surviving cells for many generations as the DNA damage memory.

Although these results shed light on a role of abnormal chromatin structure in the initiation and perpetuation of genomic instability, the mechanism(s) by which delayed effects are manifested still must be determined. One attractive explanation will be that those chromatins with abnormal structure are potentially unstable. In fact, chromosome aberrations detected in X-chromosome required DNA breaks, indicating that abnormal chromatin is likely to cause delayed DNA breaks. The possibility was further supported by the results that induction of DNA double-strand breaks was frequently observed in the progeny of surviving cells [9]. Thus, abnormal chromatin structure may be recognized by the mechanism to maintain chromatin integrity, or it may be unable to reconstitute higher-order chromatin in a replication process, which results in creating the fragile site. Future studies are expected to prove this hypothesis, which may open a new paradigm in understanding the long-term effects of ionizing radiation on human beings.

References

1. Little JB (2003) Genomic instability and bystander effects: a historical perspective. Oncogene 22:6978–6987
2. Morgan WF (2003) Non-targeted and delayed effects of exposure to ionizing radiation: I. Radiation induced genomic instability and bystander effects in vitro. Radiat Res 159: 567–580

3. Wright EG, Coates PJ (2006) Untargeted effects of ionizing radiation: implications for radiation pathology. Mutat Res 597:119–132
4. Suzuki K (1997) Multistep nature of X-ray-induced neoplastic transformation in mammalian cells: genetic alterations and instability. J Radiat Res 38:55–63
5. Chang WP, Little JB (1992) Persistently elevated frequency of spontaneous mutations in progeny of CHO clones surviving X-irradiation: association with delayed reproductive death phenotype. Mutat Res 270:191–199
6. Limoli CL, Kaplan MI, Phillips JW, et al (1997) Differential induction of chromosomal instability by DNA strand-breaking agents. Cancer Res 57:4048–4056
7. Richardson C, Jasin M (2000) Frequent chromosomal translocations induced by DNA double-strand breaks. Nature (Lond) 405:697–700
8. Suzuki K, Ojima M, Kodama S, et al (2006) Delayed activation of DNA damage checkpoint and radiation-induced genomic instability. Mutat Res 597:73–77
9. Suzuki K, Yokoyama S, Waseda S, et al (2003) Delayed reactivation of p53 in the progeny of cells surviving ionizing radiation. Cancer Res 63:936–941

p53 Dependency of Delayed and Untargeted Recombination in Mouse Embryos Fertilized by Irradiated Sperm

Ohtsura Niwa

Summary. Radiation induction of genomic instability has been demonstrated in whole-animal systems. Although the molecular mechanisms underlying the induced genomic instability are not known at present, this phenomenon could be regarded as the manifestation of a cellular fail-safe system in which fidelity of repair and replication is downregulated to tolerate DNA damage. Two features of genomic instability, namely, delayed mutation and untargeted mutation, require mechanisms for "damage memory" and for "damage sensing, signal transduction and execution" to induce mutations at a nondamaged site. In this chapter, the phenomenon of transgenerational genomic instability and possible mechanisms are discussed using mouse data collected in our laboratory as the main bases.

Key words Radiation · Sperm irradiation · Mouse embryos · p53 · Delayed recombination

Genomic Instability and Dynamic Mutations

The term dynamic mutation was originally coined to describe the expansion of the trinucleotide repeat sequences associated with human neuromuscular degenerative disorders [1]. Patients with these disorders carry an allele of the target gene that has a higher than normal number of tandem trinucleotide repeats. The trinucleotide repeat of the affected allele further changes its copy number in somatic and germ cells. The precise mechanism of trinucleotide expansion in somatic and germ cells is not known at present, but the dynamic nature of the expansion poses a challenge to the current concept of mutagenesis in which mutation is thought to arise as the result of misrepair and misreplication of DNA damage. In the case of trinucleotide expansion, there seems to be no requirement of DNA damage at the alleles. Rather, the sequence of the affected allele itself is the cause of the expansion. In fact, the boundary length of normal and affected alleles is reported to match that of the

---

National Institute of Radiological Sciences, 4-9-1 Anagawa, Inage, Chiba 263-8555, Japan

Okazaki fragment [1]. DNA replication along the entire genome is not a uniform process, and the regional sequence context together with the local chromatin configuration affect the replication fork progression, the fidelity of polymerization, and the rate of recombination. Thus, mutation can arise as a nontargeted event.

Dynamic mutations are not restricted to trinucleotide repeat expansion and, in fact, the phenomenon was already known in the 1940s in chemical mutagenesis research. In her pioneering work on *Drosophila* with mustard gas, Auerbach [2] demonstrated that treatment of parental males (P_0 generation) with this chemical induced a sex-linked recessive lethal in the F_1 progeny (scored in the F_2), but also in the F_3 generation. Mustard gas is an alkylating agent, and the resulting DNA damage can be repaired within a few hours in the treated fly. Therefore, one has to conclude that the delayed mutation occurring after three generations of reproduction cannot be caused by persisting DNA damage. Rather, the treatment must have induced a higher mutability that persisted through generations. Similarly, the classic work of Nomura clearly showed that parental irradiation increased the frequency of lung adenoma in F_1 mice [3]. The increase was observed in progeny derived from irradiated spermatozoa, spermatid, and spermatogonial stages. The magnitude of observed increases, however, is difficult to reconcile with the known induced germline mutation rates in mice. For example, the frequency of adenomas in the progeny derived from irradiated spermatozoa (5 Gy) is around 20% addition, and the figures are approximately similar in the progeny derived from the other irradiated germ cell stages. When the spontaneous frequency of 5% is taken into account, the induced rate of adenomas becomes about 3% per Gy, a value that is three orders of magnitude higher than the estimated germ cell mutation rate of 3×10^{-5}/locus/Gy in specific locus experiments [4]. This simple comparison of the rates indicates that the mutations responsible for the F_1 tumors cannot be those induced directly by radiation at tumor-related genes in the gonads of parents. Similar to the delayed mutation shown by Auerbach, the tumor-causing mutation could have arisen in somatic cells of F_1 mice born to irradiated parents.

Mutagenesis as an Active Response of Cells

The foregoing examples of delayed and high-frequency mutations suggest an interesting possibility that some mutation may occur not as a passive consequence of DNA damage, but as a result of active cellular response to DNA damage. Although genomic integrity is crucial for somatic cells, the fidelity is rather costly because it requires precision in repair and replication. Recent studies have revealed that *Escherichia coli* can downregulate the fidelity of replication and repair overprecision. This damage tolerance allows damaged cells to survive and proliferate at the cost of possible mutation [5]. Thus, damage tolerance is a mutagenic cellular response to genotoxic stress.

The active mutagenic pathway of cells can be triggered not only by DNA, but by a wide variety of stresses. In fact, it has been known for decades that mutation rate can be augmented by culturing *E. coli* cells in nutritionally poor media [6,7]. This "adaptive mutation" is thought to be the strategy of bacteria to create mutants better adapted to a harsh environment by increasing the mutation rate. Adaptive mutation can be found in nutritionally deprived yeast cells. However, it is not known whether a similar adaptive mechanism is present in mammalian cells.

Radiation-Induced Genomic Instability

Recent studies have provided evidence for the induction of dynamic mutations in mammalian cells in culture. Alpha-particle-irradiated mouse hematopoietic stem cells were found to produce chromosome aberrations even after many cycles of replication [8]. Similar chromosomal instability has also been observed in a variety of cell types, but the mechanisms remain to be elucidated [9]. In addition to chromosomal instability, radiation can also induce delayed gene mutations [10]. These phenomena are now generically termed as genomic instability, which is characterized by two features: untargeted mutation and delayed mutation. Untargeted mutation requires the "damage sensor, signal transducer and effector," and delayed mutation requires the "damage memory keeper."

Untargeted and delayed mutations are caused by radiation, if they persist through generations. A possible involvement of delayed genomic instability in radiation carcinogenesis is of particular interest. The epidemiological study of atomic bomb survivors demonstrates a linear dose response of solid tumors, and the single-hit induction of cancer contradicts the well-accepted multistep carcinogenesis mechanism [11,12]. Furthermore, solid cancer develops after a long latency period of a few decades. These facts raise the question of whether the relevant carcinogenic mutation is induced in a delayed manner as a result of genomic instability, instead of being induced by the direct mechanism, although a model constructed on the direct mutagenic action of radiation has been proposed [13].

Transgenerational Minisatellite Mutations in Mice

The induction by radiation of genomic instability in mouse germ cells in vivo has been studied using hypervariable minisatellite sequences. Minisatellite sequences are composed of a stretch of short tandem repeats that were originally discovered in the human genome [14]. These sequences are highly mutable in germ cells and to a lesser extent in somatic cells. The mutational changes manifest as changes in the number of tandem repeat cores and hence allele length. Thee postulated mutational mechanisms include slippage during replication, intraallelic recombination, unequal sister chromatid exchange, or simple deletion [15,16]. Mouse minisatellites were named expanded simple tandem repeats (ESTRs). We used Ms6hm, a hypervariable ESTR sequence, as a marker for studying germ cell mutations. The Ms6hm locus is 3 to 10 kb in length with a short GGGCA repeat and is highly variable among laboratory mouse strains [17,18].

Evidence that the progeny of irradiated males showed higher frequencies of mutations at the paternally inherited Ms6hm locus has been published [19]. While all germ cell stages respond to mutation induction, spermatids are the most sensitive. In a strict sense, mutation induction in the spermatozoa stage may not be considered as a male germline event because spermatozoa lack biochemical activity and mutation fixation takes place in fertilized zygotes. However, introduction of DNA damage into the egg via the sperm permits studies of untargeted events, namely, mutations in the nonirradiated *maternal* allele, as discussed next.

In our experiments [20], male (C56BL/6N) mice were X-irradiated (6 Gy) and mated to unirradiated (C3H/HeN) female mice, and the F_1 progeny descended from irradiated spermatozoa were used for the analysis. The results showed that the mutation frequencies were increased not only in the paternal allele (as expected) but also in the *maternally derived* allele. Mutations in the maternal allele clearly demonstrate that untargeted mutations have occurred. The inference that mutation induction at the paternal allele is also untargeted rest on the following arguments: (a) a dose of 6 Gy induces about 300 DNA double-strand breaks (DSB)s; (b) the Ms6hm sequence in the C57BL strain is about 10 kb; (c) the chance that a mutation will occur as a result of direct damage to the locus is about 10^{-3}; and (d) the observed increase in mutation frequency is of the order of 10^{-1}, which is two orders of magnitude higher than expected.

Transgenerational Mutations at the Pink-Eyed Unstable Allele Locus in Mice

The pink-eyed dilution locus has several mutant alleles. The pink-eyed unstable allele (*p-un*) has a partial tandem duplication that reverts somatically to the wild type at high frequencies [21]. Somatic reversion mutation can easily be scored in the retinal pigment epithelium (RPE) as clusters of black pigmented cells. The pink-eyed Jackson allele (*p-J*), on the other hand, is caused by a deletion, and therefore no reversion takes place for this allele. The combination of these two alleles offers yet another tool to study delayed transgenerational reversion mutation induced by radiation. Male mice homozygous for the *p-J* allele were irradiated with 6 Gy X-rays and immediately mated with the female homozygous for the *p-un* allele. The F_1 progeny were analyzed for the reversions at the maternally inherited *p-un* allele.

The data show that the reversion frequency is around 3 to 5 spots per RPE in the unirradiated control and 7 to 8 in the irradiated group [22]. As the RPE develops at day 11 to 12 in the fetus, induced mutations in this system are delayed events occurring after many cycles of replication following the introduction of damage (via sperm) to the egg. As in the case of the ESTR mutation, F_1 mice descended from irradiated spermatocytes or spermatogonia showed no evidence for induction of mutations at the maternally inherited *p-un* allele. Interestingly, the induced (but not spontaneous) reversion of the *p-un* allele was found to be p53 dependent, as no increase in the reversion was observed in $p53^{-/-}$ F_1 mice (Shiraishi, manuscript in preparation).

Genomic Cross Talk and p53-Dependent S-Phase Checkpoint in Early Mouse Embryogenesis

The observations on untargeted and delayed mutations of the maternal allele in the F_1 progeny descended from irradiated sperm support our hypothesis that a damage sensing/transducer/effector system and a damage memory-keeping system are operating for this phenomenon; the first of these senses the DNA damage in the male genome and sends a signal to the female genome. This "genomic cross talk" results in untargeted mutation in the latter.

Mouse zygotes are known to possess a high level of p53 protein. Because at this stage sperm and oocytes genomes exist as separate pronuclei in which one round of DNA synthesis occurs before the first cleavage division, we tested the pronuclear cross-talk hypothesis by microinjecting a reporter with the p53-responsible promoter into the female pronucleus of the zygote and examined its activation by irradiated sperm. Clear evidence for such cross talk between pronuclei was observed [23]. In the same experiment, we studied the S-phase progression by pulse-labeling with ^{3}H-thymidine of control zygotes and zygotes fertilized with 6 Gy irradiated sperm (sperm-irradiated zygotes). In both groups, pronuclear DNA synthesis was first detected at 8 h after fertilization, and the first cleavage division occurred 23–24 h after fertilization. This observation suggests that the p53-dependent G_1/S and G_2/M checkpoints do not operate in the zygotes. However, the amount of ^{3}H-thymidine uptake was severely suppressed by sperm irradiation. Interestingly, DNA synthesis was suppressed also in the female pronucleus to a similar extent as in the male pronucleus. The extent of suppression suggested that the p53-dependent S checkpoint operates in a low-dose region up to 2 Gy to sperm. Also, this suppression of DNA synthesis was not observed for sperm-irradiated $p53^{-/-}$ zygotes.

We are not aware of any study in which evidence for a role of p53 in the S-phase checkpoint has been found, and our observation is the first one to suggest this novel function. This p53 dependency was also observed in primary mouse fibroblasts. One of the reasons why previous studies were unable to detect the p53 dependency could be that this novel S checkpoint seems to operates only in the low-dose range below 2 Gy whereas most of the S checkpoint studies have used much higher doses, of 10 to 20 Gy.

Further analysis of sperm-irradiated $p53^{-/-}$ zygotes indicated that the suppression could be restored by microinjection of p53 protein, and this finding was further exploited for the analysis of the functional domain of p53 protein for this novel S checkpoint function [24]. Mutation in the DNA-binding domain, but not in the transactivation domain, was found to abrogate the activity, demonstrating the importance of the domain for the S-phase checkpoint. The mechanism of the suppression of DNA synthesis was studied by the iododeoxyuridine (IdUrd) and chlorodeoxyuridine (CldUrd) double-labeling method in mouse embryonic fibroblasts of p53 wild type and the $p53^{-/-}$ genotype. The results indicated that the speed of replication fork progression was slowed down in the wild-type cells after exposure to 1–2 Gy but the replication origin firing was not affected. Further analysis has shown that the p53 function in the S checkpoint is located downstream of ataxia-telangiectasia mutated (ATM) kinase and is required for phosphorylation of a yet to be identified target protein needed for the suppression (Shimura, manuscript in preparation). The preliminary working hypothesis that we have developed for the p53-dependent S-phase checkpoint is as follows: the DNA damage sensor detects and sends signals to ATM kinase, which with the help of p53 phosphorylates the third protein, which then slows down the progression of the replication fork.

p53-Dependent Enhancement of Recombination Between Sister Chromatids

The foregoing observations demonstrate that p53 is involved in retarding the replication fork progression after irradiation. This retardation is an untargeted event because we have already shown that DNA synthesis of female pronuclei was suppressed in sperm-irradiated zygotes. Since our results of untargeted and delayed mutation in the whole body system are all caused by recombination, we have studied whether the p53-dependent S checkpoint has any effect on recombinational events. In somatic cells, recombination occurs between sister chromatids and between homologous chromosomes, the latter being much less frequent in normal cells but highly frequent for some tumor cells.

In other studies, we compared the frequencies of radiation-induced sister chromatid exchanges (SCE) in $p53^{+/+}$ and $p53^{-/-}$ mouse fibroblasts. Irradiation of the fibroblasts increased the frequency of SCE in a dose-dependent manner in p53 wild-type fibroblasts. To our surprise and excitement, this increase was not observed when $p53^{-/-}$ fibroblasts were examined, suggesting that radiation induction of SCE required the functional p53 (Niwa, unpublished observation).

A Possible Mechanism for Untargeted Recombination

Our results presented in this chapter suggest that p53 slows down replication fork progression upon detection of radiation damage and that the slow movement of the replication fork is likely to increase the chance of recombination between sister chromatids. This p53-dependent elevation of recombination is the likely reason for the untargeted mutation observed in our study of transgenerational instability of the minisatellite and *p-un* alleles. Should this turn out to be correct, the resulting recombination mutations at these two marker loci represent error-free type exchange events and not error-prone instability events such as delayed chromosome instability and genomic instability.

Minisatellite sequences undergo dynamic mutation in humans and mice. This type of mutation has been the subject of intensive studies because it was thought to occur in risk-related events such as induced genomic instability [25]. In some reports, minisatellite instability was transmitted for two generations in the descendants of irradiated male mice [26]. Our unpublished study of the *p-un* allele suggests lack of transmission to the F_2 generation (Shiraishi, manuscript in preparation). Chromosome instability was not observed in the atomic bomb survivors exposed in utero [27]. Thus, some of the instability markers such as the mouse *Ms6hm* locus and the *p-un* allele of the pink-eyed dilution locus may not be suitable for the study of risk-related delayed chromosome instability and genomic instability induced by radiation. It is also likely that embryogenesis and fetal development may be well protected from radiation induction of delayed chromosome instability and genomic instability, except in rare mutant mice [28].

Acknowledgments. The author wishes to thank Dr. Sankaranarayanan for critically reading the manuscript. Also, thanks are due to M. Toyoshima, N. Uematsu, S.K. Adiga, T. Shimura, K. Shiraishi, M. Taga, J. Takeda, and H. Nagai. This work is supported by a grant-in-aid from the Ministry of Education, Culture, Sports, Science and Technology of Japan, and by a grant from the Nuclear Safety Research Association.

References

1. Richards RI (2001) Dynamic mutations: a decade of unstable expanded repeats in human genetic disease. Hum Mol Genet 10:2187–2194
2. Auerbach C (1943) The induction by mustard gas of chromosomal instability in *Drosophila melanogaster*. Proc R Soc Edinb B 62:307–320
3. Nomura T (1982) Parental exposure to X rays and chemicals induces heritable tumours and anomalies in mice. Nature (Lond) 296:575–577
4. Russell WL, Kelly EM (1982) Specific-locus mutation frequencies in mouse stem-cell spermatogonia at very low radiation dose rates. Proc Natl Acad Sci U S A 79:539–541
5. Radman M (2001) Fidelity and infidelity. Nature (Lond) 413:115
6. Cairns J, Foster PL (1991) Adaptive reversion of a frameshift mutation in *Escherichia coli*. Genetics 128:695–701
7. Bjedov I, Tenaillon O, Gerard B, et al (2003) Stress-induced mutagenesis in bacteria. Science 300:1404–1409
8. Kadhim MA, Macdonald DA, Goodhead DT, et al (1992) Transmission of chromosomal instability after plutonium alpha-particle irradiation. Nature (Lond) 355:738–740
9. Morgan WF (2003) Non-targeted and delayed effects of exposure to ionizing radiation: I. Radiation-induced genomic instability and bystander effects in vitro. Radiat Res 159: 567–581
10. Little JB (2003) Genomic instability and bystander effects: a historical perspective. Oncogene 22:6978–6987
11. Preston DL, Shimizu Y, Pierce DA, et al (2003) Studies of mortality of atomic bomb survivors. Report 13: Solid cancer and noncancer disease mortality: 1950–1997. Radiat Res 160:381–407

12. Vogelstein B, Kinzler KW (1993) The multistep nature of cancer. Trends Genet 9:138–141
13. Pierce DA, Vaeth M (2003) Age-time patterns of cancer to be anticipated from exposure to general mutagens. Biostatistics 4:231–248
14. Jeffreys AJ, Wilson V, Tein SL (1985) Hypervariable 'minisatellite' regions in human DNA. Nature (Lond) 314:67–73
15. Yauk CL, Dubrova YE, Grant GR, et al (2002) A novel single molecule analysis of spontaneous and radiation-induced mutation at a mouse tandem repeat locus. Mutat Res 500:147–156
16. Jeffreys AJ, Neumann R (1997) Somatic mutation processes at a human minisatellite. Hum Mol Genet 6:129–132
17. Kelly R, Bulfield G, Collick A, et al (1989) Characterization of a highly unstable mouse minisatellite locus: evidence for somatic mutation during early development. Genomics 5:844–856
18. Mitani K, Takahashi Y, Kominami R (1990) A GGCAGG motif in minisatellites affecting their germline instability. J Biol Chem 256:15203–15210
19. Niwa O (2003) Induced genomic instability in irradiated germ cells and in the offspring; reconciling discrepancies among the human and animal studies. Oncogene 22:7078–7086
20. Niwa O, Kominami R (2001) Untargeted mutation of the maternally derived mouse hypervariable minisatellite allele in F_1 mice born to irradiated spermatozoa. Proc Natl Acad Sci U S A 98:1705–1710
21. Gondo Y, Gardner JM, Nakatsu Y, et al (1993) High-frequency genetic reversion mediated by a DNA duplication: the mouse pink-eyed unstable mutation. Proc Natl Acad Sci U S A 90:297–301
22. Shiraishi K, Shimura T, Taga M, et al (2002) Persistent induction of somatic reversions of the pink-eyed unstable mutation in F_1 mice born to fathers irradiated at the spermatozoa stage. Radiat Res 157:661–667
23. Shimura T, Inoue M, Taga M, et al (2002) p53-dependent S-phase damage checkpoint and pronuclear cross talk in mouse zygotes with X-irradiated sperm. Mol Cell Biol 22:2220–2228
24. Toyoshima M, Shimura T, Adiga SK, et al (2005) Transcription-independent suppression of DNA synthesis by p53 in sperm-irradiated mouse zygotes. Oncogene 24:3229–3235
25. Dubrova YE (2003) Long-term genetic effects of radiation exposure. Mutat Res 544:433–439
26. Dubrova YE, Plumb MA (2002) Ionising radiation and mutation induction at mouse minisatellite loci. The story of the two generations. Mutat Res 499:143–150
27. Ohtaki K, Kodama Y, Nakano M, et al (2004) Human fetuses do not register chromosome damage inflicted by radiation exposure in lymphoid precursor cells except for a small but significant effect at low doses. Radiat Res 161:373–379
28. Pampfer S, Streffer C (1989) Increased chromosome aberration levels in cells from mouse fetuses after zygote X-irradiation. Int J Radiat Biol 55:85–92

The Yin and Yang of Low-Dose Radiobiology

Tom K. Hei[1,2], Hongning Zhou[1], and Vladimir N. Ivanov[2]

Summary. Two conflicting phenomena, bystander effect and adaptive response, are important in determining the biological responses at low doses of radiation and have the potential to impact the shape of the dose–response relationship. Using the Columbia University charged-particle microbeam and the highly sensitive human–hamster hybrid (A_L) cells mutagenic assay, we show here that nonirradiated cells acquire mutagenesis through direct contact with cells whose nuclei have been traversed with a lethal dose of 20 alpha (α-)particles each. Pretreatment of cells with a low dose of X-rays 4 h before α-particle irradiation significantly decreased this bystander mutagenic response. Although adaptive response is largely protective in nature and the bystander response, in general, signifies detrimental effects, the two processes share many common characteristics. There is evidence that extracellular signal-related kinase (ERK), nuclear factor-κB, cytokines, and mitochondrial functions play an important role in the bystander effects. However, all these signaling events are applicable to the adaptive response as well. These data suggest a common lineage between these two stress-related phenomena. A better understanding of how these two effects interact at the cellular, tissue, and organ levels will address some of the pressing issues on target size, radiation dose response, and, ultimately, low dose risk assessment.

Key words Bystander effects · Adaptive response · Mitochondrial function · Nuclear factor-κB · Signaling events

Introduction

Radiation is a two-edged sword: on the one hand, it is an effective therapeutic modality for the treatment of many types of human cancers, and on the other hand it is a well-known human carcinogen. The estimated lifetime cancer mortality risk

---

[1]Center for Radiological Research, College of Physicians and Surgeons, and
[2]Department of Environmental Health Sciences, Mailman School of Public Health, Columbia University, New York, NY 10032, USA

from low-dose/low-dose-rate radiation exposure, based on epidemiological data from the Japanese atomic bomb survivors, is estimated to be 0.05 per sievert (Sv) for the whole population [1]. However, direct characterization of risk at low doses is at or beyond the limits of epidemiology. Cancer risk from exposure to ionizing radiation clearly increases at a dose above 10 cGy, and no obvious threshold dose is detectable. At doses below 10 cGy, the radiobiological effects are rather complex and are subjected to modulations by various competing forces, including bystander effects and adaptive response.

Radiation-induced bystander effect is defined as the induction of biological effects in cells that are not directly traversed by a charged particle, but are in close proximity to cells which are. Interest in this effect was sparked by earlier reports demonstrating that, following a low dose of alpha (α)-particles, a larger proportion of cells showed biological damage than was estimated, based on microdosimetric principle, to have been hit by an α-particle [2]. To demonstrate the induction of a radiation-induced bystander effect unequivocally, studies were conducted using a microbeam in which a defined proportion of cells in a confluent monolayer were irradiated individually with a defined number of α-particles [3,4]. These studies provided the first clear-cut indication of a radiation-induced bystander phenomenon.

Adaptive response is characterized by a reduction in radiobiological response in cells pretreated with a low dose of ionizing radiation (generally ≤ 10 cGy) followed by exposure to a challenging, higher dose. Since the original experiments reported in 1984 [5], numerous data have shown the existence of such a response with a variety of endpoints in various cell types [6]. Although bystander effect and adaptive response are important parameters for low-dose radiation response, there are only limited data available comparing the two effects [7–9].

Adaptive Response on Bystander Mutagenesis

To define the interaction between adaptive response and bystander effects, human–hamster hybrid (A_L) cells were used together with the Columbia University single-particle microbeam. For determining the adaptive response, cells were irradiated with a low dose of X-rays (10 cGy) 4 h before the α-particle irradiation. To examine the response of bystander cells to the subsequent challenging dose, 10% of the cells were randomly irradiated with a lethal dose of 20 α-particles each directed at the nuclear centroids. Mutant fractions at the CD59 locus of the A_L cells were scored using an antibody-complement cytotoxic assay as previously described [10,11]. Western blots were used to identify various signaling proteins, and an electrophoretic mobility shift assay (EMSA) was used to detect the DNA-binding activities of various bystander signaling molecules.

A_L cells irradiated with a 10 cGy dose of X-rays resulted in a low but significant induction of mutations at the *CD59* locus (Fig. 1). The background *CD59*⁻ mutant fraction among the population of A_L cells used in these experiments averaged 61 ± 19. Consistent with our previously published data, irradiation of 10% of a

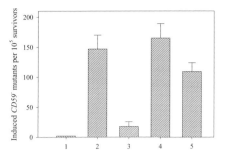

Fig. 1. Induced mutant fraction of human–hamster hybrid (A$_L$) cells in which 10% had been irradiated with 20 α-particles through the nucleus with or without pretreatment with a 10-cGy dose of X-rays. *1*, Control; *2*, 20 α-particles, 10%; *3*, X-rays alone, 10 cGy; *4*, assuming an additive effect between the two effects; *5*, actual mutant fraction of cells pretreated with 10 cGy dose of X-rays followed by targeting 10% of cells with a lethal dose of 20 α-particles. Data are pooled from three independent experiments. *Bars* ±SD

confluent cell population with a lethal dose of 20 α-particles each through the nuclei resulted in a mutant yield that was about three times higher than the background among the nonirradiated neighboring cells [3]. Pretreatment of cells with a 10-cGy dose of X-rays significantly reduced this bystander mutagenesis ($P < 0.05$, Fig. 1) [12]. These results implied that, in the presence of low-dose radiation stress, the bystander mutagenesis is suppressed by the adaptive response, although the mechanism (or mechanisms) is unclear.

Parameters Affecting the Adaptive Response and the Bystander Effect

Table 1 summarizes the similarity and difference in various parameters that can modulate radiation-induced adaptive response and the bystander effect. In general, there are more similarities than differences between the two phenomena. Both are primarily low-dose phenomena, and neither shows a dose–response induction of effects. Both the adaptive response and the bystander effect have been demonstrated by a range of biological endpoints including cell killing, oncogenic transformation, mutagenesis, chromosomal aberrations, induction of p53 protein, and DNA repair foci. Although bystander effects are not p53 dependent, there are reports that adaptive response, in some studies, is related to p53 function [13]. It should be noted that cancer cells with mutated p53 protein can also demonstrate an adaptive response [14]. Both phenomena involve signals that mediate through either gap junctions or soluble mediators [15,16].

Table 1. A comparison of radiation-induced bystander effect versus adaptive response

Parameter	Bystander	Adaptive response
Low-dose phenomenon	+	+
Dose–response relationship	–	–
LET* dependence	–	–
Endpoints examined	Many	Many
Biological consequence	Harmful/protective	Protective
p53 dependence	–	±
Individual variability	–	+
Involves gap junctions	+	+
Involves soluble mediator(s)	+	+
Involves ROS/RNS	+	+
Requires protein synthesis	+	+
Genomic instability	+	+

*Linear Energy Transfer

Table 2. Signaling events that are common to both the adaptive response and the bystander effect

Reactive radical species
Mitochondrial function
NFκB activities
MAPK/ERK kinase activities
Cytokine activities

Signaling Events Common to Both the Adaptive Response and the Bystander Effect

Table 2 lists several signaling events that are common to both these low-dose phenomena and suggest that the adaptive response and the bystander effect share a common stress-related signaling lineage. These events include reactive radical species such as superoxide anions, hydroxyl radicals, hydrogen peroxide, nitric oxide, and peroxynitrite anions. The observations that extracellularly applied antioxidants, such as superoxide dismutase [17] and catalase [18], can inhibit medium-mediated bystander responses suggest a role of reactive radical species in the bystander signaling scheme. Because mitochondria are the main source of energy production as well as generators of free radicals in cells, it is consistent with the recent observation that mitochondrial DNA-deficient cells exhibit a lower bystander response in the presence of wild-type cells [19]. Similarly, reactive radical species can presumably damage DNA to initiate an adaptive response. The observation that nitric oxide, secreted from irradiated donor cells, can induce an adaptive response in bystander cells [20] provides strong evidence that nitric oxide plays an important role in both these low-dose responses.

Activation of Mitogen-Activated Protein Kinase (MAPK)/ Extracellular Signal-Related Kinase (ERK) Signaling Pathways in Bystander and Adaptive Responses

Previous studies have shown that cyclooxygenase 2 (COX-2) is an important signaling molecule for radiation-induced bystander effects [21]. It is known that insulin growth factor activates the mitogen-activated protein kinase (MAPK) signaling cascade, and activation of extracellular signal-related kinase (ERK) by phosphorylation is a critical upstream event preceding *COX-2* expression. Using Western blot analyses, it was evident that a strong upregulation of phospho-ERK levels in both α-irradiated and bystander normal human fibroblasts occurred 4 h after irradiation [21]. In fact, increased levels of phospho-ERK could even be detected 16 h after treatment, indicating a persistent response to the bystander signaling. In contrast, activity of MAPK p38 kinase was found to be increased 4 h after treatment and was not detectable 16 h after irradiation. It should be noted that, when compared with the controls, the ratio of phosphorylated ERK to native ERK increased from 2 to 13 among the bystander cells. If activation of the MAPK signaling cascade and ERK phosphorylation are essential in mediating the bystander effect, it should be possible to mitigate the later response by using a specific inhibitor of the MEK-ERK signaling cascade. In fact, pretreatment of cells with a non-cytotoxic dose of PD 98059 (50 μM), a specific inhibitor of MEK-ERK kinase, completely suppressed bystander toxicity observed in the human fibroblast cultures [21].

The role of MAPK/ERK pathways in radiation-induced adaptive response was previously demonstrated in mammalian cells. A low priming dose of X-rays (2 cGy) induced translocation of protein kinase C-alpha (PKC-α) from cytosol to membrane. On subsequent exposure to a challenging dose of X-rays (3 Gy), a lower incidence of chromosomal translocation was observed in preirradiated cultures that could be correlated with activation of p38 MAPK kinase activities [22].

Role of Nuclear Factor Kappa B (NFκB) in Bystander and Adaptive Responses

As NFκB is an important transcription factor for many signaling genes including COX-2, it is likely that NFκB participates in the bystander response. There is clear evidence that α-particle irradiation upregulates NFκB-binding activity in both directly irradiated and bystander cells, whereas Bay 11–7082, a pharmacological inhibitor of IKK/NFκB, efficiently suppresses this upregulation and also reduces levels below the basal amount [19]. This inhibitor of NFκB activity also efficiently downregulates COX-2 and inducible nitric oxide synthase (iNOS) expression levels in both directly irradiated and bystander fibroblasts. Earlier studies using confluent human skin fibroblasts exposed to low fluences of α-particles have demonstrated a rapid upregulation of NFκB, JNK, and ERK in the exposed population [23] and suggest activation of these stress-inducible signaling pathways in bystander cells. As induction of NFκB-binding activity can be found in both directly irradiated and bystander cells, its role in the bystander response in this study is, therefore, equivocal.

In contrast, there is recent evidence that NFκB plays an important function in the adaptive response [24]. Pretreatment of mouse epidermal cells with a 10-cGy dose of X-rays increased survival of the cells to a subsequent, challenging dose of 2 Gy, and the response was abrogated by pretreatment with the NFκB inhibitor, IMD 0354 [25].

Effects of Cytokines on Radiation-Induced Bystander and Adaptive Responses

There is recent evidence that exogenous tumor necrosis factor-alpha (TNF-α) in concert with interleukin 1-beta (IL-1β) directly controls COX-2 expression in human lung fibroblast (NHLF) cultures [19]. Both TNF-α and IL-1β were found to be induced following α-irradiation of NHLF. The inhibitory monoclonal antibody (mAb) against TNF-α, which was introduced into the cell media, substantially decreased levels of NF-κB and JNK, which was accompanied by a well-pronounced decrease in COX-2 expression in both irradiated and, especially, in bystander NHLF [19]. These studies provide a clear link of the binding of cell-surface receptors for the various cytokines with the downstream activation of NF-κB and mitogen-activated protein kinases in bystander effects.

Because NFκB can be activated by several pathways involving TNF-α and IL-1, and NF-κB activities have been linked to radiation-induced adaptive response, it is no surprise that cytokines have a profound effect on the radioadaptive behavior of cells. Earlier studies by Cong et al. have demonstrated that mice pretreated with interferon from extracted human liver RNA showed significant protective effects in bone marrow and germ cells upon exposure to X-rays [26].

Conclusion

Radiation-induced bystander effect and adaptive response are two conflicting phenomena that are stress related and are observed mainly at the low-dose region. At high radiation doses, direct damage to the cells or tissues would dwarf these low-dose effects. Although many of the bystander responses reported thus far have been detrimental in nature, there are reported protective effects as well, for example, induction of apoptosis of potentially damaged cells [27]. On the other hand, there is evidence that bystander cells also show increase in genomic instability, a predisposing factor for carcinogenesis. Hence, the contribution of bystander effects in radiation risk assessment has to be evaluated in terms of tissue context, the phenotypic behavior of their progeny, and the presence of other competing, low-dose effects that include adaptive response.

Adaptive response generally signifies protective effects. The two phenomena share many common parameters as well as signaling events. A better understanding of the mechanisms involved in the two processes and how they interact will be important in obtaining a better and more accurate assessment of low-dose radiation risk.

Acknowledgments. Work was supported by funding from the National Institutes of Health grants CA 49062, ES 11804, NIH Resource Center Grant RR 11623, Environmental Center grant ES 09089, and from the U.S. Department of Energy DEFG-ER63441.

References

1. International Commission on Radiological Protection (1990) Recommendations of the ICRP. ICRP Publication 60. Pergamon Press, Oxford, England
2. Nagasawa H, Little J (1992) Induction of sister chromatid exchanges by extremely low doses of α-particles. Cancer Res 52:6394–6396
3. Zhou H, Randers-Pehrson G, Waldren CA, et al (2000) Induction of a bystander mutagenic effect of alpha particles in mammalian cells. Proc Natl Acad Sci U S A 97:2099–2104
4. Belyakov OV, Malcolmson AM, Folkard M, et al (2001) Direct evidence for a bystander effect of ionizing radiation in primary human fibroblasts. Br J Cancer 84:674–679
5. Olivieri G, Bodycote J, Wolff S (1984) Adaptive response of human lymphocytes to low concentrations of radioactive thymidine. Science 223:594–597
6. Rigaud O, Moustacchi E (1996) Radioadaptation for gene mutation and the possible molecular mechanisms of the adaptive response (review). Mutat Res 358:127–134
7. Sawant SG, Randers-Pehrson G, Metting NF, et al (2001) Adaptive response and the bystander effect induced by radiation in C3H10T1/2 cells in culture. Radiat Res 156:177–180
8. Iyer R, Lehnert BE (2002) Low dose, low-LET ionizing radiation-induced radioadaptation and associated early responses in unirradiated cells. Mutat Res 503:1–9
9. Iyer R, Lehnert BE (2002) Alpha-particle-induced increases in the radioresistance of normal human bystander cells. Radiat Res 157:3–7
10. Waldren CA, Jones C, Puck TT (1979) Measurement of mutagenesis in mammalian cells. Proc Natl Acad Sci U S A 76:1358–1362
11. Hei TK, Waldren CA, Hall EJ (1988) Mutation induction and relative biological effectiveness of neutrons in mammalian cells. Radiat Res 115:281–291
12. Zhou H, Randers-Pehrson G, Geard CR, et al (2003) Interaction between radiation induced adaptive response and bystander mutagenesis in mammalian cells. Radiat Res 160:512–516
13. Wang X, Ohnishi T (1997) p53 dependent signal transduction induced by stress. J Radiat Res 38:179–194
14. Boothman DA, Meyers M, Odegaard E, et al (1996) Altered G1 checkpoint control determines adaptive responses to ionizing radiation. Mutat Res 358:143–154
15. Kadhim MA, Moore SR, Goodwin EH (2004) Interrelationships amongst radiation induced genomic instability, bystander effects and the adaptive response. Mutat Res 568:21–32
16. Matsumoto H, Hamada N, Takahashi A, et al (2007) Vanguards of paradigm shift in radiation biology: radiation induced adaptive and bystander responses. J Radiat Res 48:97–106
17. Yang H, Asaad N, Held KD (2005) Medium-mediated intercellular communication is involved in bystander responses of X-ray-irradiated normal human fibroblasts. Oncogene 24:2096–2103

18. Lyng FM, Maquire P, McClean B, et al (2006) The involvement of calcium and MAP kinase signaling pathways in the production of radiation induced bystander effects. Radiat Res 165:400–409
19. Zhou H, Ivanov HN, Lien YC, et al (2008) Mitochondrial function and NF-κB mediated signaling in radiation induced bystander effects. Cancer Res 68:2233–2240
20. Matsumoto H, Hayashi S, Hatashita M, et al (2001) Induction of radio-resistance by a nitric oxide mediated bystander effect. Radiat Res 155:387–396
21. Zhou H, Ivanov VN, Gillespie J, et al (2005) Mechanism of radiation-induced bystander effect: role of the cyclooxygenase-2 signaling pathway. Proc Natl Acad Sci U S A 41:14641–14646
22. Shimizu T, Kato T Jr, Tachibana A, et al (1999) Coordinated regulation of radioadaptive response by protein kinase C and p38 mitogen activated protein kinase. Exp Cell Res 251:424–432
23. Azzam EI, DeToledo SM, Spitz DR, et al (2002) Oxidative metabolism modulates signal transduction and micronucleus formation in bystander cells from alpha particle irradiated normal human fibroblast cultures. Cancer Res 62:5426–5442
24. Ahmed KM, Li JJ (2008) NF-κB mediated adaptive resistance to ionizing radiation. Free Radic Biol Med 44:1–13
25. Fan M, Ahmed KM, Coleman MC, et al (2007) NFκB and MnSOD mediate adaptive radio-resistance in low dose irradiated mouse skin epithelial cells. Cancer Res 67:3220–3228
26. Cong XL, Wang XL, Su Q, et al (1998) Protective effects of extracted human liver RNA, a known interferon inducer, against radiation induced cytogenetic damage in male mice. Toxicol Lett 95:189–198
27. Coates PJ, Lorimore SA, Wright EG (2004) Damaging and protective cell signaling in the untargeted effects of ionizing radiation. Mutat Res 568:5–20

Induction and Persistence of Cytogenetic Damage in Mouse Splenocytes Following Whole-Body X-Irradiation Analysed by Fluorescence In Situ Hybridisation. V. Heterogeneity/Chromosome Specificity

M. Prakash Hande[1] and A.T. Natarajan[2]

Summary. To determine the chromosome specificity and heterogeneity for retrospective biological dosimetry for estimation of absorbed dose, the kinetics of induction and persistence of chromosome aberrations involving chromosomes 2, X, and 3 following X-irradiation were analysed in mouse splenocytes. Female Swiss albino mice were whole-body exposed to 0, 0.5, 1.0, 2.0, or 3.0 Gy X-rays. Fluorescence in situ hybridisation using painting probes for chromosomes 2, 3, and X was performed on metaphase chromosomes from isolated splenocytes at 0, 7, 28, 56, 112, and 224 days postirradiation to detect chromosome aberrations. Dose–response curves for dicentrics and translocations were fitted well with either linear quadratic model. The frequency for dicentrics decayed exponentially with time, and none could be detected at 112 days postexposure for all the doses except 3 Gy. Translocation frequency for the three chromosomes tested declined in a dose-dependent fashion during the first 3 months after irradiation, beyond which translocations exhibited stability. Complex chromosome aberrations were also detected at the last time point studied here. The different chromosomes tested here, 2, 3, and X, involved in aberrations with similar frequencies immediately after irradiation, and their persistence was not significantly different. The results indicate that there was no chromosome specificity in the induction or persistence of chromosome translocations in mice following exposure to different doses of X-rays. The data on the decay of translocations and their later stability have implications on the use of translocations in retrospective biological dosimetry for estimating absorbed dose in case of accidents.

Key words Retrospective dosimetry · Ionizing radiation · Biodosimetry molecular cytogenetics · Fluorescence in situ hybridization · Chromosome alteration

---

[1]Department of Physiology, Yong Loo Lin School of Medicine, National University of Singapore, 2 Medical Drive, Singapore 117597
[2]Department of Agrobiology and Agrochemistry, University of Tuscia, Viterbo, Italy

Introduction

Radiation-induced chromosome aberrations, especially translocations, can be easily visualised and quantified following fluorescence in situ hybridisation (FISH) technique, using chromosome-specific DNA libraries. Based on the DNA content of the individual chromosomes used in FISH, a multiplication factor is applied to estimate the aberration frequency for the whole genome. Using this technology, we have studied the induction and persistence of chromosome aberrations, both stable and unstable alterations, in mouse splenocytes up to 224 days after in vivo X-irradiation to develop a mouse model for retrospective dosimetry [1,2]. We have seen a rapid decline of dicentric frequency and a moderate decay in chromosome translocations in mice with time after irradiation. In these earlier studies, we used a composite library of mouse chromosomes 1, 11, and 13 in single-colour FISH. In a study from a different laboratory, Spruill et al. [3] have shown that translocations decreased during the first 3 months after irradiation and then stabilised for another year.

Although use of a cocktail of several chromosome-specific probes increases the efficacy of the assay [4,5], exchanges between the painted chromosomes go unnoticed or cannot be detected accurately. Recent evidence shows that certain human chromosomes may be preferentially involved in aberration induction [6,7]. It has also been proposed that induction of aberration after irradiation is non-DNA proportional. To evaluate this speculation, we have used three different chromosomes, 2, 3, and X, either singly (chromosome 3) or in combination (chromosomes 2 and X) in single-colour or two-colour FISH, respectively, on the same samples used in our earlier study [2]. Briefly, mice exposed to different doses of X-rays (0.5, 1.0, 2.0, or 3.0 Gy) were followed up to 224 days postirradiation to detect chromosome aberrations such as dicentrics and translocations (reciprocal, nonreciprocal). The results are presented here, and the incidence of chromosome-specific induction of aberration is discussed.

Materials and Methods

Animals

Random-bred Swiss albino female mice, 8 weeks of age and weighing 20–25 g, were used. They were housed in an air displacement room with controlled temperature and humidity and fed with standard laboratory chow and water ad libitum. These experiments have been approved by the appropriate ethical committee of the University.

X-Ray Exposure

Seventy-two mice were whole-body exposed to 0.5, 1.0, 2.0, or 3.0 Gy X-rays (Andrex X-ray machine; 4.0 mA, 200 kV, SSD ~45 cm) at 1.0 Gy/min. Three mice from each dose group were killed by cervical dislocation and their spleens removed within 30 min after irradiation; the remaining ones were housed for later analysis. Twelve unirradiated animals served as controls.

Isolation of Splenocytes, Cell Harvest, and Slide Preparation

Following the initial sample collection (day 0) within 30 m after X-ray exposure, spleens were aseptically removed from each of three animals of each dose group on days 7, 28, 56, 112, and 224 following irradiation. The methods for isolation of splenocytes and culture are explained in detail in earlier publications [1,2].

In Situ Hybridisation

Mouse chromosome-specific DNA libraries for chromosomes 2, 3, and X (Cambio, Cambridge, UK) were used for in situ hybridisation. The procedure was essentially the same as described in our earlier reports [1,8–10].

Scoring of Aberrations

Slides were observed using a Zeiss Axioplan microscope equipped with filters for observation for DAPI (blue), FITC (green), and TRITC (red) filters. Translocations between painted and unpainted chromosomes were scored. Dicentrics and fragments were scored for the whole genome using a DAPI filter in the same metaphases.

Statistics

Standard errors of aberration frequencies were based on data for individual animals. Fitting of the dose–response data employed linear-quadratic functions, which is the appropriate dose–response model for acute exposures to low linear energy transfer (low-LET) radiation [11]. Best-fit curves for the decay of each class of aberration for different doses were calculated by the maximum-likelihood method or least squares method. Statistical analysis of the data was done using the software Microsoft Excel (Ver. 5.0a).

Results and Discussion

In our previous studies [1,2], it was observed that dicentrics decay over time with none seen at about 3 months after irradiation in mice, whereas translocations remained stable over time with initial decay during the first 3 months post radiation exposure. In the present investigation, chromosome specificity in the production of chromosome aberrations was studied using chromosome-specific probes for 2, 3, and X. The dose–response curve for dicentric and translocation frequencies for individual chromosomes obtained immediately after X-irradiation is given in Fig. 1. Although the data are in agreement with our previous studies [1,2] for genomic frequencies, translocation frequencies were slightly higher in this study (ratio ranging from 1.0 to 1.4). Metaphase chromosomes with translocations (reciprocal translocation involving the X-chromosome and an unpainted chromosome is displayed as a representative chromosome aberration) and dicentrics are shown in Fig. 2C, D. Dicentric frequency declined in an exponential manner over time after

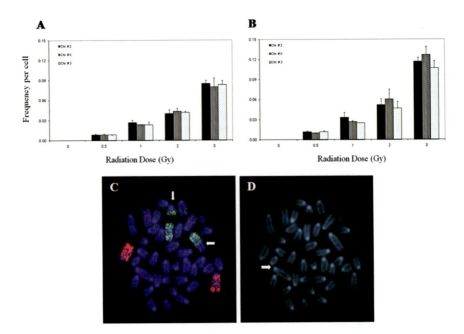

Fig. 1. Dose–response data for frequencies of (**A**) dicentrics and (**B**) translocations per cell in mouse splenocytes following X-irradiation. The dose–response data are well fitted by a linear quadratic function of the form $c + \alpha D + \beta D^2$ where c is the y-intercept, α is the linear coefficient, β is the quadratic coefficient, and D is the dose (Gy). **C** Fluorescence in situ hybridisation using chromosomes 2 (*red*) and X (*green*) on metaphase of mouse splenocytes following irradiation with X-rays. *Arrows* point to a reciprocal translocation involving chromosome X and an unpainted chromosome. **D** The same metaphase as in **C** observed under DAPI filter. *Arrows* point to dicentric chromosomes

Fig. 2. Persistence of chromosome translocations in mouse splenocytes following in vivo exposure to X-rays. **A** Translocations involving chromosome 2. **B** Translocations involving chromosome 3. **C** Translocations involving X-chromosome

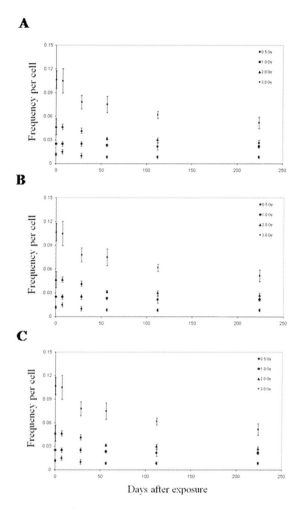

exposure in a dose-dependent manner, which is in agreement with our earlier studies [1,2] and data from other laboratories [3]. On the other hand, translocations involving chromosomes 2, 3, and X decayed initially up to 3 months of age and then remained relatively constant until 224 days, which was the last time point studied (Fig. 2A–C). The decay in translocation frequency may have occurred because of loss of cells bearing one or more aberrations [2]. Some of the earlier reports point to the stability of translocations with time after exposure to radiation and clonal expansion of cells carrying translocations [3]. Chromosome insertions were also found to be stable in mice 6 months after X-irradiation (data not shown). This finding is in line with our earlier studies on the presence of complex chromosome aberrations in blood lymphocytes of individuals occupationally exposed to plutonium in the Mayak facility [12–14]. Interestingly, we did not find any chromosome specificity in the occurrence or persistence of chromosome aberrations induced by X-irradiation in mice (Fig. 2A–C), in contrast to the earlier in vitro studies on human lymphocytes where chromosome-specific induction of chromosome translocations was detected [6,7]. Similarly, chromosome-specific alterations were not detected in Mayak workers (Hande, unpublished).

We have demonstrated here long persistence of chromosome translocations induced in vivo by ionising radiation. In our study, we did not observe any chromosome specificity in the production and stability of chromosome translocations. The presence of nonreciprocal and complex chromosome aberrations even after 6 months postirradiation suggests that these distinct classes of translocations should not be ignored in biological dosimetric studies. By recognising the loss of translocations during the early period following irradiation [1–3] and the important role of clonal expansion and ageing [3], caution should be exercised in using such chromosome aberrations in retrospective biological dosimetry of absorbed doses in case of past radiation exposures.

Acknowledgments. M.P.H. acknowledges the grant support from Defence Innovative Research Programme, Defence Science and Technology Agency, Singapore.

References

1. Hande MP, Boei JJ, Granath F, et al (1996) Induction and persistence of cytogenetic damage in mouse splenocytes following whole-body X-irradiation analysed by fluorescence in situ hybridization. I. Dicentrics and translocations. Int J Radiat Biol 69:437–446
2. Hande MP, Natarajan AT (1998) Induction and persistence of cytogenetic damage in mouse splenocytes following whole-body X-irradiation analysed by fluorescence in situ hybridization. IV. Dose response. Int J Radiat Biol 74:441–448
3. Spruill MD, Nelson DO, Ramsey MJ, et al (2000) Lifetime persistence and clonality of chromosome aberrations in the peripheral blood of mice acutely exposed to ionizing radiation. Radiat Res 153:110–121
4. Lucas JN, Awa A, Straume T, et al (1992) Rapid translocation frequency analysis in humans decades after exposure to ionizing radiation. Int J Radiat Biol 62:53–63
5. Lucas JN, Hill FS, Burk CE, et al (1996) Stability of the translocation frequency following whole-body irradiation measured in rhesus monkeys. Int J Radiat Biol 70:309–318
6. Knehr S, Zitzelsberger H, Braselmann H, et al (1994) Analysis of DNA-proportional distribution of radiation-induced chromosome aberrations in various triple combinations of human chromosomes using fluorescence in situ hybridisation. Int J Radiat Biol 65:683–690
7. Boei JJ, Vermeulen S, Natarajan AT (1997) Differential involvement of chromosomes 1 and 4 in the formation of chromosomal aberrations in human lymphocytes after X-irradiation. Int J Radiat Biol 72:139–145
8. Hande MP, Boei JJ, Natarajan AT (1996) Induction and persistence of cytogenetic damage in mouse splenocytes following whole-body X-irradiation analysed by fluorescence in situ hybridization. II. Micronuclei. Int J Radiat Biol 70:375–383
9. Hande MP, Boei JJ, Natarajan AT (1997) Induction and persistence of cytogenetic damage in mouse splenocytes following whole-body X-irradiation analysed by fluorescence in situ hybridization. III. Chromosome malsegregation/aneuploidy. Mutagenesis 12:125–131
10. Boei JJ, Balajee AS, de Boer P, et al (1994) Construction of mouse chromosome-specific DNA libraries and their use for the detection of X-ray-induced aberrations. Int J Radiat Biol 65:583–590

11. Lloyd D, Edwards AA, Prosser JS (1986) Chromosome aberrations induced in human lymphocyte by in vitro acute X and gamma radiation. Radiat Prot Dosim 15:191–196
12. Hande MP, Azizova TV, Geard CR, et al (2003) Past exposure to densely ionizing radiation leaves a unique permanent signature in the genome. Am J Hum Genet 72:1162–1170
13. Mitchell CR, Azizova TV, Hande MP, et al (2004) Stable intrachromosomal biomarkers of past exposure to densely ionizing radiation in several chromosomes of exposed individuals. Radiat Res 162:257–263
14. Hande MP, Azizova TV, Burak LE, et al (2005) Complex chromosome aberrations persist in individuals many years after occupational exposure to densely ionizing radiation: an mFISH study. Genes Chromosomes Cancer 44:1–9

Cancer Research

Molecular Understanding of RET/PTC-Mediated Thyroid Carcinogenesis

Young Suk Jo, Dong Wook Kim, Min Hee Lee, Soung Jung Kim,
Jung Hwan Hwang, and Minho Shong

Summary. Differentiated thyroid cancers, including papillary and follicular carcinomas, frequently develop as a result of genetic alterations. Papillary thyroid cancers (PTC) show balanced inversions or translocations that usually involve the 3.0-kb intron 11 of the tyrosine kinase receptor protein RET. These rearrangements result in the formation of *RET/PTC* through the fusion of the tyrosine kinase domain of the *RET* proto-oncogene with the 5′-end of activating heterologous sequences belonging to the *RET*-fused genes. RET/PTC has been reported to be a constitutively active kinase in thyroid epithelial cells. Although RET/PTC has intrinsic tyrosine kinase activity, the direct substrates of RET/PTC in thyroid cells are largely unknown. We have examined the interaction of RET/PTC and Signal transducer and activator of transcription-3 (STAT3), and the phosphorylation activity of RET/PTC on the Y705 residue of STAT3. STAT3 is a direct substrate for RET/PTC tyrosine kinase, and Y705 phosphorylation in STAT3 by RET/PTC is a critical signaling pathway for the specific induction of genes in the RET/PTC-mediated transformation process. Here we show that LKB1 act as a suppressor of *STAT3* in RET/PTC-mediated processes of transformation. The mutations of LKB1 protein kinase in humans results in a disorder termed Peutz–Jeghers syndrome (PJS), which predisposes to a wide spectrum of benign and malignant tumors. LKB1+/− heterozygous mice develop tumors resembling those found in human PJS. The overexpression of LKB1 in LKB1-deficient cancer cells induced a G_1 cell-cycle arrest, and genetic studies in *Caenorhabditis elegans*, *Drosophila*, and *Xenopus* have indicated that the LKB1 homologue in these organisms plays a role in regulating cell polarity. We have reported that RET/PTC is able to activate STAT3 and that it is involved in transformation in thyroid carcinogenesis. The wild-type and kinase dead mutant LKB1 decreased *STAT3* transcriptional activity in RET/PTC-transfected cells. LKB1 showed interactions with STAT3 in immunoprecipitation experiments. The LKB1 and activated STAT3 colocalized within the nucleus. The GAL4-fused LKB1 showed intrinsic repressor activities. However, the repressor activities were not affected by treatment of HDAC inhibitors. The LKB1-mediated suppression of *STAT3* transcription was not dependent on S727 residue in the

---

Department of Internal Medicine, Laboratory of Endocrine Cell Biology, Chungnam National University School of Medicine, 640 Daesadong, Junggu, Daejeon, Korea 301-721

transactivation domain of STAT3. These observations indicate that LKB1 is a transcriptional co-repressor of *STAT3* that is activated by thyroid-specific oncogenic tyrosine kinase, RET/PTC. In addition, we showed that the 2-indolinone compounds SU5416, SU6668, and SU11248 (sunitinib) showed variable activities in the inhibition of RET/PTC tyrosine kinases. SU11248 showed the most potent and very specific properties for the inhibition of RET/PTC. These findings suggest that 2-indolinone derivates, such as SU11248, might be a potential therapeutic candidate by inhibiting RET/PTC in papillary thyroid cancer.

Key words Thyroid · RET/PTC · STAT3 · LKB1 · Thyroid cancer

Introduction

Differentiated thyroid cancers, including papillary and follicular carcinomas, frequently develop as a result of genetic alterations. Follicular thyroid carcinomas show a translocation, t(2;3)(q13;p25), that results in the fusion of the DNA-binding domains of the thyroid transcription factor PAX8 to domains A to F of the peroxisome proliferator-activated receptor 1. Papillary thyroid carcinomas (PTCs) show balanced inversions or translocations that usually involve the 3.0-kb intron 11 of the tyrosine kinase receptor protein RET (rearranged in transformation) [1]. These rearrangements result in the formation of RET/PTC through the fusion of the tyrosine kinase domain of the *RET* proto-oncogene with the 5′-end of activating heterologous sequences belonging to the *RET*-fused genes [2,3]. To date, at least 15 such chimeric mRNAs involving 10 different genes have been reported, of which RET/PTC1 (fused to H4) and RET/PTC3 (fused to ELE1) are by far the most common in papillary thyroid cancer. RET/PTC has been reported to be a constitutively active kinase in thyroid epithelial cells. In a transgenic mouse model, the targeted expression of RET/PTC in the thyroid gland causes PTCs [4]. However, a thyroid-targeted RET/PTC carrying mutations in the kinase domain does not cause changes in follicular morphology. These findings suggest that a kinase domain with intrinsic kinase activity that can interact with signaling molecules by binding to phosphotyrosine residues is critical for cellular transformation in vivo.

RET has been shown to activate diverse signaling pathways through the interaction of several signaling molecules. The autophosphorylated RET interacts with Grb2/Grb7/Grb10/Grb14, phospholipase C, and FRS2. These interactions consequently activate the Ras/ERK, c-Jun NH2-terminal protein kinase, and phosphatidylinositol 3-kinase signaling pathways [5–7]. Although RET and RET/PTC share common kinase domains, the cellular distributions of RET and RET/PTC are different: RET is present in the plasma membrane, whereas RET/PTC is confined to the cytoplasm. This difference in subcellular location may result in differences in signaling activation because of disparities in substrate proximity. Recent studies have suggested that RET/PTC and MEN2A-RET, a gain-of-function point mutation of RET, have different cellular effects: RET/PTC1 induces stress fiber formation in PC Cl 3 cells, but MEN2A-RET does not. Furthermore, the induction of stress fibers by RET/PTC1 is restricted to thyroid cells, indicating that the actions of RET/PTC1 are cell type specific.

Although RET/PTC has intrinsic tyrosine kinase activity, the direct substrates of RET/PTC in thyroid cells are largely unknown. Signal transducer and activator of transcription-3 (STAT3) is a latent cytoplasmic transcription factor that mediates several cellular mechanisms during transformation in cultured cell models [8–10]. The cellular transformation by STAT3 requires constitutive activation, and the activity of STAT3 is regulated mainly by specific phosphorylation of the tyrosine 705 (Y705) residue [11]. The oncogenic tyrosine kinase v-*src* phosphorylates Y705 in STAT3 and induces cellular transformation in a STAT3-dependent manner [12,13]. Several human tumors, including leukemias, lymphomas, breast cancers, and head and neck cancers, show constitutive activation of STAT3. Several downstream target genes, including *cyclin D1, D2, D3, A, cdc25A*, and *bcl-xL*, have been suggested as candidate genes involved in STAT3-mediated transformation.

Gene expression studies in LKB1-null fibroblasts show multiple changes, including increased expression of matrix metalloproteinase 2 (MMP-2), matrix metalloproteinase 9 (MMP-9), vascular endothelial growth factor (VEGF), insulin-like growth factor-binding protein 5 (IGFBP-5), and prostaglandin-endoperoxide synthase 2 (COX-2) [14,15]. Interestingly, these genes are all regulated by STAT3 and play roles in cell growth, tumorigenesis, and angiogenesis. STAT3 is a latent cytoplasmic transcription factor that performs a variety of functions in regulating cell growth, inflammation, and early embryonic development. STAT3 is frequently constitutively activated in cancer cells, and it is classified as an oncogene. Expression of a constitutively active dimer of STAT3 transforms cultured cells and promotes tumor formation in nude mice. Several nonreceptor tyrosine kinases that activate STAT3 stimulate malignant transformation of cultured cells. In addition, the constitutively active RET/PTC tyrosine kinase, found in papillary thyroid cancer (PTC) cells, phosphorylates tyrosine 705 of STAT3 and promotes dimerization and translocation and stimulates transactivation activity of STAT3. Cells expressing RET/PTC or RET/PTC-activated STAT3 exhibit elevated rates of transformation, proliferation, migration, and invasion [16]. Taken together, these findings suggest that the tumor suppressor function of LKB1 may be mediated by its ability to suppress RET/PTC-dependent activation of STAT3 and STAT3-mediated oncogenesis.

As knowledge of thyroid cancer biology improves, a number of molecular components that could be targeted for treatment of thyroid cancers, which do not respond to conventional therapies, have been investigated [17]. Several compounds that alter pathways involved in thyroid cancer are currently being evaluated in clinical trials, and several of these agents have been tested in thyroid cancer both in vitro and in vivo [18,19]. SU11248 (sunitinib) is a selective, orally administered, receptor tyrosine kinase (RTK) inhibitor that targets platelet-derived growth factor receptor (PDGFR), vascular endothelial growth factor receptor (VEGFR), and *fms*-related tyrosine kinase 3 (FLT3) with IC_{50} values of 5–50 nM in cellular autophosphorylation assays [20,21]. SU11248 was also designed to target KIT and is predicted to inhibit KIT kinase activity in cells. SU11248 has been shown to possess antitumor activity correlated with inhibition of RTKs expressed on tumor cells. For example, SU11248 blocks the activity of wild-type and activated FLT3 expressed by acute myelogenous leukemia-derived cell lines. SU11248 also blocks tumor proliferation and survival by inhibiting RTKs expressed on endothelial or stromal cells. For example, SU11248 has been shown to inhibit VEGFR, FLK/KDR, and PDGFR-β, each of which plays a prominent role in angiogenesis [22].

Materials and Methods

Materials

Media and cell culture reagents and materials were purchased from Life Technologies (Gaithersburg, MD, USA), Sigma (St. Louis, MO, USA), Fisher Scientific (Fairlawn, NJ, USA), Corning (Corning, NY, USA), and HyClone Laboratories (Logan, UT, USA). Antibodies for RET were from Santa Cruz Biotechnology (Santa Cruz, CA, USA); STAT3 total, phosphorylated STAT3 (Y705, S727), was from Cell Signaling Technology; and antiphosphotyrosine antibody (4G10) was from Upstate Biotechnology (Lake Placid, NY, USA).

Plasmids

The pcDNA3-RET/PTC3, pcDNA3.1-RET/PTC1, pcDNA3.1-RET/PTC1-Y141F, and pcDNA3.1-RET/PTC1-Y317F mutants were constructed by site-directed mutagenesis using Ex Taq polymerase (TaKaRa) with proofreading activity and the following primer pairs: RET/PTC1 forward, 5'-CCCTCTAGAATGGCGGACAG-3' and RET/PTC1 Y141F reverse, 5'-ACCGTGGTGAACCCTGCTC-3'; and RET/PTC1 Y141F forward, 5'-GAGCAGGGTTCACCACGGT-3' and RET/PTC1 reverse, 5'-CCCAAGCTTCTAGAATCTAGTAAATG-3'. The two polymerase chain reaction (PCR) fragments generated were then used in a new PCR reaction with the RET/PTC1 forward and RET/PTC1 reverse primers. The PCR fragment generated from this reaction was digested with *Xba*I and *Hin*dIII, and the *Xba*I and *Hin*dIII fragment of pcDNA3.1-RET/PTC1 was replaced with the *Xba*I and *Hin*dIII mutant fragment. Similarly, the RET/PTC1 Y317F mutant was constructed by PCR using Ex Taq polymerase and the following primer pairs: RET/PTC1 forward and RET/PTC1 Y317F reverse, 5'-CACTTTGCGTGGTGAAGATATGAT-3'; and RET/PTC1 Y317F forward, 5'-ATCATATCTTCACCACGCAAAGTG-3' and RET/PTC1 reverse primers. The two PCR fragments generated were then used in a new PCR reaction with the RET/PTC1 forward and RET/PTC1 reverse primers. The PCR fragment generated was digested with *Xba*I and *Hin*dIII, and the *Xba*I and *Hin*dIII mutant fragment of pcDNA3.1-RET/PTC1 was replaced with the *Xba*I and *Hin*dIII mutant fragment. The conditions for all PCR reactions were predenaturation at 94°C for 5 min, followed by 32 cycles of denaturation at 94°C for 30 s, annealing at 56°C for 30 s, and elongation at 72°C for 60 s.

pEGFP-LKB1-WT, pEGFP-LKB1-R304W, pEGFP-LKB1-I177N, pEGFP-LKB1-K175-D176del, and GFP-LKB1 E98-G155del were provided [23]. pcDNA3.1-flag-STAT3, pCMV2-flag-LKB1-ΔNK, pCMV2-flag-STAT3-ΔTAD, pCMV2-flag-STAT3-ΔSH2, pCMV2-flag-STAT3-ΔLK, pCMV2-flag-STAT3-ΔDBD, and pCMV2-flag-NTD were also provided [24]. Myc-tagged LKB1-WT was generated by PCR using pCMV6-HA-LKB1 as a template; and the point mutant LKB1-K78M was constructed using the QuikChange II XL Site-Directed Mutagenesis kit (Stratagene, La Jolla, CA, USA) and the following primers: sense, 5′-CGCAGGGCGGTCATGATCCTCAAGAAG-3′; and antisense, 5′-CTTCT TGAGGAT-CATGAC CGCCCTGCG-3′. pCMV6-HA-LKB1-ΔN, pCMV6-HA-LKB1-ΔNK, and pCMV6-HA-LKB1-ΔC were constructed by PCR amplification of the respective regions from pCMV6-LKB1. The amplified fragments were digested with *Xba*I and *Eco*RI and ligated to the expression vector pCMV6-HA. All plasmid constructs generated in this study were confirmed by automated DNA sequencing.

Compounds

The indolinone derivatives including SU11248, SU5416, and SU6668 were synthesized in research scale in LG Life Science (Seoul, Korea) with previously established synthetic methods [20,25,26]. We used these compounds in vitro and into cells with high purity (>99.5%). Stock solutions (50 mM) were made in 100% dimethyl sulfoxide (DMSO). Equivalent DMSO concentrations served as vehicle controls.

Cell Culture, Transfection, and Promoter Activity Assay

Murine fibroblasts (NIH3T3), human kidney fibroblasts (HEK293), human breast cancer cells (MCF-7 and MDA-BA-435), human cervical adenoma cells (HeLa), LKB1 knockout murine embryo fibroblasts (LKB1−/−MEF) [14], and papillary thyroid carcinoma cells (TPC-1) were cultured in Dulbecco's modified Eagle's medium. Human thyroid carcinoma cells (ARO, NPA) and human hepatocellular carcinoma cells (HepG2) were cultured in RPMI 1640. Media were supplemented with 10% fetal bovine serum (FBS), 100 U/ml penicillin, and 100 g/ml streptomycin in a humidified chamber containing a 5% CO_2 atmosphere at 37°C.

Cells were transfected by the LipofectAMINE method (Invitrogen, San Diego, CA, USA) according to the manufacturer's instructions. Briefly, 1 μg RET/PTC1 plasmid was incubated with 6 μl LipofectAMINE Plus reagent at room temperature for 15 min, 2 μl LipofectAMINE reagent was added, and the mixture was incubated at room temperature. After 15 min, the semiconfluent cells were washed twice with 1× phosphate-buffered saline (PBS) and then incubated with DNA-LipofectAMINE Plus reagent complexes at 37°C in a humidified chamber containing 5% CO_2 for 4 h. After transfection, the mixture was aspirated, and cells were cultured in DMEM with 15% fetal bovine serum for an additional 12, 24, or 48 h.

ARO cells were cotransfected with various combinations of the following constructs: RET/PTC1, wild-STAT1, wild-STAT3, mutant STAT1S, mutant STAT1Y, mutant STAT3S, and mutant STAT3Y (300 ng plasmid each) in association with the m67 luciferase reporter construct (all gifts from Dr. J. Bromberg, Memorial Sloan-Kettering Cancer Institute, New York, NY, USA); the VEGF reporter construct containing −2.7 kb of the VEGF promoter region, the cyclin D1 reporter construct containing −1745 bp of the cyclin D1 promoter region, and the intracellular adhesion molecule (ICAM)-1 reporter construct (pCAM-1822) [27,28] containing − 1800 bp drove the expression of the luciferase gene. After transfection for the indicated time, the cells were lysed and the luciferase assay was performed using a Dual-Luciferase Reporter assay system (Promega, Madison, WI, USA). The transfection efficiency was normalized by the value of cotransfected *Renilla* luciferase.

Western Blot Analysis

Cells were centrifuged, washed with PBS, and lysed at 0°C for 30 min in lysis buffer [20 mM HEPES, pH 7.4; 2 mM ethylenediaminetetraacetic acid (EDTA); 50 mM β-glycerol phosphate; 1% Triton X-100; 10% β-glycerol, 1 mM dithiothreitol; 1 mM phenylmethylsulfonyl fluoride; 10 µg/ml leupeptin; 10 µg/ml aprotinin; 1 mM Na3VO4; 5 mM NaF]. The protein content was determined using the Bio-Rad dye binding microassay (Bio-Rad Laboratories, Hercules, CA, USA), and 20 µg protein per lane was electrophoresed on a 10% sodium dodecyl sulfate (SDS)-polyacrylamide gel after boiling for 5 min in SDS sample buffer. Proteins were blotted onto Hybond enhanced luminescence membranes (Amersham Pharmacia Biotech, Arlington Heights, IL, USA). After electroblotting, the membranes were blocked with Tris-buffered saline and Tween 20 (10 mM Tris-HCl, pH 7.4; 150 mM NaCl; 0.1% Tween 20) containing 5% milk and incubated with the primary antibody diluted in blocking buffer for 1 h. The primary antibody dilutions were those recommended by the manufacturer. Membranes were then washed, incubated with the appropriate second antibody (1:3000) in blocking buffer for 1 h, and rewashed. Blotted proteins were detected using the enhanced chemiluminescence detection system (New England Biolabs, Beverly, MA, USA).

Immunoprecipitations

The following immunoprecipitation procedures were carried out at 4°C. Cells grown on 100-mm dishes were washed with phosphate-buffered saline (PBS) twice before lysis. Radioimmunoprecipitation assay (RIPA) buffer containing protease inhibitors (20 µg/ml leupeptin, 10 µg/ml pepstatin A, 10 µg/ml chymostatin, 2 µg/ml aprotinin, 1 mM phenylmethylsulfonyl fluoride) was added for cell lysis and incubated for 30 min. The cell lysate was collected, triturated, and centrifuged at 1000 g for 10 min. To preclear the cell lysate, the supernatant was mixed with 20 µl protein A/G beads (Santa Cruz Biotechnology), incubated for 30 min while rocking, and centrifuged for 15 min at 1000 g. Precleared samples were incubated with a primary antibody for 2 h with rocking, and then protein A beads were added, incubated for 1 h, and centrifuged at 1000 g. The immunoprecipitates were collected and washed three times with RIPA buffer.

MTT Assay

Cell viability assays were carried out using the 3-(4,5-dimethylthiazol-2-yl)-2,5-diphenyltetrazolium bromide (MTT) dye conversion assay in 96-well plates. After exposure to SU5416 or SU11248, MTT (25 µl 5 mg/ml MTT in sterile PBS) was added to 100 µl cell suspension and allowed to incubate for 2 h at 37°C. The reaction was stopped, and the cells were lysed with the addition of 100 µl lysis buffer consisting of 20% SDS in a water/DMF (1:1) solution at pH 4.7. Cell lysates were placed at 37°C overnight to allow cell lysis and dye solubilization. The optical density (OD) was read at 595 nm using a THERMOmax microplate reader (Molecular Devices, Menlo Park, CA, USA). Data are expressed as a percentage of vehicle-treated (water) control values. MTT assays were carried out three independent experiments done in triplicate.

Statistics

The data were expressed as the mean ± SE unless noted otherwise. Statistics were analyzed by one-way repeated-measures analysis of variance (ANOVA) with a significance level of 0.05.

Results

Association and Tyrosine Phosphorylation of STAT3 by RET/PTC

To investigate target proteins that are tyrosine phosphorylated by RET/PTC within cells, we expressed RET/PTC1 in ARO cells and analyzed the expression by Western blot using an antiphosphotyrosine antibody. We found that a number of

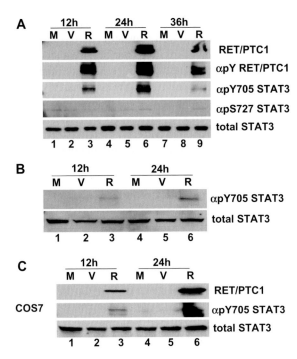

Fig. 1. Tyrosine phosphorylation of endogenous STAT3 by RET/PTCs. A Whole-cell lysates of ARO cells transfected with 1 μg RET/PTC1 expression plasmids were analyzed by Western blot using antibodies against phosphorylated Signal transducer and activator of transcription-3 (STAT3) (Y705 and S727), a phosphotyrosine-specific antibody (4G10), and an anti-RET antibody. B Whole-cell lysates of ARO cells transfected with 1 μg RET/PTC3 expression plasmids were analyzed by Western blot using an antibody against phosphorylated STAT3 (Y705). C The whole-cell lysates of the COS7 cells transfected with 1 μg RET/PTC1 expression plasmids were prepared and analyzed using Western blot using antibodies against RET and phosphorylated STAT3 (Y705). To confirm equal loading of lysates, each of the blots in A–C was reprobed using an antibody against total STAT3. The results are representative of a minimum of three (usually five) independent experiments. *PTC*, papillary thyroid cancer; *M*, mock transfected; *V*, pcDNA3.1 (**A**, **C**) or pcDNA3 (**B**) empty plasmid transfected; *R*, pcDNA3.1-RET/PTC1 (**A**, **C**) or pcDNA3-RET/PTC3 (**B**) transfected

intracellular proteins are tyrosine phosphorylated by RET/PTC1; in particular, we observed the appearance of a phosphotyrosine band when RET/PTC and STAT3 were coexpressed in ARO cells (data not shown). To test whether RET/PTC phosphorylates endogenous STAT3, we expressed RET/PTC1 in ARO cells and observed Y705 phosphorylation of STAT3 using phospho-specific antibodies. We could detect the autophosphorylated forms of RET/PTC in ARO cells 12 h after transfection with RET/PTC (Fig. 1A). The cells transfected with empty vector and mock transfected cells did not show tyrosine phosphorylation of STAT3. The lysates obtained from cells expressing RET/PTC1 for 12, 24, and 36 h showed autophosphorylation of RET/PTC and Y705 phosphorylation of STAT3 (Fig. 1A, lanes 3, 6, and 9). Phosphospecific antibodies specifically recognizing the phosphorylated S727 residue of STAT3 did not bind to lysates of RET/PTC-expressing cells. To see the effects of other variants of RET/PTC, we expressed RET/PTC3 instead of RET/PTC1 in ARO cells and again observed the Y705 phosphorylation of endogenous STAT3 (Fig. 1B). We also observed Y705 phosphorylation of endogenous STAT3 in COS7 cells expressing RET/PTC1 (Fig. 1C), indicating that the phosphorylation is not cell specific.

To investigate the association of STAT3 with RET/PTC, we transiently expressed RET/PTC1 and performed a coimmunoprecipitation experiment (data not shown). The cell lysates obtained from mock, empty vector, and RET/PTC1 transfection were immunoprecipitated with antibodies against RET. The immunoprecipitates were separated by sodium dodecyl sulfate-polyacrylamide gel electrophoresis (SDS-PAGE), transferred to a membrane, and blotted with an antibody against STAT3. We were able to detect endogenous STAT3 (data not shown), but not endogenous JAK2 (data not shown), in RET/PTC1 immunoprecipitates.

Association Between STAT3 and RET/PTC1

STAT3 is known to bind the YXXQ/V motif in the intracellular domain of cytokine receptors. RET/PTC1 has two potential sites for STAT3 binding, at positions ^{141}YXXV and ^{317}YXXQ. To determine whether these residues indeed serve as STAT3 docking sites, the tyrosine 141 and 317 residues were mutated into phenylalanine (Fig. 2A). To investigate whether STAT3 is phosphorylated by the RET/PTC1-Y141F and RET/PTC1-Y317F mutants, we transiently transfected ARO cells with wild-type RET/PTC1, RET/PTC1-Y141F, or RET/PTC1-Y317F, and performed Western blot analysis with antibodies against RET, STAT3, phosphospecific STAT3 (pY705), and phosphotyrosine (4G10). All three forms of RET/PTC were adequately expressed (Fig. 2B). Wild-type RET/PTC1 and RET/PTC1-Y141F showed tyrosine phosphorylation; however, RET/PTC1 Y317F showed a markedly decreased level of tyrosine phosphorylation (Fig. 2B, lane 4). RET/PTC1 Y317F significantly lost its ability to induce the STAT3-mediated transactivation of the m67 luciferase reporter gene compared to the wild type and RET/PTC1Y141F (Fig. 2D). These observations suggest that Y317 residue of RET/PTC1 is important for its autophosphorylation and for the Y705 phosphorylation of STAT3.

In a parallel experiment, we used coimmunoprecipitation to observe the interactions between RET/PTC1 and STAT3. Wild-type and mutant RET/PTC1 were expressed in ARO cells, and the lysates were immunoprecipitated with anti-RET antibodies. The wild-type RET, RET/PTC1 Y141F, and RET/PTC1 Y317F all interacted with endogenous STAT3 (Fig. 2C).

Regulation of Cyclin D1, VEGF, and ICAM-1 Gene Transcription by RET/PTC

STAT3 has been shown to regulate the transcription of cyclin D1, VEGF, and ICAM-1, which have been reported to be involved in tumorigenesis, angiogenesis,

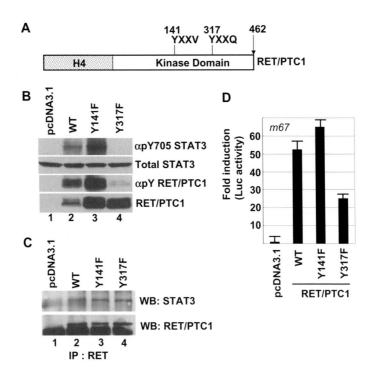

Fig. 2. Roles of the [141]YXXV and [317]YXXQ motifs in RET/PTC1-mediated STAT3 activation and interaction. **A** The pcDNA3.1-RET/PTC1-Y141F and pcDNA3.1-RET/PTC1-Y317F mutants were constructed by site-directed mutagenesis as described in Materials and Methods. **B** ARO cells cultured in 6-cm dishes were transfected with wild-type RET/PTC1 (1 μg), mutant RET/PTC1Y141F (1 μg), or RET/PTCY317F (1 μg) plasmids for 24 h. Whole-cell lysates were analyzed by Western blot using antibodies against phosphorylated STAT3 (Y705), phosphotyrosine-specific antibody (4G10), and RET. To confirm equal loading of lysates, the blots were reprobed using an antibody against total STAT3. **C** ARO cells cultured in 10-cm dishes were transiently transfected with pcDNA3.1 (4 μg), wild-RET/PTC1 (4 μg), mutant RET/PTC1Y141F (4 μg), or RET/PTC1Y317F (4 μg) for 24 h. After cell lysis, 500 μg each lysate was precipitated with an anti-RET antibody and then detected with an antibody against total STAT3 and RET. **D** ARO cells cultured in 6-cm dishes were cotransfected with the m67 reporter construct (100 ng) and pcDNA3.1 (1 μg), wild-RET/PTC1 (1 μg), mutant RET/PTC1Y141F (1 μg), or RET/PTC1Y317F (1 μg) for 24 h, and luciferase activities were measured and normalized to *Renilla* luciferase activity. Data are expressed as mean ± SD of three independent experiments

and metastasis. To investigate whether RET/PTC activates the transcription of cyclin D1, VEGF, and ICAM-1 through the activation of STAT3, we performed a promoter assay using cyclin D1, VEGF, and ICAM-1 promoter reporter constructs. We transiently transfected RET/PTC1 into ARO cells, along with reporter constructs fused to VEGF (−2.7 kb), cyclin D1 (−1745 bp), and ICAM-1 (−1822 bp) promoter fragments. RET/PTC1 expression increased the promoter activities of cyclin D1 about threefold compared to control (Fig. 3A). This RET/PTC1-induced transactivation of the cyclin D1 promoter was completely inhibited by

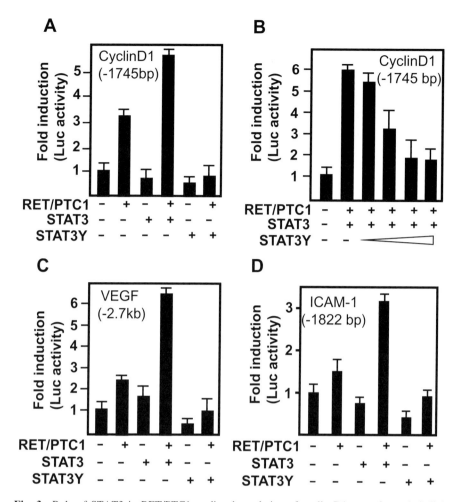

Fig. 3. Role of STAT3 in RET/PTC1-mediated regulation of cyclin D1, vascular endothelial growth factor (VEGF), and intracellular adhesion molecule (ICAM)-1. **A, C** In a reporter assay, ARO cells cultured in 6-cm dishes were transiently cotransfected with a cyclin D1 reporter construct (300 ng/ml) containing a 2.7-kb upstream promoter sequence and a VEGF reporter construct (300 ng/ml) containing a 1745-bp promoter together with the pcDNA3.1 (300 ng), RET/PTC1 (300 ng), STAT3 (300 ng), STAT3Y (300 ng), RET/PTC1 (300 ng) plus STAT3 (300 ng), and RET/PTC1 (300 ng) plus STAT3Y (300 ng) constructs. Transfected ARO cells were maintained in RPMI-1640 media with 10% fetal bovine serum (FBS) for 24 h. The luciferase activity from pcDNA3.1-transfected cells was used as the control. **B** ARO cells cultured in 6-cm dishes were cotransfected with the cyclin D1 reporter construct and RET/PTC1 (300 ng/ml), wild-type STAT3 (300 ng/ml), and increasing amounts of STAT3Y mutant (from *left*: 50 ng, 100 ng, 300 ng, 500 ng). Transfected ARO cells were maintained in RPMI 1640 media with 10% FBS for 24 h. The luciferase activity from pcDNA3.1-transfected cells was used as a control. **D** ARO cells cultured in 6-cm dishes were transiently cotransfected with the pCAM-1822 reporter construct (300 ng) together with the pcDNA3.1 (300 ng), RET/PTC1 (300 ng), STAT3 (300 ng), STAT3Y (300 ng), RET/PTC1 (300 ng) plus STAT3 (300 ng), or RET/PTC1 (300 ng) plus STAT3Y (300 ng) construct. Transfected ARO cells were maintained in RPMI 1640 media with 10% FBS for 24 h. The luciferase activity from pcDNA3.1-transfected cells was used as the control. All experiments were repeated at least three times. Data are normalized for transfection efficiency and are shown as the mean ± SE. Significance ($P < 0.005$) was determined by two-way analysis of variance

cotransfection of the STAT3Y plasmid, suggesting that RET/PTC1-mediated induction of cyclin D1 transcription results from the activation of endogenous STAT3. Coexpression of STAT3 and RET/PTC1 yielded a much higher increase in the cyclin D1 promoter activity than did control or RET/PTC1 alone. To confirm the effect of RET/PTC1, STAT3, and STAT3Y on the induction of cyclin D1, we transfected cyclin D1 together with RET/PTC1, STAT3, and STAT3Y. The induction of cyclin D1 transactivation by RET/PTC1-mediated STAT3 activation was decreased in a dose-dependent manner by the addition of STAT3Y (Fig. 3B). A similar pattern of regulation by RET/PTC1 and STAT3 was observed for the VEGF and ICAM-1 promoters (Fig. 3C,D). The VEGF promoter luciferase construct, which contains about 2.7 kb of the 5′-flanking region of the VEGF gene, showed increased promoter activity when cotransfected with RET/PTC1 and/or STAT3, but the dominant-negative STAT3Y inhibited the RET/PTC1-induced VEGF promoter activity (Fig. 3B). The ICAM-1 promoter was also responsive to RET/PTC1 expression via STAT3 activation (Fig. 3D). A mutation (delGAS) of the STAT-binding element in the ICAM-1 promoter abolished RET/PTC1-mediated induction of ICAM-1 (data not shown).

We performed semiquantitative reverse transcriptase (RT)-PCR in two different lines of NIH3T3 cells, which were stably transfected with RET/PTC1 (data not shown), to observe the changes in the endogenous cyclin D1, VEGF, and ICAM-1 levels by RET/PTC. The level of the cyclin D1, VEGF, and ICAM-1 products were significantly higher in the RET/PTC-expressing cells than in the vector control in repeated experiments (data not shown).

LKB1 Suppresses RET/PTC-Dependent Activation of STAT3

The ability of LKB1 to regulate activation of STAT3 was examined in transiently transfected NIH3T3 cells carrying the *m67-Luc* reporter plasmid. MCF7 cells were transiently transfected with plasmids expressing RET/PTC3 (Fig. 4A), TEL-JAK2 (Fig. 4B), and STAT3, in the absence or presence of vectors expressing Myc-tagged LKB1. Expression of wild-type LKB1 suppressed RET/PTC3- and TEL-JAK2-dependent activation of STAT3. Unexpectedly, Myc-LKB1-K78M, which lacks serine/threonine kinase activity, also suppressed activation of STAT3 (Fig. 4A,B). Similarly, induction of luciferase activity stimulated by IL-6 and STAT3c (the constitutively active form of STAT3) was equivalently reduced by both wild-type and kinase-deficient Myc-LKB1 proteins (Fig. 4C,D).

Because NIH3T3 and MCF-7 cells express endogenous LKB1, the foregoing experiments were repeated in LKB1−/− mouse embryo fibroblasts (MEFs) and in the LKB1-deficient cell line NPA (inset, Fig. 4E). The results confirmed our previous results, indicating that wild type-LKB1 and Myc-LKB1-K78M suppressed RET/PTC-dependent activation of STAT3 in NPA and LKB1−/−MEFs (Fig. 4E,F). In addition, RET/PTC-dependent activation of STAT3 was significantly higher in LKB1−/−MEFs than in wild-type MEFs (Fig. 4G), and siRNA-mediated

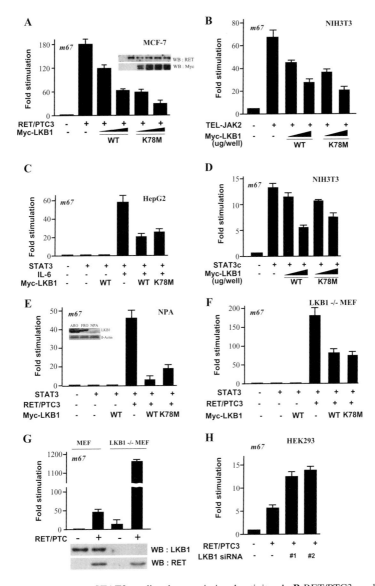

Fig. 4. LKB1 suppresses STAT3-mediated transcriptional activity. A, B RET/PTC3- and TEL-JAK2-mediated STAT3 transcriptional activity is decreased by wild-type and kinase-deficient LKB1. MCF-7 and NIH3T3 cells were transiently cotransfected with 0.1 μg of the following plasmids: m67-Luc alone or m67-Luc and plasmids expressing RET/PTC3 (A), TEL-JAK2 and Myc-LKB1 (B), or Myc-LKB1-K78M (0.2 or 0.5 μg each). C Interleukin (IL)-6 activation of STAT3 is reduced by LKB1. HepG2 cells were transiently cotransfected with 0.1 μg of the following plasmids: m67-Luc and plasmids expressing STAT3 and Myc-LKB1 or Myc-LKB1-K78M. Cells were transferred to serum-free media 12 h after transfection, then treated with IL-6 (20 ng/ml) for 6 h. D LKB1 suppresses the activity of constitutively active STAT3c. NIH3T3 cells were transiently cotransfected with 0.1 μg of the following plasmids: m67-Luc (0.1 μg) and vectors expressing STAT3c (0.1 μg) and Myc-LKB1 or Myc-LKB1-K78M (0.1 or 0.2 μg each). E, F Exogenous expression of LKB1 suppresses activation of STAT3 in NPA and LKB1–/–MEFs. NPA, and LKB1–/–MEFs were transiently cotransfected with 0.1 μg of the following plasmids: m67-Luc and plasmids expressing STAT3, RET/PTC3, and Myc-LKB1 or Myc-LKB1-K78M. G RET/PTC-dependent activation of STAT3 in LKB1–/–MEF cells. LKB1–/–MEF cells were transfected with 0.5 μg RET/PTC3. H Effect of downregulation of LKB1 on activation of STAT3. HEK293 cells were transiently cotransfected with plasmid expressing RET/PTC3 (0.1 μg) and 20 nM LKB1 siRNA

downregulation of LKB1 stimulated transcriptional transactivation by STAT3 (Fig. 4H). These results indicate that LKB1 negatively regulates RET/PTC-dependent activation of STAT3, and that this effect does not require LKB1 kinase activity.

The LKB1 Kinase Domain Interacts with the STAT3 Linker Domain In Vivo

The results just described suggest that LKB1 may inhibit STAT3 by direct binding, independent of its kinase function. This idea was tested by immunoprecipitating extracts of HEK293 cells cotransfected with plasmids expressing Flag-tagged STAT3 and Myc-tagged LKB. Immunoprecipitation analyses were carried out with anti-Flag and anti-Myc antibodies (data not shown). Flag immunoprecipitates were analyzed by Western blot using anti-Myc antibodies, and Myc immunoprecipitates were analyzed by Western blot with anti-Flag antibodies. LKB1 and STAT3 were detected in both immunoprecipitates, indicating that LKB1 and STAT3 interact physically with each other. Furthermore, by using confocal microscopy, we observed that Myc-LKB1 and endogenous STAT3 colocalize in the nucleus (data not shown). This observation was confirmed by treating cells with IL-6 to induce translocation of STAT3 to the nucleus. Figure 5D shows that IL-6 also induced nuclear localization of LKB1. This result suggests that STAT3 and LKB1 form a complex after migrating to the nucleus and that the activity of STAT3 in the nucleus is suppressed by LKB1.

To identify the domains required for the protein–protein interaction between STAT3 and LKB1, immunoprecipitation experiments were performed using truncated forms of STAT3 and LKB1 (Fig. 5A,B). In cells expressing Myc-LKB1 and wild-type or truncated STAT3, wild-type STAT3, STAT3-ΔTAD, and STAT3-ΔSH2 were competent to bind Myc-LKB1, but STAT3-ΔLK, STAT3-ΔDBD, and STAT3-NTD were not (Fig. 5A). In cells expressing Flag-STAT3 and wild-type or truncated LKB1, wild-type LKB1, HA-LKB1-ΔN, and HA-LKB1-ΔC were competent to bind Flag-STAT3, but HA-LKB1-ΔNK, which lacks both the N-terminal and kinase domains, was not (Fig. 5B). These results suggest that the kinase domain of LKB1 interacts with the linker domain of STAT3.

LKB1 Suppresses STAT3-Mediated Gene Expression

LKB1 appears to suppress binding of STAT3 to its target promoters and STAT3-dependent transcription of the *m67-Luc* reporter gene. Thus, experiments were performed to test the effect of LKB1 on expression of STAT3 target genes and on cell proliferation. The promoters of genes encoding cyclin D1 and VEGF are induced by STAT3; thus, cyclin D1- and VEGF-*Luc* reporter gene constructs were used to measure activation of STAT3. In NIH3T3 cells, STAT3-dependent transcriptional activation was significantly higher in cells expressing RET/PTC

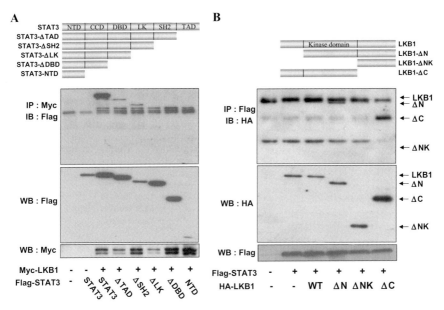

Fig. 5. Interaction between STAT3 linker domain and LKB1 kinase domain. **A** The LKB1 kinase domain interacts with the STAT3 linker domain. HEK293 cells were grown in 100-mm dishes and transiently cotransfected with plasmids expressing STAT3 deletion constructs (2 μg), Myc-LKB1 (2 μg), and control vector (4 μg). Protein (1 mg) was immunoprecipitated with anti-Myc antibody and separated by SDS-PAGE, followed by immunoblotting. Blots were probed with anti-Flag antibody. Total LKB1 expression (*bottom*) and the STAT3 deletions (*middle*) were detected using the antibodies indicated. *TAD*, transactivating domain; *SH2*, Src homology 2 domain; *LK*, linker domain; *DBD*, DNA-binding domain; *NTD*, N-terminal domain. **B** STAT3 interacts with the LKB1 kinase domain. HEK293 cells were grown in 100-mm dishes and transiently cotransfected with plasmids expressing Flag-STAT3 (2 μg) and LKB1 deletion constructs (2 μg) or control vector (4 μg). Proteins (1 mg) were immunoprecipitated with the anti-Flag antibody and separated by SDS-PAGE, followed by immunoblotting. Blots were probed with the anti-Myc antibody. Levels of STAT3 (*bottom*) and LKB1 (*middle*) were detected with the antibodies indicated. Δ*N*, N-terminal deletion; Δ*NK*, N-terminal and kinase domain deletion; Δ*C*, C-terminal deletion

(Fig. 6A,B). However, RET/PTC-dependent activation of STAT3 was suppressed by wild-type and kinase-deficient LKB1 (Fig. 6A,B). The effect of LKB1 overexpression on expression of endogenous cyclin D1 and bcl-xL was examined in MDA-MB-435 cells, in which STAT3 is activated constitutively (Fig. 6C). In these cells, overexpression of LKB1 significantly suppressed expression of endogenous cyclin D1 and bcl-xL protein.

The effect of siRNA-mediated knockdown of LKB1 on cellular proliferation was examined in TPC-1 human thyroid cancer cells. TPC-1 cells have a rearrangement

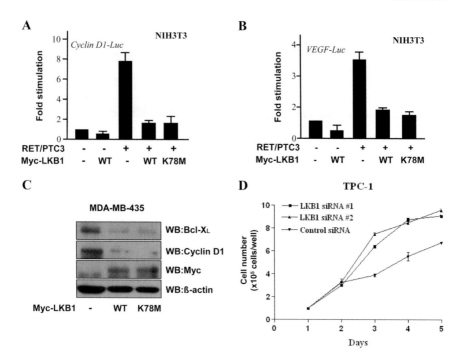

Fig. 6. LKB1 suppresses STAT3-mediated gene expression. **A, B** LKB1 suppresses transcription of cyclin D1-Luc and VEGF-Luc. NIH3T3 cells were grown in 12-well plates and transiently cotransfected with plasmids (0.1 µg) expressing cyclin D1-Luc (**A**), VEGF1-Luc (**B**), and RET/PTC3 and Myc-LKB1 or Myc-LKB1-K78M. Cells were lysed 24 h following transfection, and luciferase activity was measured. **C, D** LKB1 decreases cyclin D1 and Bcl-xL protein levels. MDA-MB-435 (**C**) cells were transiently transfected with plasmids (0.5 µg) expressing Myc-LKB1 or Myc-LKB1-K78M and control vector. TPC-1 cells (**D**) were transfected with LKB1 siRNA or control siRNA. Cell numbers were counted daily

of the endogenous RET/PTC1 gene, and the growth of these cells is dependent on activation of STAT3 by RET/PTC [29]. As shown in Fig. 6D, transfection with LKB1 targeted siRNA stimulated proliferation of TPC-1 cells, whereas control siRNA did not. These results suggest that LKB1 modulates RET/PTC- and STAT3-dependent proliferation of TPC-1 cells.

The Indolinone Compounds SU5416, SU6668, and SU11248 Inhibit the RET/PTC Kinase In Vitro

The indolinone derivatives SU5416, SU6668, and SU11248 are potent antiangiogenic small molecule inhibitors of RTKs, including those of the VEGFR family. These compounds were designed to have broad selectivity for the split kinase family of RTKs as well. We measured the effects of SU5416, SU6668, and SU11248 on the RET/PTC tyrosine kinase. We produced active RET/PTC3 protein using a baculovirus expression system. The RET/PTC3 kinase assay (data not shown) revealed that SU5416, SU6668, and SU11248 inhibited phosphorylation of the synthetic E4Y polypeptide tyrosine kinase substrate in a dose-dependent manner with an IC_{50} of approximately 944 nM for SU5416, 562 nM for SU6668, and 224 nM for SU11248. These results indicate that SU11248 is the most active indolinone compound for the in vitro inhibition of RET/PTC kinase.

SU11248 Inhibits Proliferation of TPC-1 Cells

In NIH-RET/PTC cells, SU11248 treatment was accompanied by a remarkable reduction in RET/PTC autophosphorylation levels. To further investigate, we measured the proliferation of TPC-1 cells harboring endogenous RET/PTC1 rearrangement in the presence of SU5416, SU6668, or SU11248 in cultures treated for 1 to 3 days with various doses (0.02–1 µM) of SU5416, SU6668, or SU11248 (Fig. 7). Although SU5416 and SU6668 did not significantly affect the growth of TPC-1

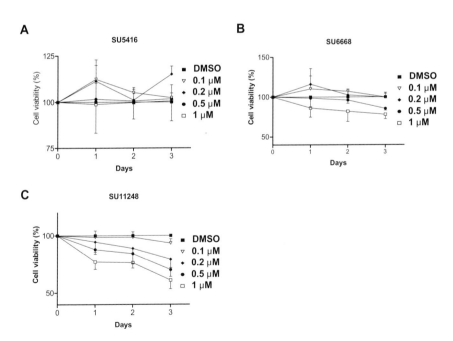

Fig. 7. SU11248 causes growth inhibition of TPC-1 cells. Cell viability assays were carried out using the MTT dye conversion assay in 96-well cell culture plates after exposure to SU5416, SU6668, or SU11248. Data are expressed as a percentage of dimethyl sulfoxide (*DMSO*) control. MTT assays were carried out in three independent experiments done in triplicate. Cell viability was reduced in SU11248-treated TPC-1 cells compared to DMSO-, SU5416-, and SU6668-treated cultures. As a negative control, K-*ras*- and H-*ras*-transformed cells were used. Neither Rat2-K-Ras nor Rat2-H-Ras cells were affected by SU11248 and SU5416 (data not shown)

cells, SU11248 treatment resulted in dose-dependent suppression of TPC-1 proliferation.

Discussion

The restriction of RET/PTC expression to thyroid tumors of the papillary subtype suggests that RET/PTC kinase is linked to specific signaling pathways in thyroid epithelial cells and that these signaling pathways can lead to cell transformation, growth, and proliferation in vivo and in vitro. For the past few years, many investigators have studied RET/PTC-mediated signaling pathways involved in tumorigenesis, and recent reports have shown that RET/PTC triggers the formation of stress fibers, a process that is dependent on Rho GTPase in RET/PTC-transfected thyroid cells [30]. However, the molecular mechanisms responsible for RET/PTC-mediated tumorigenesis are still generally poorly known.

Evidence is accumulating that constitutively activated STAT3 is involved in cellular transformation and the malignant progression of human cancers [11]. Constitutively active STAT3 has been found in several malignancies, including acute myeloid leukemia (AML), multiple myeloma, and head and neck cancers, among many others. In some cases, oncogenic tyrosine kinases, including v-Src, v-Eyk, and v-Ros, activate STAT3 in the absence of extracellular ligand stimulation, whereas in other cases disturbed cytokine production in malignant cells has been identified as the cause of aberrant STAT3 signaling. Recently, Schuringa et al. reported that MEN2A-RET, a germline mutant of RET with a changed cysteine residue in the extracellular domain, activates exogenous STAT3 by phosphorylating the Y705 and S727 residues in NIH3T3 and COS7 cells [31]. MEN2A-RET is a constitutively active membrane-inserted receptor tyrosine kinase; in contrast, RET/PTCs are not located in the membrane but are present exclusively in cytoplasm [32]. This difference in cellular distribution may result in MEN2A-RET and RET/PTC having different proximity to substrates. However, our studies suggest that cytoplasmic RET/PTC1 and RET/PTC3 are able to induce tyrosine phosphorylation of the Y705 residue in endogenous and exogenous STAT3.

Two different RET/PTC variants, RET/PTC1 and RET/PTC3, showed the same ability to phosphorylate the Y705 residue of STAT3. These observations suggest that the N-terminal RET-fused genes, H4 in RET/PTC1 and ELE1 in RET/PTC3, do not determine the substrate specificity of RET/PTC-mediated Y705 phosphorylation of STAT3. In addition, it may suggest that RET-fused genes are not involved in the association between STAT3 and RET/PTC.

RET/PTC1 transfection with the m67 reporter, which is induced by activated STAT3, resulted in a marked increase in reporter activity. These observations again suggest that (1) RET/PTC1 is able to activate endogenous STAT3, and (2) RET/PTC1-mediated Y705 phosphorylation functionally activates STAT3 for gene transcription. From coexpression experiments, we found that STAT3Y, a dominant-negative mutant construct of STAT3, specifically attenuates the RET/PTC1-mediated increase of m67 reporter activities, indicating that Y705 phosphorylation of STAT3 is specifically modified by RET/PTC during STAT3-mediated gene regulation. STAT3S, which has a mutation in the S727 residue located in the transactivation domain of STAT3, also decreased the RET/PTC-induced m67 reporter activity. This effect may be caused by its inhibition of endogenously activated Y705-phosphorylated STAT3-mediated transcription, although we did not observe any changes in S727 phosphorylation status in RET/PTC1-transfected cells.

Several tyrosine kinases phosphorylate STAT3 [33]. JAKs mediate STAT3 phosphorylation in cytokine signaling, and c-Src kinases are able to induce tyrosine phosphorylation of STAT3 in cellular transformation. However, the JAK2 inhibitor AG490 and the c-Src inhibitor PP1 did not block the RET/PTC1-mediated Y705 phosphorylation of STAT3, and these inhibitors did not alter the RET/PTC1-induced increase of m67 luciferase reporter activity [34]. Together, these results suggest that STAT3 is a direct substrate of RET/PTC tyrosine kinase in vivo. This finding is supported by the ability of immunoprecipitated RET/PTC to induce tyrosine phosphorylation of STAT3 in vitro.

The intracellular domains of cytokine receptors offer docking sites for STAT3 for recruitment and activation. The YXXQ motif has been identified in gp130 as a binding motif for STAT3 activation in IL-6 signaling. Schuringa et al. reported that MEN2A-RET activates STAT3 through two YXXV/Q motifs, Y752 and Y928 (homologous residues to the Y141 and Y317 sites on RET/PTC1, respectively) [31]. However, our observations of the interactions between STAT3 and two mutant RET/PTC1s that have mutated tyrosine motifs in the kinase domain, [141]YXXV and [317]YXXQ, suggest that these two sequences of RET/PTC1 are not critical motifs for interactions with STAT3. The Y317 residue of RET/PTC1 is important for autophosphorylation and also plays a critical role in the induction of the Y705 phosphorylation of STAT3. The mutant construct RET/PTC1 Y317F was not able to induce cellular transformation in NIH3T3 cells (data not shown), and activated the m67 luciferase promoter to a lesser degree. These observations suggest that interactions between RET/PTC and STAT3 may not require the consensus YXXQ/V motif in RET/PTC1. Because multiple tyrosine residues in RET/PTC are phosphorylated constitutively, the SH2 domains in STAT3 may bind to other phosphotyrosine residues. Although cytoplasmic Src kinase is known to phosphorylate the Y705 residue of STAT3, the YXXQ motif was not found in Src. These findings suggest that the YXXQ motif is unnecessary in cytoplasmic tyrosine kinase such as Src and RET/PTC for the phosphorylation of Y705 residue on STAT3.

Although STAT3 is known to be a transcription factor and an oncogene that can transform cells with oncogenic tyrosine kinases, the downstream target genes that are activated during STAT3-mediated oncogenesis have not been identified. Cyclin D1, VEGF, and ICAM-1 are candidate genes because they contain the STAT3-binding elements in their promoter regions and may play important roles in cell-cycle progression, angiogenesis, and cellular migration, which are important in tumor development and progression. All these genes are induced by RET/PTC1-mediated STAT3 activation. We also found that Y705 phosphorylation of STAT3 is critical for the transformation of NIH3T3 cells by RET/PTC1 and their proliferation thereafter. All these observations suggest that STAT3 activation is not only involved in RET/PTC-mediated transformation but is also important for the maintenance of the proliferative potential of transformed cells. Physiological STAT3 activation is important for the regulation of cell proliferation and self-tolerance in thyroid cells. However, constitutive activation of RET/PTC may result in prolonged activation of STAT3 and in the uncontrolled induction of STAT3 downstream genes for cellular transformation.

The change in the STAT3 expression level in human papillary thyroid cancer has not been reported. Furthermore, there is no information on the differences in the level of tyrosine-phosphorylated STAT3 between the RET/PTC-positive and -negative human papillary thyroid carcinomas. It was necessary to examine the in vivo level of activated STAT3 in papillary thyroid cancer, which has rearranged RET/PTC tyrosine kinase.

In sum, we have shown that RET/PTC associates with STAT3 and activates it through the specific phosphorylation of the tyrosine 705 residue. Y705 phosphorylation of STAT3 requires the intrinsic kinase activity of RET/PTC and turns on the cyclin D1, VEGF, and ICAM-1 genes. In addition, RET/PTC-mediated cellular transformation and the proliferation of transformed cells require tyrosine 705 phosphorylation of STAT3 in NIH3T3 cells. We conclude that STAT3 activation by the RET/PTC tyrosine kinase is one of the critical signaling pathways for the regulation of specific genes, such as cyclin D1, VEGF, and ICAM-1, and for cellular transformation.

LKB1 is a tumor suppressor with intrinsic serine/threonine kinase activity, defects in which cause PJS, an autosomal dominant human disease characterized by a high incidence of benign and malignant intestinal tumors [35]. The gene expression signature of LKB1-null fibroblasts includes significantly elevated expression of STAT3 target genes such as *MMP2*, *MMP9*, *VEGF*, *IGFBP5*, and *COX-2*. Previous studies reported that RET/PTC tyrosine kinase phosphorylates and activates STAT3 [16]. This study demonstrates that the ability of RET/PTC to activate endogenous and exogenous STAT3 is suppressed by wild-type and kinase-deficient LKB1. It is unlikely that LKB1 acts through an upstream activator of STAT3, because it suppresses STAT3 transcriptional activity in the presence of Tel-JAK2 [36] and IL-6, and it also stimulates the constitutively active STAT3c. This study also shows that LKB1-mediated suppression of STAT3 transcriptional activity is independent of the phosphorylation status of STAT3.

LKB1 has been reported to cause G_1 growth arrest in cultured cells via induction of p21$^{WAF1/CIP1}$ [37,38] and stimulation of Brg1 ATPase [39]. LKB1 kinase activity is required for p21$^{WAF1/CIP1}$ induction, and overexpression of LKB1 causes p21$^{WAF1/CIP1}$-induced growth arrest in cells with undetectable or low levels of endogenous LKB1. In contrast, although Brg1-associated growth arrest also requires LKB1 kinase activity, wild-type LKB1 and the kinase-deficient form LKB1-SL26 both stimulate Brg1 ATPase. This finding suggests that some regulatory functions of LKB1 may not require its kinase activity. This finding is also consistent with our observation that several naturally occurring and recombinant kinase-deficient forms of LKB1 retain the ability to suppress activation of STAT3. One exception to this is LKB1-ΔNK, a recombinant form of LKB1 that lacks the N-terminal region and the kinase domain, and which does not suppress RET/PTC-dependent activation of STAT3. These results support the conclusion that the LKB1 kinase domain, but not its kinase activity, is essential for suppressing activation of STAT3.

STAT3 is also regulated by the phosphorylation status of tyrosine 705 and serine 727, although tyrosine 705 appears to be more important in this regard than serine 727. Nevertheless, some regulators of STAT3, including PIAS3 and Grim-19, suppress STAT3 transcriptional activity via direct binding, and have no effect on tyrosine phosphorylation of STAT3 [40,41]. Similarly, wild-type and kinase-deficient forms of LKB1 bind to STAT3 and modulate its activity independent of tyrosine 705 phosphorylation. Furthermore, the LKB1 kinase domain and the STAT3 linker domain are required for binding of LKB1 and STAT3. Thus, there are similarities in the mechanism by which LKB1, PIAS3, and Grim-19 interact with STAT3. STAT3 regulates transcription of many downstream target genes, including many oncogenesis-related genes, by binding to and activating the promoter of the target genes. Furthermore, expression of exogenous LKB1 reduced expression of cyclin D1 and bcl-xL protein and transcription of a luciferase reporter gene driven by the cyclin D1 or VEGF promoters. Last, siRNA-mediated knockdown of LKB1 siRNA stimulated proliferation of TPC-1 cells.

In conclusion, this study shows that LKB1 suppresses RET/PTC-dependent activation of STAT3 by interacting with the STAT3 linker domain, leading to decreased expression of downstream targets of STAT3. Thus, we propose here a novel mechanism by which LKB1 acts as tumor suppressor and counteracts oncogenic STAT3.

The compounds SU11248, SU5416, and SU6668 are derivatives of indolinone and have a wide spectrum of inhibitory actions on tyrosine kinases [42]. The compounds were developed as inhibitors of the ATP-binding site of tyrosine kinases and have entered preclinical and clinical trials. Administered orally, SU11248 is a small organic molecule with antitumor and antiangiogenic activity that acts through selectively targeting PDGFR, VEGFR, KIT, and FLT3. By inhibiting the activity of these RTKs, SU11248 directly targets tumor cell proliferation and survival in cancers where these receptors are involved. SU11248 has been demonstrated to inhibit both FLK/KDR and PDGFR-β phosphorylation in vivo and has exhibited antitumor activity in a large number of preclinical xenograft tumor models, including leukemia expressing FLT3-activating mutations.

The kinase domain of RET/PTC shows 50% overall homology to the kinase domains of KIT, FLT3, PDGFR, and VEGFR. Most tyrosine kinase inhibitors that bind to ATP-binding pockets showed significant inhibitory activities on multiple classes of tyrosine kinases, which show relatively low homology in the kinase domain. We have shown that SU11248 inhibits the RET/PTC3 kinase with an IC_{50} of 224 nM in vitro. This IC_{50} is very similar to the IC_{50} (250 nM) for inhibition of the wild-type *fms*-related tyrosine kinase/Flk2/Stk-2 (FLT3). FLT3 belongs to the type III split-kinase domain family of RTKs and is primarily expressed on immature hematopoietic progenitors, but it is also found on some mature myeloid and lymphoid cells. Two classes of mutations activating FLT3 have been identified in AML patients: internal tandem duplication (ITD) mutations in the juxta-membrane region expressed in 25% to 30% of AML patients, and point mutations in the activation loop of the kinase domain found in approximately 7% of patients. SU11248 inhibits phosphorylation of FLT3 and causes regression of subcutaneous FLT3 tumors.

SU11248 is a potent (IC_{50} of 224 nM) inhibitor of RET/PTC oncoproteins. SU11248-mediated block of RET/PTC inhibited RET/PTC signaling, decreased RET/PTC autophosphorylation and STAT3 activation, and blocked the transforming capacity of RET/PTC. Furthermore, SU11248 exerted a powerful growth-inhibitory effect on thyroid carcinoma cell lines (TPC1) that spontaneously harbor a RET/PTC rearrangement. Because these carcinoma cells do not express detectable levels of KDR and SU5416 and SU6668 did not inhibit proliferation, our data suggest that the SU11248 effects are mediated by RET/PTC1 inhibition, and the possibility that they are mediated by KDR inhibition can be excluded. SU11248 has several possible advantages over previously developed compounds in the treatment of RET/PTC-associated PTC, including its antiangiogenic effects, low toxicity, and the possibility of oral administration. Furthermore, a recent phase I trial reported that potentially active target plasma concentrations between 50 and 100 ng/ml (250 nM) can be achieved with moderate interpatient variability and a long half-life compatible with a single daily dosing. Our IC_{50} value of SU11248 was 224 nM, so this dose is projected into an effective concentration in vivo.

SU11248 is currently undergoing phase III clinical trials for treatment of renal cell carcinoma, lung cancer, and gastrointestinal stromal tumor, and our current evidence of SU11248 inhibition of RET/PTC in vitro provides basic information to initiate in vivo studies with animal models of PTC and subsequent clinical trials.

Acknowledgments. This work was supported in part by the second phase of the Brain Korea 21 program of the Ministry of Education and by the Research Program for New Drug Target Discovery (M10748000319-07N4800-31910) grant from the Ministry of Science & Technology, South Korea.

References

1. Santoro M, Melillo RM, Carlomagno F, et al (2002) Molecular mechanisms of RET activation in human cancer. Ann N Y Acad Sci 963:116–121
2. Grieco M, Santoro M, Berlingieri MT, et al (1990) PTC is a novel rearranged form of the ret proto-oncogene and is frequently detected in vivo in human thyroid papillary carcinomas. Cell 60:557–563
3. Pierotti MA, Bongarzone I, Borello MG, et al (1996) Cytogenetics and molecular genetics of carcinomas arising from thyroid epithelial follicular cells. Genes Chromosomes Cancer 16:1–14
4. Santoro M, Chiappetta G, Cerrato A, et al (1996) Development of thyroid papillary carcinomas secondary to tissue-specific expression of the RET/PTC1 oncogene in transgenic mice. Oncogene 12:1821–1826
5. Besset V, Scott RP, Ibanez CF (2000) Signaling complexes and protein-protein interactions involved in the activation of the Ras and phosphatidylinositol 3-kinase pathways by the c-Ret receptor tyrosine kinase. J Biol Chem 275:39159–39166

6. Chiariello M, Visconti R, Carlomagno F, et al (1998) Signalling of the Ret receptor tyrosine kinase through the c-Jun NH2-terminal protein kinases (JNKS): evidence for a divergence of the ERKs and JNKs pathways induced by Ret. Oncogene 16:2435–2445
7. Segouffin-Cariou C, Billaud M (2000) Transforming ability of MEN2A-RET requires activation of the phosphatidylinositol 3-kinase/AKT signaling pathway. J Biol Chem 275:3568–3576
8. Zhong Z, Wen Z, Darnell JE Jr (1994) Stat3: a STAT family member activated by tyrosine phosphorylation in response to epidermal growth factor and interleukin-6. Science 264: 95–98
9. Bromberg JF (2001) Activation of STAT proteins and growth control. Bioessays 23: 161–169
10. Bromberg J, Darnell JE Jr (2000) The role of STATs in transcriptional control and their impact on cellular function. Oncogene 19:2468–2473
11. Bromberg JF, Wrzeszczynska MH, Devgan G, et al (1999) Stat3 as an oncogene. Cell 98:295–303
12. Cao X, Tay A, Guy GR, et al (1996) Activation and association of Stat3 with Src in v-Src-transformed cell lines. Mol Cell Biol 16:1595–1603
13. Bromberg JF, Horvath CM, Besser D, et al (1998) Stat3 activation is required for cellular transformation by v-src. Mol Cell Biol 18:2553–2558
14. Bardeesy N, Sinha M, Hezel AF, et al (2002) Loss of the Lkb1 tumour suppressor provokes intestinal polyposis but resistance to transformation. Nature (Lond) 419:162–167
15. Rossi DJ, Ylikorkala A, Korsisaari N, et al (2002) Induction of cyclooxygenase-2 in a mouse model of Peutz–Jeghers polyposis. Proc Natl Acad Sci U S A 99:12327–12332
16. Hwang JH, Kim DW, Suh JM, et al (2003) Activation of signal transducer and activator of transcription 3 by oncogenic RET/PTC (rearranged in transformation/papillary thyroid carcinoma) tyrosine kinase: roles in specific gene regulation and cellular transformation. Mol Endocrinol 17:1155–1166
17. Braga-Basaria M, Ringel MD (2003) Clinical review 158. Beyond radioiodine: a review of potential new therapeutic approaches for thyroid cancer. J Clin Endocrinol Metab 88: 1947–1960
18. Carlomagno F, Vitagliano D, Guida T, et al (2002) ZD6474, an orally available inhibitor of KDR tyrosine kinase activity, efficiently blocks oncogenic RET kinases. Cancer Res 62: 7284–7290
19. Fagin JA (2002) Perspective: lessons learned from molecular genetic studies of thyroid cancer. Insights into pathogenesis and tumor-specific therapeutic targets. Endocrinology 143: 2025–2028
20. Mendel DB, Laird AD, Xin X, et al (2003) In vivo antitumor activity of SU11248, a novel tyrosine kinase inhibitor targeting vascular endothelial growth factor and platelet-derived growth factor receptors: determination of a pharmacokinetic/pharmacodynamic relationship. Clin Cancer Res 9:327–337
21. O'Farrell AM, Abrams TJ, Yuen HA, et al (2003) SU11248 is a novel FLT3 tyrosine kinase inhibitor with potent activity in vitro and in vivo. Blood 101:3597–3605
22. Turner HE, Harris AL, Melmed S, et al (2003) Angiogenesis in endocrine tumors. Endocr Rev 24:600–632
23. Boudeau J, Kieloch A, Alessi DR, et al (2003) Functional analysis of LKB1/STK11 mutants and two aberrant isoforms found in Peutz–Jeghers syndrome patients. Hum Mutat 21:172
24. Zhang J, Yang J, Roy SK, et al (2003) The cell death regulator GRIM-19 is an inhibitor of signal transducer and activator of transcription 3. Proc Natl Acad Sci U S A 100:9342–9347
25. Sun L, Tran N, Liang C, et al (1999) Design, synthesis, and evaluations of substituted 3-[(3- or 4-carboxyethylpyrrol-2-yl)methylidenyl]indolin-2-ones as inhibitors of VEGF, FGF, and PDGF receptor tyrosine kinases. J Med Chem 42:5120–5130
26. Smolich BD, Yuen HA, West KA, et al (2001) The antiangiogenic protein kinase inhibitors SU5416 and SU6668 inhibit the SCF receptor (*c-kit*) in a human myeloid leukemia cell line and in acute myeloid leukemia blasts. Blood 97:1413–1421

27. Chung J, Park ES, Kim D, et al (2000) Thyrotropin modulates interferon-gamma-mediated intercellular adhesion molecule-1 gene expression by inhibiting Janus kinase-1 and signal transducer and activator of transcription-1 activation in thyroid cells. Endocrinology 141:2090–2097
28. Park ES, Kim H, Suh JM, et al (2000) Thyrotropin induces SOCS-1 (suppressor of cytokine signaling-1) and SOCS-3 in FRTL-5 thyroid cells. Mol Endocrinol 14:440–448
29. Kim DW, Jo YS, Jung HS, et al (2006) An orally administered multitarget tyrosine kinase inhibitor, SU11248, is a novel potent inhibitor of thyroid oncogenic RET/papillary thyroid cancer kinases. J Clin Endocrinol Metab 91:4070–4076
30. Barone MV, Sepe L, Melillo RM, et al (2001) RET/PTC1 oncogene signaling in PC Cl 3 thyroid cells requires the small GTP-binding protein Rho. Oncogene 20:6973–6982
31. Schuringa JJ, Wojtachnio K, Hagens W, et al (2001) MEN2A-RET-induced cellular transformation by activation of STAT3. Oncogene 20:5350–5358
32. Kim DW, Hwang JH, Suh JM, et al (2003) RET/PTC (rearranged in transformation/papillary thyroid carcinomas) tyrosine kinase phosphorylates and activates phosphoinositide-dependent kinase 1 (PDK1): an alternative phosphatidylinositol 3-kinase-independent pathway to activate PDK1. Mol Endocrinol 17:1382–1394
33. Aaronson DS, Horvath CM (2002) A road map for those who don't know JAK-STAT. Science 296:1653–1655
34. Hwang ES, Kim DW, Hwang JH, et al (2004) Regulation of signal transducer and activator of transcription 1 (STAT1) and STAT1-dependent genes by RET/PTC (rearranged in transformation/papillary thyroid carcinoma) oncogenic tyrosine kinases. Mol Endocrinol 18:2672–2684
35. Hemminki A, Markie D, Tomlinson I, et al (1998) A serine/threonine kinase gene defective in Peutz–Jeghers syndrome. Nature (Lond) 391:184–187
36. Ho JM, Beattie BK, Squire JA, et al (1999) Fusion of the ets transcription factor TEL to Jak2 results in constitutive Jak-Stat signaling. Blood 93:4354–4364
37. Tiainen M, Vaahtomeri K, Ylikorkala A, et al (2002) Growth arrest by the LKB1 tumor suppressor: induction of p21(WAF1/CIP1). Hum Mol Genet 11:497–1504
38. Tiainen M, Ylikorkala A, Makela TP (1999) Growth suppression by Lkb1 is mediated by a G(1) cell cycle arrest. Proc Natl Acad Sci U S A 96:9248–9251
39. Marignani PA, Kanai F, Carpenter CL (2001) LKB1 associates with Brg1 and is necessary for Brg1-induced growth arrest. J Biol Chem 276:32415–32418
40. Lufei C, Ma J, Huang G, et al (2003) GRIM-19, a death-regulatory gene product, suppresses Stat3 activity via functional interaction. EMBO J 22:1325–1335
41. Chung CD, Liao J, Liu B, et al (1997) Specific inhibition of Stat3 signal transduction by PIAS3. Science 278:1803–1805
42. Smith JK, Mamoon NM, Duhe RJ (2004) Emerging roles of targeted small molecule protein-tyrosine kinase inhibitors in cancer therapy. Oncol Res 14:175–225

Molecular Prediction of Therapeutic Response and Adverse Effect of Chemotherapy in Breast Cancer

Yoshio Miki

Summary. Breast cancer is considered to be relatively sensitive to chemotherapy, and multiple combinations of cytotoxic agents are used as standard therapy. Chemotherapy is applied empirically despite the observation that not all regimens are equally effective across the population of patients. Up-to-date clinical tests for predicting cancer chemotherapy response are not available, and individual markers have shown little predictive value. A number of microarray studies have demonstrated the use of genomic data, particularly gene expression signatures, as clinical prognostic factors in breast cancer. The identification of patient subpopulations most likely to respond to therapy is a central goal of recent personalized medicine. We have designed experiments to identify gene sets that will predict treatment-specific response in breast cancer. Taken together with our recent trial of construction of a high-throughput functional screening system for chemosensitivity-related genes, studies for drug sensitivity will provide rational strategies for establishment of the prediction system with high accuracy and identification of ideal targets for drug intervention.

Key words Breast cancer · Gene expression profile · Microarray · Personalized medicine · Drug sensitivity

Introduction

The suboptimal efficacy of most drugs for cancer therapy may be viewed as a result of our failure to account for individual differences in cancer etiology and drug response. Full understanding of the factors underlying these individual characteristics should allow the development of more specific diagnoses and therapeutics. Breast cancer ranks first in incidence among gynecological cancers. According to

---

Department of Molecular Genetics, Medical Research Institute, Tokyo Medical and Dental University, 1-5-45 Yushima, Bunkyo-ku, Tokyo 113-8510, Japan
Department of Molecular Diagnosis, The Cancer Institute of JFCR, 3-10-6 Ariake, Koto-ku, Tokyo 135-8550, Japan

the 2003 vital statistics records on the Japanese population, the mortality rate from breast cancer (15.2%) is increasing. For the treatment of breast cancer, surgery and several different chemotherapy regimens are used. The development of optimal consensus treatment guidelines for breast cancer requires comprehensive analysis of the results of randomized clinical trials and the interpretation of their clinical, biological, and personal relevance for individual patients. Recent recommendations (St. Gallen [1,2]; NIH Consensus [3]) based on clinical tests in large-scale, randomized control trials in the United States and Europe focused on the implications of evidence for patient treatment selection. They promoted the standardization of therapies in hospitals or regions, avoiding any divergent therapies. Breast cancer is considered to be relatively sensitive to chemotherapy, as compared to other solid tumors. Multiple combinations of cytotoxic drugs are used as standard therapy. The most effective combination regimens include anthracyclines (epirubicine or doxorubicin), which are topoisomerase II inhibitors. The taxanes (paclitaxel and docetaxel) and capecitabine are a new class of antimicrotubule agents that are more effective than older drugs such as anthracyclines and are often used in patients with advanced breast cancer with tumor cells that are resistant to anthracyclines [4–6]. Therefore, it is hoped that the addition of paclitaxel to anthracycline-containing chemotherapy will improve treatment efficacy for a subset of patients. However, not all regimens may be equally effective for all patients. It is not yet possible to select the most effective regimen for a particular individual, because there are no clinically useful predictive markers of a patient's response to chemotherapy. Now the question is "Is it possible to personalized chemotherapy and select the single best regimen for an individual?"

Paclitaxel and docetaxel are taxoid drugs, and are now the most active agents for breast cancer. They both work by interfering with mitosis, but they each do it a little differently, and the sensitivity is heterogeneous. To avoid unnecessary treatment, identification of a predictive marker is desired to distinguish between patients who are likely to respond and those who are not. We report the discovery of a gene expression profile that predicts response to paclitaxel or docetaxel in breast cancer patients. Second, to predict the probability of adverse effect on paclitaxel treatment, we conducted genotyping analysis on breast cancer patients enrolled in neoadjuvant paclitaxel therapy.

Materials and Methods

Patients and Tissues

Tumor samples from 74 patients with primary breast cancer who received neoadjuvant chemotherapy were accessed from the Cancer Institute Hospital of JFCR. We took core needle samples from patients with primary breast cancer before treatment and then assessed tumor response to neoadjuvant under Informed Consent.

Patients were divided into five groups according to pathological response (grade 0, extremely resistant; grade 1a, resistant; grade 1b, moderate responder; grade 2, responder; grade 3, high responder).

Gene Expression Analysis

We used the procedures of gene expression profiling using oligo microarrays described previously [7]. Briefly speaking, laser-captured microdissection (LCM) is applied to obtain purified cell populations. RNA from a tumor sample and reference RNA from normal cells are reverse transcribed, amplified, and labeled with different fluorescent dyes. The mixture is hybridized to an array. Genes whose expressions differ between the samples are identifiable by scanning the microarray with a laser-based detection system. To identify the gene set for the prediction of therapeutic response, gene expression analyses were performed using DNA microarray and quantitative reverse transcription-polymerase chain reaction (Q-RT-PCR) (Fig. 1). DNA microarray is an excellent experimental tool to analyze gene expression comprehensively. Although individual microarray studies can be highly informative, there are inconsistencies between various microarray platforms, making it

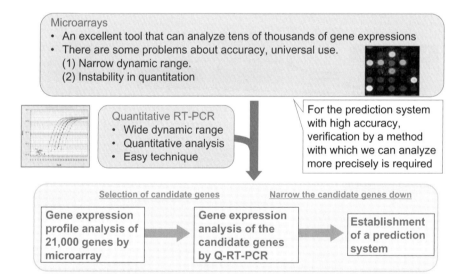

Fig. 1. Gene expression analysis by microarrays and quantitative reverse transcriptase-polymerase chain reaction (*Q-RT-PCR*). Patients were divided into two groups, responder (sensitive) and nonresponder (resistant), based on clinical and pathological response. Differentially expressed genes were statistically selected based on microarray data between responder and nonresponder groups. Expression of selected genes was quantified in all cases by real-time RT-PCR. Selection of the candidate genes for discriminating between nonresponder and responder was based on the RT-PCR data for establishment of a prediction system

difficult to compare independently obtained data addressing the same biological problem [8,9]. Also, there are some problems about dynamic range, accuracy, universal use. On the other hand, Q-RT-PCR is widely recognized to be the gold standard method for quantifying gene expression. However, studies using RT-PCR technology as a discovery tool have historically been limited to relatively small gene sets compared to other gene expression platforms such as microarrays. For the development of a prediction system with high accuracy, verification by a method that we can analyze more precisely is required. Therefore, our strategy is that first we performed gene expression profiling of 21 000 genes by DNA microarray for selection of candidate genes. Then, differentially expressed genes were selected between a drug-resistant group and a drug-sensitive group based on DNA microarray data. Next, expression of selected candidate genes was quantified by Q-RT-PCR for confirming the array data, increasing reliability, and narrowing down the candidate genes to establish a prediction system based on RT-PCR data.

Results

The scheme of identifying genetic markers for neoadjuvant chemotherapy is shown in Fig. 2. Specimens were obtained by core needle biopsy before treatment began, and pure populations of tumor cells were collected by LCM. After RNA extraction,

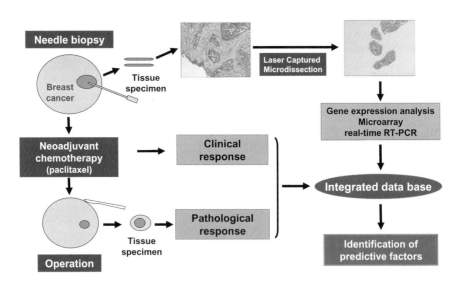

Fig. 2. Study of identifying genetic markers for neoadjuvant chemotherapy. We have combined the laser-captured microdissection (LCM) method with microarray technology. Tumor cells were selectively collected by LCM to exclude most of the stromal tissues to analyze cancer cells and assess gene expression. Clinical and pathological responses are evaluated at completion of treatment. Differentially expressed genes were selected for discriminating between nonresponders and responders

Table 1. Effects of cancer chemotherapy and gene selection for response prediction

Pathological effect	Nonresponder			Responder		Total
	Grade 0[a]	Grade 1a	Grade 1b	Grade 2[a]	Grade 3[a]	
Number of selected genes	7	22	7	14	1	51

Grade 0, not effective; grade 1a, high response in less than 1/3 cancer cells; grade 1b, high response in 1/3–2/3 cancer cells; grade 2, high response in more than 2/3 cancer cells; grade 3, complete response

[a] Fifty genes were selected for response prediction from 21 000 genes from highly sensitive group (grades 2, 3), and extremely resistant group (grade 0) by Mann–Whitney U test ($P < 0.05$).

gene expression analyses were performed using microarray or real-time RT-PCR. On the other hand, a patient receives chemotherapy treatment, and clinical response is evaluated at completion of treatment. Furthermore, surgical specimens were examined to determine the pathological response to chemotherapy. All clinical and genomic data are entered into an integrated database and analyzed for identification of predictive factors. We have identified several sets of genes that predict patient response to several different types of neoadjuvant chemotherapy such as paclitaxel, epirubicine, and docetaxel. Before clinical application, independent validation of the prediction system is required, and we have started a validation study for prediction of the therapeutic response to preoperative paclitaxel on new cases. These kinds of findings bring oncologists one step closer to being able to select the most effective regimen for a particular individual.

Approximately 50 differentially expressed genes between responder (grades 2 and 3) and extremely resistant (grade 0) groups were selected by Mann–Whitney U test (Table 1). Second, correlation between RNA expression measured by the arrays and semiquantitative RT-PCR was ascertained on the selected genes. Using the semiquantitative RT-PCR data of selected genes, we performed the machine learning method (AdaBoost) to determine the greatest estimated accuracy between responders (grades 2 and 3) and nonresponders (grades 0, 1a, and 1b), and high-scored predictive sets were selected.

Discussion

Chang et al. reported the application of DNA microarray analysis in the identification of predictive factors of response to docetaxel in 24 breast cancer patients [10]. They identified differential expression patterns of 92 genes correlated with docetaxel response. In leave-one-out cross-validation analysis, 10 of 11 sensitive tumors (responders) and 11 of 13 resistant tumors (nonresponders) were correctly classified, with an accuracy of 88%. On the other hand, Ayers et al. identified a set of key genetic markers (74 genes) that predict whether patients are likely to be cured (pathological complete response, pCR) by a chemotherapy regimen commonly given before surgery (neoadjuvant chemotherapy). It was reported that the markers predicted, with 75% accuracy, whether chemotherapy would completely eradicate tumor cells in 24 patients with early-stage breast cancer treated with neoadjuvant chemotherapy (paclitaxel followed by 5-fluorouracil, doxorubicin, and cyclophosphamide: T/FAC) [11]. These findings need to be validated in large-scale clinical trials before a test to predict patient response to chemotherapy can be routinely used.

DNA microarray analysis is a revolutionary experimental tool for analyzing gene expression comprehensively, and gene expression profiling has created new possibilities for the molecular characterization of cancer. A number of microarray studies have reported candidate genes for prediction of therapeutic response or clinical outcome. However, there are not many clinically useful systems showing that the method is highly precise, because it is not easy to identify true target genes by mathematical (statistical) algorithms. Functional analyses for their characterization of candidate genes are required. These kinds of findings bring oncologists one step closer to being able to select the most effective regimen for a particular individual.

References

1. Rabaglio M, Aebi S, Castiglione-Gertsch M (2007) Controversies of adjuvant endocrine treatment for breast cancer and recommendations of the 2007 St. Gallen conference. Lancet Oncol 8:940–949
2. Cinieri S, Orlando L, Fedele P, et al (2007) Adjuvant strategies in breast cancer: new prospectives, questions and reflections at the end of 2007 St. Gallen International Expert Consensus Conference. Ann Oncol 18(suppl):63–65
3. Eifel P, Axelson JA, Costa J, et al (2001) National Institutes of Health Consensus Development Conference Statement: adjuvant therapy for breast cancer, November 1–3, 2000. J Natl Cancer Inst 93:979–989
4. Fisher B, Bryant J, Wolmark N, et al (1998) Effect of preoperative chemotherapy on the outcome of women with operable breast cancer. J Clin Oncol 16:2672–2685
5. Rivera E, Holmes FA, Frye D, et al (2000) Phase II study of paclitaxel in patients with metastatic breast carcinoma refractory to standard chemotherapy. Cancer (Phila) 89:2195–2201
6. Wolmark N, Wang J, Mamounas E, et al (2001) Preoperative chemotherapy in patients with operable breast cancer: nine-year results from National Surgical Adjuvant Breast and Bowel Project B-18. J Natl Cancer Inst Monogr 30:96–102
7. Oishi Y, Nagasaki K, Miyata S, et al (2007) Functional pathway characterized by gene expression analysis of supraclavicular lymph node metastasis-positive breast cancer. J Hum Genet 52:271–279
8. Sorlie T, Tibshirani R, Parker J, et al (2003) Repeated observation of breast tumor subtypes in independent gene expression data sets. Proc Natl Acad Sci U S A 100:8418–8423
9. Kruse JJ, Stewart FA (2007) Gene expression arrays as a tool to unravel mechanisms of normal tissue radiation injury and prediction of response. World J Gastroenterol 13:2669–2674
10. Chang JC, Wooten EC, Tsimelzon A, et al (2003) Gene expression profiling for the prediction of therapeutic response to docetaxel in patients with breast cancer. Lancet 362:362–369
11. Ayers M, Symmans WF, Stec J, et al (2004) Gene expression profiles predict complete pathologic response to neoadjuvant paclitaxel and fluorouracil, doxorubicin, and cyclophosphamide chemotherapy in breast cancer. J Clin Oncol 22:2284–2293

Multiple Roles of NBS1 for Genotoxic and Nongenotoxic Stresses

Kenshi Komatsu, Mikio Shimada, Ken Tsuchida, Kyosuke Nakamura, Hiromi Yanagihara, and Junya Kobayashi

Summary. Nijmegen breakage syndrome (NBS) is characterized by genome instability and microcephaly. We show here that NBS human cells are severely sensitive to mitomycin C, similar to Fanconi anemia (FA). To study the details of interstrand cross-link (ICL) repair in NBS and FA, a highly sensitive psoralen–PEO–biotin (PPB) dot blot assay was developed to provide sensitive quantitative measurements of ICLs during the removal process. Studies utilizing this assay demonstrated a decreased rate of ICL removal in cells belonging to the FA core complex group (e.g., groups A and G), but ICL removal was restored to normal levels after these cells were complemented with wt-FANCA and wt-FANCG. In addition, a defect in ICL removal was also observed in cells with a mutated FANCD2 protein. Conversely, FA-D1 cells with a defective BRCA2 protein display normal ICL removal, although they are compromised with respect to recombination. We also show that cells from patients with NBS were defective in ICL removal, whereas they are impaired in recombination, similar to that of BRCA/XRCC3-defective cells. On the other hand, NBS1 is implicated in a response to nongenotoxic stress. We show here that the subpopulation of NBS1 is localized at the centrosomes and has a crucial role for maintenance of the centrosomes. Downregulation of NBS1 by siRNA induces supernumerary centrosomes, and this was confirmed by experiments using NBS1 knockout mouse cells. Although introduction of wt-NBS1 cDNA into knockout mouse cells restores the number of centrosomes to normal levels, it is abolished after the introduction of NBS1 mutated at the FHA domain and at a serine residue of 343, both of which are essential regions for ataxia-telangiectasia and Rad3-related protein (ATR) activation. The present results indicate the involvement of NBS1 in a response to genotoxic stress and in maintenance of centrosome through the ATR pathway.

Key words NBS1 · ICL removal · Mitomycin C · Centrosome

Radiation Biology Center, Kyoto University, Yoshida-Konoe, Sakyo, Kyoto 606-8501, Japan

Introduction

Nijmegen breakage syndrome (NBS) is a rare recessive genetic disorder, characterized by birdlike facial appearance, early growth retardation, congenital microcephaly, immunodeficiency, and a high frequency of malignancies. NBS belongs to the so-called chromosome instability syndromes; in fact, NBS cells display spontaneous chromosomal aberrations and are hypersensitive to DNA double-strand break-inducing agents, such as ionizing radiation. The disease appeared to be prevalent in Eastern and Central European populations where more than 90% of patients are homozygous for the founder mutation 657del5, leading to a truncated variant of the protein. NBS1 forms a multimeric complex with MRE11/RAD50 nuclease at the C-terminus, and retains or recruits them at the vicinity of sites of DNA damage by direct binding to histone H2AX [1], which is phosphorylated by the PI3-kinase family, such as ataxia-telangiectasia mutated protein (ATM), in response to DNA damage. Thereafter, the NBS-1 complex proceeds to rejoin double-strand breaks (DSB) by either homologous recombination (HR) repair [2] or nonhomologous end-joining (HNEJ).

We measured the ability of several NBS cells and A-T cells to regulate HR repair using the DR-GFP or SCneo system [3]. ATM deficiency did not reduce the HR repair frequency of an induced DSB, and it was confirmed by findings that HR frequencies are only slightly affected by deletion of the ATM-binding site at the extreme C-terminus NBS-1. In contrast, the HR-regulating ability is dramatically reduced by deletion of the MRE11-binding domain at the C-terminus of NBS-1 and markedly inhibited by mutations in the FHA/BRCT domains at the N-terminus. This impaired capability in HR is consistent with a failure to observe MRE11 foci formation. These results suggested that the N- and C-terminal domains of NBS1 are the major regulatory domains for HR pathways, very likely through the recruitment and retention of the MRE11 nuclease to DSB sites in an ATM-independent fashion.

MRE11 are human homologues of bacterial SbcC, which is a regulatory protein for RecA-homologous recombination, and their defect causes high sensitivity to mitomycin C cross-linking agents. We showed here that NBS1 knockdown human cells were severely sensitive to mitomycin C [4]. On the other hand, NBS-1 is implicated in prevention of DNA rereplication, and the cells mutated in NBS1 protein lead to genomic instability (Shimada et al., in preparation). We show here that the subpopulation of NBS-1 localized at the centrosomes and has a crucial role for maintenance of the centrosomes.

Materials and Methods

Cell Culture and Transfection

A31-1 cells were derived from NBS1 knockout mice [5]. Human HeLa S3 cells, U2OS cells, BJ cells, MCF7, and mouse NIH3T3 cells were used as control cell lines. BRCA1–/– ES cells and WT ES cells were kind gifts from Dr. Moynahan. H94-38 (a FA group G cell line), H9-38 + FANCG (complemented with human wt-FANCG), FAD423 (a FA group D1 cell line), and FAD423 + BRCA2 (complemented with human wt-BRCA2) were gifts from Dr. H. Joenje (Free University, Amsterdam), and RB520 (a FA group A lymphoid cell line). GM07116 (a NBS cell line) and GM07116 + NBS1 (complemented with human wt-NBS1) were established by our laboratory. All cell lines were cultured in Dulbecco's modified Eagle's medium (Sigma Chemical) supplemented with 10% fetal bovine serum (HyClone) at 37°C in a humidified atmosphere containing 10% CO_2.

In Vitro Assay for Interstrand Cross Links (ICLs)

The psoralen–PEO–biotin (PPB) compound was used as obtained from the manufacturer (Pierce Biotechnology, Rockford, IL, USA). PPB was dissolved in water to form a stock solution and was stored at 4°C. Various concentration of PPB was added to *Eco*RI (Toyobo, Tokyo, Japan) -digested pBR322 plasmid DNA (4.4 kb). After a 10-min incubation in the dark, DNA samples were irradiated with UVA light (365 nm) with a dose of 12 J/m^2 using a transilluminator, FUNA-UV-LINKER FS-1500 (Funakoshi, Tokyo, Japan). PPB/UVA-treated DNA samples were denatured in 0.2 N NaOH at 55°C for 10 min. To eliminate furan-side monoadducts, DNA samples were incubated with 0.2 N NaOH at 80°C for 30 min. The DNA samples were then loaded onto a 0.7% agarose gel in TBE buffer and electrophoresed for 4 h at 25 V. To blot the DNA, the agarose gels were treated with 0.25 N HCl for 30 min and 0.4 N NaOH for 20 min, and then transferred to nitrocellulose membranes over 16 h. Nitrocellulose membranes were baked at 80°C for 4 h and treated with blocking buffer (0.2% casein, 0.9% NaCl, 0.2 mg/ml KCl, 1.44 vmg/ml Na_2HPO_4, 0.24 mg/ml KH_2PO_4, pH 7.4) for 30 min. Streptavidin horseradish peroxidase (Amersham, UK) and chemiluminescence were used for the detection of PPB adducts. Quantification of PPB adducts was done as follows: the film was imaged with Open lab software. After transformation into gray-scale images, the total intensity was calculated with ImageJ software (NIH).

RNA-Mediated Interference

A siTrio RNA oligonucleotides that inhibit mouse NBS1 (NM 013752), human NBS1 (NM 002485), mouse BRCA1 (NM 009764), GFP as a control, and nontargeting short interfering RNA (B-Bridge International) were transfected into cells by using Lipofectamin 2000 (Invitrogen).

Immunostaining

Cells on cover glasses were washed with phosphate-buffered saline (PBS), fixed in cold methanol (−20°C) for 10 min, and incubated with a detergent solution (4°C) for 5 min. The cells were incubated with a blocking solution for 30 min, and then subjected to the following primary antibodies: anti-NBS1 (Novus Biologicals), MRE11 (Novus Biologicals), BRCA1 (Santa Cruz Biotechnology), γ-tubulin (Sigma Chemical), and secondary antibodies: Alexa488-conjugated antirabbit IgG (Molecular Probes) and Alexa-546-conjugated antirabbit IgG (Molecular Probes). Fluorescence from the Alexa-488 or -546 was visualized with a laser-scanning microscope (Olympus). At least 200 cells in each sample were examined for centrosome number and nuclear morphology.

Results

ICL Removal Capabilities of NBS1

ICL removal capacity in FA core complex group cells was next examined with the PPB dot blot assay. The FA core complex group cells examined here are characterized by a high sensitivity to ICL-inducing agents such as mitomycin C. The FA-G cell line, H94-38, showed defects in ICL removal, but normal levels of ICL removal were restored in cells complemented with the wt-FANCG gene. Similarly, defects in ICL repair were observed in the FA-A lymphoblast cell line, RB520. ICL removal in both FA cell lines was seen at levels that were similar to those observed in XP-F cells. Subsequently, FA-ID complex group cells were examined to determine their ICL removal capability. PD20 cells from a patient classified as belonging to subgroup D2 showed a decreased ability to remove ICLs, although the cell line defects were marginal.

Cells from patients belonging to the FA-BRCA group are highly sensitive to mitomycin C, and their ability to remove ICLs was next measured with the PPB dot blot assay. BRCA2-defective FAD423 cells, belonging to group FA-D1, showed normal ICL removal, with a time-course similar to that observed in control cells. ICL removal kinetics remained constant, even after the introduction of wt-BRCA2, although cellular sensitivity was restored to normal levels. These results were also seen in an experiment using Chinese hamster Irs1SF cells, which are deficient in the recombination protein XRCC3, and a member of the RAD51 paralogue. These cells and the corresponding complemented cells displayed levels of ICL removal similar to those seen in control cells, although their sensitivity to ICLs was restored to normal cell survival levels in complemented cells. These results clearly indicated that FA core complex group cells are defective in ICL removal, whereas recombination-defective BRCA group cells showed normal

ICL removal. FA-ID complex cells had an intermediate ability to remove ICLs, which was between that of the FA core complex group cells and the BRCA group cells. Similar to the BRCA-defective group, NBS cells are significantly defective in homologous recombination, and show a high sensitivity to the ICL agent [2]. Unexpectedly, however, the NBS cell line, GM07116, showed a defect in ICL removal, while normal level of ICL removal was restored in cells complemented with wt-NBS1 gene. This result is in contrast to ICL removal in BRCA-defective cells, indicating the functional similarity of NBS to the FA core complex group.

Centrosome Localization and the Phenotypes in the Absence of NBS1

NBS1 and γ-tubulin were immunostained in mouse NIH3T3 cells, human HeLa S3 cells, MCF7 cells, and BJ cells by using antibodies for both proteins. All cells showed one or two clear discrete foci (focus) for NBS1, and they colocalized with γ-tubulin, a main component of the centrosome. This colocalization was also observed during mitosis. To confirm the immunostaining results, cell lysates from HeLa S3 cells and NIH3T3 cells were fractionated by sucrose gradient centrifugation, and each fraction was analyzed by Western blot. Our analysis revealed that NBS1 and MRE11, a component of the NBS1 complex, coelute with γ-tubulin from fraction 21 to fraction 24 in HeLa cells and NIH3T3 cells. These findings are consistent with the finding that NBS1 is immunoprecipitated with γ-tubulin and MRE11.

To further examine whether NBS1 is involved in the maintenance of centrosomes, NBS1 protein in NIH3T3 and U2OS cells was knocked down by siRNA, and the number of centrosomes was scored with immunostaining for γ-tubulin. Our results shows that disruption of NBS1 significantly induced supernumerary centrosomes, defined as cells having three or fewer centrosomes per cell, and the frequencies were four to five times higher in both NIH3T3 cells and U2OS cells than in untreated cells. Furthermore, NBS1-deficient cells were prepared from knockout mouse cells and examined for centrosome instability. NBS1 knockout mouse cells similarly showed supernumerary centrosomes, whereas they were restored to normal levels after introduction of wild-type NBS1 cDNA. Subsequently, we generated NBS1 mutations in the FHA domain at serine residues of 278 and 343, and deletions in the MRE11-binding region, although the FHA and S278/343 are essential for ataxia-telangiectasia and Rad3-related protein (ATR) activation after DNA damage. Interestingly, no restoration was observed after the introduction of the NBS1 mutants FHA-2D and S278/343A. On the other hand, the MRE11-binding region was dispensable for centrosome maintenance, and the frequency of supernumerary centrosomes remained unchanged after the introduction of this deletion mutant protein. These results indicated that NBS1 is localized to centrosomes and may play a role in centrosome maintenance through ATR activation.

Discussion

Present results indicate that the defect in FA core complex and NBS cells in the ICL removal process occurs at an earlier repair step before the BRCA-mediated recombination. On the other hand, the comet assay failed to detect a defect in ICL repair in FA cells, whereas defects in ICL repair were clearly seen in incision-deficient XP-F cells. The present observations, taken together with those from the comet assay, suggest the involvement of FA core complex proteins and NBS1 protein in a late step of the ICL repair process rather than in the steps involving ICL recognition and incision, because the comet assay recognizes the unhooking process during the first incision by the XPF endonuclease. Therefore, analyses of ICL removal kinetics revealed that a deficient step in the FA core complex groups and NBS is located between the XPF-mediated incision step and the BRCA-mediated recombination. This finding is consistent with evidence that the FA core complex cells might be defective in TLS, which occurs over the base of unhooked ssDNA harboring ICL adducts at a step before the second incision.

Centrosome duplication is highly reminiscent of DNA replication, because the centrosome must be duplicated only once in each cell cycle. Although DNA replication is strictly regulated to prevent the rereplication of chromosomes by licensing the control mechanism, NBS1-knockdown cells enhanced the rereplication of chromosomal DNA when induced by SV40 large T antigen or by the overexpression of licensing factor Cdt1. NBS1 is required for the suppression of rereplication through a mechanism by which NBS1 activates ATR and thereby phosphorylates downstream proteins such as RPA. Similar to observations in DNA rereplication, the present results showed that deficiency in NBS1 causes supernumerary centrosomes. Our NBS1 mutation experiments showed that domains of NBS1 essential for ATR activation [6], such as FHA and S278/343, are crucial for centrosome maintenance. This determination is consistent with a recent report indicating that cells from patients with PNCT-Seckel syndrome with mutations in pericentrin are deficient in ATR signaling and show supernumerary centrosomes. Furthermore, centrosomal defects in ATR signaling have a causative effect on the growth of the brain, which is clinically observed as microcephaly. This model is supported by evidence that cells from patients with ATR-Seckel syndrome with mutations in ATR show supernumerary centrosomes and clinical phenotypes with microcephaly. Based on a clinical phenotype of microcephaly in NBS and the present results, NBS1 could cooperatively function with ATR in centrosome maintenance, similar to nuclear ATR signal activation by NBS1 in response to DNA damage.

References

1. Kobayashi J, Tauchi H, Sakamoto S, et al (2002) NBS1 localizes to γ-H2AX foci through interaction with the FHA/BRCT domain. Curr Biol 12:1846–1851
2. Tauchi H, Kobayashi J, Morishima K, et al (2002) Nbs is essential for DNA repair by homologous recombination in higher vertebrate cells. Nature (Lond) 420:93–98
3. Sakamoto S, Iijima K, Mochizuki D, et al (2007) Homologous recombination repair is regulated by domains at the C-terminus of NBS1 and is independent of ATM. Oncogene 26:6002–6009
4. Tsuchida K, Komatsu K. Impaired removal of DNA interstrand cross-link in Nijmegen breakage syndrome and Fanconi anemia other than BRCA-defective group. Cancer Sci., in press.
5. Matsuura, S, Kobayashi J, Tauchi H, et al (2004) Nijmegen breakage syndrome and DNA double strand break repair by NBS1 complex. Adv Biophys 38:65–80
6. Morishima K, Sakamoto S, Kobayashi J, et al (2007) TopBP1 associates with NBS1 and is involved in homologous recombination repair. Biochem Biophys Res Commun 362:872–879

Radiation Basic Life Sciences, Part 2

The DNA Damage Response in Nontargeted Cells

Kevin M. Prise, Giuseppe Schettino, and Susanne Burdak-Rothkamm

Summary. Cells have evolved complex processes to maintain the stability of their genomes. In response to genotoxic stress, the DNA damage response (DDR) is activated whereby a series of interlinked sensor processes signal to a panel of repair pathways, which can attempt to repair the damage. Recent studies have shown compelling evidence for the activation of DDR by ionising radiation even when radiation is not directly deposited in the DNA within the nucleus via bystander responses. Several groups have reported activation of a DDR response in bystander cells involving γ-H2AX formation and the potential formation of DNA double-strand breaks leading to mutations, chromosomal aberrations, and cell death. Earlier studies by Little and colleagues have proposed that clustering of damage including base damage at DNA replication forks may be important in bystander cells. In further studies, we now have evidence in bystander cells that the initial phosphorylation of H2AX is performed by the ataxia-telangiectasia and Rad3-related protein (ATR) rather that ataxia-telangiectasia mutated protein (ATM) or DNA-dependent protein kinase (DNA-PK). This action occurs predominantly in S-phase cells and supports the assertion that damage accumulation in bystander cells leads to stalled replication forks. As well as responses in bystander cells, DDR is also observed in cells where only the cytoplasm has been irradiated using microbeam approaches. Despite the historical dogma that DNA within the nucleus is the critical target, it is clear that cytoplasmic irradiation, involving mitochondrial responses, can lead to downstream biological consequences in terms of DDR, mutation formation cell killing, and apoptosis.

Key words DNA damage · DNA repair · Radiation · Bystander effect

---

Centre for Cancer Research and Cell Biology, Queen's University Belfast, 97 Lisburn Road, Belfast BT9 7BL, UK

Introduction

Our understanding of processes involved in genomic maintenance after radiation damage has been driven by an increasing elucidation of the DNA damage response (DDR). Cells have evolved complex processes to maintain the stability of their genomes in response to genotoxic stress. DDR is activated by a series of interlinked sensor processes signalling to a panel of repair pathways that can attempt to repair the genomic damage [1,2]. For direct ionising radiation damage to DNA, complex lesions consisting of localised clusters of base damages and strand breaks pose significant challenges for the repair machinery and lead to a high probability of chromosomal damage and cell killing [3].

Recent studies have shown compelling evidence for the activation of DDR by ionising radiation even when radiation is not directly deposited in the DNA within the nucleus. A key approach to this has been the use of microbeams where precise doses of radiation can be delivered to individual cells within a population [4]. For example, bystander responses have been observed where cells that have not been directly irradiated respond to the fact that their neighbours have been exposed. Several groups have reported activation of a DDR response in bystander cells involving γ-H2AX formation and the potential formation of DNA double-strand breaks (DSB) leading to mutations, chromosomal aberrations, and cell death. Our own studies, using both charged-particle and X-ray microbeams, have shown that these bystander responses are activated even when cells are not directly irradiated through the nucleus. Interestingly, the level of bystander response induced is of the same magnitude independent of whether nucleus or cytoplasm is targeted [5].

The Induction of γ-H2AX Foci in Bystander Cells

We and others have previously reported the induction of γ-H2AX foci in nontargeted bystander cells [6–10]. Bystander γ-H2AX foci induction occurred as early as 30 min and up to 48 h after irradiation, and the involvement of reactive oxygen species (ROS) and transforming growth factor (TGF)-$β_1$ in the induction of γ-H2AX foci was shown in primary human astrocytes and T98G glioma cells [7]. The study of ataxia-telangiectasia and Rad3-related (ATR) mutated Seckel cells and matched normal fibroblasts could identify ATR as a central figure within the bystander signalling cascade leading to γ-H2AX foci formation. In contrast, the inhibition of ataxia-telangiectasia mutated (ATM) and DNA-dependent protein kinase (DNA-PK) could not suppress the induction of bystander γ-H2AX foci. ATR, ATM, and DNA-PK are members of the phosphoinositol 3-kinase-like kinase (PIKK) family which act as sensors of DNA damage and translate the signal into responses of cell-cycle arrest and DNA repair [11]. ATR is associated with an activating subunit, ATRIP, which responds to single-stranded DNA-RPA complexes [12] and is recruited to sites of stalled replication and ultraviolet (UV) damage independent of ATM. The phosphorylation and activation of ATM in response to UV treatment or replication fork stalling is ATR dependent [13].

On analysis of the cell-cycle position, it was observed that γ-H2AX bystander foci were restricted to S-phase cells, supporting the hypothesis of an accumulation of DNA damage at stalled replication forks in bystander cells that induces γ-H2AX foci in an ATR-dependent manner.

This hypothesis is strengthened by the recent report of H2AX phosphorylation at sites of gemcitabine-induced stalled replication forks [14] and agrees with the earlier studies of Little et al. [15] pointing to an accumulation of oxidative damage at stalled replication forks as being a key event in bystander responses.

Reduced Clonogenic Survival in Bystander Cells

Our most recent results [16] have demonstrated the radiation-induced decrease in clonogenic survival in ATR/ATM-proficient bystander cells and a complete abrogation of this effect in ATR/ATM- but not DNA-PK-deficient cells. We conclude that both ATR and ATM participate in bystander signalling, leading to decreased survival in nontargeted cells. In contrast, in directly targeted cells survival decreased upon ATR, ATM, and DNA-PK inhibition, suggesting the possibility of a differential modulation of targeted and nontargeted effects through ATM and ATR inhibitors. We could also demonstrate an ATR-dependent phosphorylation of ATM (S1981) in bystander cells, placing ATM downstream of ATR in the radiation-induced bystander signalling network. Further work is required to elucidate the interaction of these damage-sensing and signalling pathways with DNA repair. What is clear from several studies is that the nonhomologous end-joining pathway plays a major role in the bystander response, because if this route is inhibited or knocked down, increased yields of DSB are observed, leading to increased mutations [17] and chromosome aberrations [15]. The role of homologous recombination in the bystander response is not yet clear and requires further investigation.

Cytoplasmic Responses to Radiation Exposure

It has long been assumed that direct interaction of radiation with nuclear DNA drives downstream biological responses. For bystander responses, doses as low as 5 mGy of low linear energy transfer (low-LET) X-rays have been shown to trigger the response [18]. At this dose, the initial level of DNA damage within the irradiated (targeted) cell will be very low with around 5 single-strand breaks, 10–15 base damages, and only 1 DSB in every five cells induced. In a review in 2002 [19], Ward speculated as to likely mechanisms involved in the initiation of damage in irradiated cells which lead to the bystander effect. He postulated a potential role for hydrated electrons produced by radiation interaction with water [20], low-energy electrons produced from individual electron tracks [21], and autooxidation processes leading to changes in spontaneous levels of damage within targeted cells [22]. Each of these roles invoked a requirement for direct damage to DNA within the irradiated cell. Other potential candidates could be the production of long-lived DNA or protein radicals, which have half-lives extending to several hours and have been shown to be capable of producing mutations and cell transformation [23,24].

Against this background, an important observation has been the recent evidence that direct irradiation of the cell nucleus is not required for the triggering of the bystander response. In our own studies, we exposed radioresistant glioma cells to precise numbers of helium ions delivered from the Gray Cancer Institute Charged Particle Microbeam [5]. We found that micronuclei, which are indicative of chromosome damage, were induced in bystander cells even when only the cell cytoplasm had been targeted. Crucially, the yield of micronuclei was independent of whether energy was deposited only in the cytoplasm or through the nucleus (which includes the underlying and overlying layers of cytoplasm). This observation means that direct energy deposition within DNA is not required to trigger a bystander response. Similar effects have been observed in exposed V79 hamster cells and primary human fibroblasts (Schettino, personal communication). Other cellular targets could thus play a role in triggering a bystander response. It is already known that irradiation of the cytoplasm in every cell using α-particles from a microbeam induces mutations and that ROS play a role under these conditions [25]. Our own studies have compared the effect of irradiating every cell, or selected cells through the cytoplasm, measuring a bystander effect as chromosomal damage. Surprisingly, we found no difference in the yield of cells with micronuclei, irrespective of the number of cells targeted [5]. In recent experiments, we have also shown evidence for early induction of DNA damage markers after cytoplasmic irradiation. In particular, we have followed the formation of nuclear foci of the DNA damage-sensing protein 53BP1 [26]. Irradiation of every cell only through the cytoplasm leads to increased 53BP1 foci formation in cells 3 h later. Significantly, when bystander cells were monitored after just a fraction of cells had been irradiated only through the cytoplasm, a similar level of 53BP1 foci induction was observed. This finding suggests that there may be commonality between the cellular response to nonnuclear damage and bystander signals.

These studies also substantiate the assumption that targets outside the nucleus play a role in the response to radiation exposure. A potential site could be the cell membrane, where ceramide-dependent signalling has been reported after irradiation [27]; additionally, initiation of free radical processes via activation of plasma membrane-bound NADPH oxidase could play a role [28,29]. Other subcellular organelles could be targets; for example, radiation-induced activation of mitochondria-dependent pathways [30] has been implicated in the induction of apoptosis, but this has not been proven in cellular systems. Potentially, damage to mitochondria may lead to leakage of ROS or changes in calcium fluxes leading to increased ROS [31,32] and downstream induction of DNA damage via oxidative processes.

Recent studies from our own group suggest a role for TGF-β_1 in the induction of DNA damage in bystander cells presumably linked to ROS production [7,33]. In our recent work it has become clear that mitochondria are involved in the production of both cytoplasmic and bystander responses and thus may be key targets of radiation exposure [26].

Conclusion

Overall, these studies are changing our views of radiation responses in cells and tissues, leading to a more comprehensive appreciation of DDR in the maintenance of genomic stability. It is clear that multiple signalling pathways interact with DDR and that unravelling these processes may provide new insights into mechanisms underpinning risk after low-dose radiation exposure.

Acknowledgments. The author acknowledges the support of Cancer Research UK [CUK] grant number C1513/A7047, the European NOTE project (FI6R 036465), and the U.S. National Institutes of Health (5P01CA095227-02).

References

1. Jackson SP (2002) Sensing and repairing DNA double-strand breaks. Carcinogenesis (Oxf) 23:687–696
2. Harper JW, Elledge SJ (2007) The DNA damage response: ten years after. Mol Cell 28:739–745
3. Hall EJ, Giaccia AJ (2006) Radiobiology for the radiologist. Lippincott William & Wilkins, Philadelphia
4. Folkard M, Prise KM, Michette AG (2007) The use of radiation microbeams to investigate the bystander effect in cells and tissues. Nucl Instrum Methods Phys Res Sect A–Accelerators Spectrometers Detectors Assoc Equip 580:446–450
5. Shao C, Folkard M, Michael BD, et al (2004) Targeted cytoplasmic irradiation induces bystander responses. Proc Natl Acad Sci U S A 101:13495–13500
6. Sokolov MV, Smilenov LB, Hall EJ, et al (2005) Ionizing radiation induces DNA double-strand breaks in bystander primary human fibroblasts. Oncogene 24:7257–7265
7. Burdak-Rothkamm S, Short SC, Folkard M, et al (2007) ATR-dependent radiation-induced gamma-H2AX foci in bystander primary human astrocytes and glioma cells. Oncogene 26:993–1002
8. Han W, Wu L, Chen S, et al (2007) Constitutive nitric oxide acting as a possible intercellular signaling molecule in the initiation of radiation-induced DNA double strand breaks in non-irradiated bystander cells. Oncogene 26:2330–2339
9. Yang H, Asaad N, Held KD (2005) Medium-mediated intercellular communication is involved in bystander responses of X-ray-irradiated normal human fibroblasts. Oncogene 24:2096–2103
10. Hu B, Wu L, Han W, et al (2006) The time and spatial effects of bystander response in mammalian cells induced by low dose radiation. Carcinogenesis (Oxf) 27:245–251
11. Rouse J, Jackson SP (2002) Interfaces between the detection, signaling, and repair of DNA damage. Science 297:547–551

12. Zou L, Elledge SJ (2003) Sensing DNA damage through ATRIP recognition of RPA-ssDNA complexes. Science 300:1542–1548
13. Stiff T, Walker SA, Cerosaletti K, et al (2006) ATR-dependent phosphorylation and activation of ATM in response to UV treatment or replication fork stalling. EMBO J 25:5775–5782
14. Ewald B, Sampath D, Plunkett W (2007) H2AX phosphorylation marks gemcitabine-induced stalled replication forks and their collapse upon S-phase checkpoint abrogation. Mol Cancer Ther 6:1239–1248
15. Little JB, Nagasawa H, Li GC, et al (2003) Involvement of the nonhomologous end joining DNA repair pathway in the bystander effect for chromosomal aberrations. Radiat Res 159:262–267
16. Burdak-Rothkamm S, Rothkamm K, Prise KM (2008) ATM acts downstream of ATR in the DNA damage response signaling of bystander cells. Cancer Res 68:7059–7065
17. Zhang Y, Zhou J, Held KD, et al (2008) Deficiencies of double-strand break repair factors and effects on mutagenesis in directly gamma-irradiated and medium-mediated bystander human lymphoblastoid cells. Radiat Res 169:197–206
18. Mothersill C, Seymour CB (2002) Bystander and delayed effects after fractionated radiation exposure. Radiat Res 158:626–633
19. Ward JF (2002) The radiation induced lesions which trigger the bystander effect. Mutat Res 499:151–154
20. Willson RL (1970) The reaction of oxygen with radiation-induced free radicals in DNA and related compounds. Int J Radiat Biol Relat Stud Phys Chem Med 17:349–358
21. Boudaiffa B, Cloutier P, Hunting D, et al (2000) Resonant formation of DNA strand breaks by low-energy (3 to 20 eV) electrons. Science 287:1658–1660
22. Ward JF (1995) Radiation mutagenesis: the initial DNA lesions responsible. Radiat Res 142:362–368
23. Koyama S, Kodama S, Suzuki K, et al (1998) Radiation-induced long-lived radicals which cause mutation and transformation. Mutat Res 421:45–54
24. Kumagai J, Masui K, Itagaki Y, et al (2003) Long-lived mutagenic radicals induced in mammalian cells by ionizing radiation are mainly localized to proteins. Radiat Res 160:95–102
25. Wu LJ, Randers-Pehrson G, Xu A, et al (1999) Targeted cytoplasmic irradiation with alpha particles induces mutations in mammalian cells. Proc Natl Acad Sci U S A 96:4959–4964
26. Tartier L, Gilchrist S, Burdak-Rothkamm S, et al (2007) Cytoplasmic irradiation induces mitochondrial-dependent 53BP1 protein relocalization in irradiated and bystander cells. Cancer Res 67:5872–5879
27. Haimovitz-Friedman A, Kan CC, Ehleiter D, et al (1994) Ionizing radiation acts on cellular membranes to generate ceramide and initiate apoptosis. J Exp Med 180:525–535
28. Narayanan PK, Goodwin EH, Lehnert BE (1997) Alpha-particles initiate biological production of superoxide anions and hydrogen peroxide in human cells. Cancer Res 57:3963–3971
29. Spitz DR, Azzam EI, Li JJ, et al (2004) Metabolic oxidation/reduction reactions and cellular responses to ionizing radiation: a unifying concept in stress response biology. Cancer Metastasis Rev 23:311–322
30. Taneja N, Tjalkens R, Philbert MA, et al (2001) Irradiation of mitochondria initiates apoptosis in a cell free system. Oncogene 20:167–177
31. Leach JK, Van Tuyle G, Lin PS, et al (2001) Ionizing radiation-induced, mitochondria-dependent generation of reactive oxygen/nitrogen. Cancer Res 61:3894–3901
32. Shao C, Lyng FM, Folkard M, et al (2006) Calcium fluxes modulate the radiation-induced bystander responses in targeted glioma and fibroblast cells. Radiat Res 166:479–487
33. Shao C, Folkard M, Prise KM (2008) Role of TGF-beta-1 and nitric oxide in the bystander response of irradiated glioma cells. Oncogene 27:434–440

The Role of Telomere Dysfunction in Driving Genomic Instability

Susan M. Bailey[1,2,3], Eli S. Williams[2], and Robert L. Ullrich[1,2,3]

Summary. The mechanistic role of radiation-induced genomic instability in radiation carcinogenesis is an attractive hypothesis that remains to be rigorously tested. There are few in vivo studies on which to base judgments, but work in our laboratory with mouse models of radiogenic mammary neoplasia provided the first indications that certain forms of genetically predisposed radiation-induced genomic instability may contribute to tumor development. Most recently, we have focused on the induction of telomere dysfunction following exposure to ionizing radiation and the role of DNA-PKcs in this process. In the present studies, characterization of dysfunctional telomeres in DNA-PKcs-deficient backgrounds, including BALB/c, provides evidence supporting our model that these uncapped telomeres behave as double-strand breaks (DSBs), despite the presence of an ample telomeric sequence. Further, we demonstrate that inappropriate interstitial telomeric sequence at sites of DSBs involves the nonhomologous end-joining (NHEJ) pathway and that autophosphorylation of DNA-PKcs plays an important role. Thus, impaired telomere function, as a significant source of spontaneous and radiation-induced chromosomal instability, has the potential to contribute to the cancer-prone phenotype associated with even partial DSB repair deficiency.

Key words Carcinogenesis · Radiation · Telomeres · Genomic instability · DNA repair

Introduction

The mechanistic role of radiation-induced genomic instability in radiation carcinogenesis is an attractive hypothesis that remains to be rigorously tested. There are few in vivo studies on which to base judgments, but work in our laboratory with

---

[1]Cancer SuperCluster, Colorado State University, Fort Collins, CO 80523, USA
[2]Cell and Molecular Biology Program, Colorado State University, Fort Collins, CO, USA
[3]Department of Environmental and Radiological Health, College of Veterinary Medicine and Biological Sciences, Colorado State University, Fort Collins, CO, USA

the BALB/c mouse model of radiogenic mammary neoplasia provided the first indications that certain forms of genetically predisposed radiation-induced genomic instability may contribute to tumor development.

The central goal of this research project is to more firmly establish the mechanistic basis of this radiation-associated genomic instability and, from this, to assess whether such induced instability might play a major role in tumorigenesis at low doses of low linear energy transfer (low-LET) radiation. In the case of BALB/c mouse mammary tumors, susceptibility to induced instability is expressed as an autosomal recessive trait in mammary epithelial cells and is manifest largely as excess chromatid damage [1]. Published studies associate this form of instability with DNA repair deficiency, polymorphic variation in the gene encoding DNA-PKcs (*Prkdc*), and mammary-associated susceptibility [2,3]. The underlying hypothesis being tested in this project is that tumor-associated genomic instability is preferentially expressed in certain recombinogenic genomic domains and that these may be cell lineage- or individual specific.

Our studies have focused on the induction of telomere dysfunction following exposure to ionizing radiation and the role of DNA-PKcs in this process. Telomeres consist of tandem arrays of short, repetitive G-rich sequence bound by a variety of telomere-associated proteins that together form a dynamic terminal structure that "caps" the ends of linear chromosomes, providing protection from illegitimate recombination, exonucleolytic attack and degradation [4]. The cellular importance of functional telomeres is evidenced by the fact that they are essential for continuous cellular proliferation, an observation that has profound implications in our understanding of aging and cancer.

Subjects and Methods

In striking contrast to natural chromosomal termini, broken chromosome ends produced by DNA double-strand breaks (DSBs) are highly recombinogenic, and represent a major threat to the integrity of the cell's genome. As potent inducers of mutations and cell death, DSBs are arguably the most dangerous form of DNA damage. The correct repair of DSBs is essential for maintaining the genetic integrity of the cell, as erroneous repair can lead to chromosomal rearrangements such as translocations, which produce novel juxtapositions of DNA sequences at the exchange breakpoints. Cancer is frequently associated with such chromosomal abnormalities [5].

We have demonstrated that effective telomeric end capping of mammalian chromosomes unexpectedly requires proteins more commonly associated with DNA DSB repair [6]. Ku70/Ku80 and DNA-PKcs all participate in DSB repair through nonhomologous end joining (NHEJ). Mutations in any of these genes cause spontaneous chromosomal end-to-end fusions that maintain large blocks of telomeric sequence at the points of fusion. The fusions, which contribute significantly to the background level of chromosomal aberrations, are not a consequence of telomere shortening, nor are they telomere associations. We have also demonstrated that nascent telomeres produced via leading-strand DNA synthesis are especially susceptible to these end-to-end fusions, suggesting a crucial difference in postreplicative processing of telomeres that is linked to their mode of replication [7].

We have found that impaired end capping in DNA-PKcs-deficient genetic backgrounds not only allows dysfunctional telomeres to join to one another (telomere–telomere fusion), but also to broken chromosome ends created by radiation-induced DSBs (telomere–DSB fusion) [8]. In initial studies, DNA-PKcs-deficient cells from mice having the *scid* mutation were exposed to graded doses of γ-rays, a potent inducer of DSBs. The strand-specific molecular cytogenetic technique of chromosome-orientation fluorescence in situ hybridization (CO-FISH) was utilized to distinguish true telomere–DSB events from telomere–telomere fusions [9]. Both types of end-joining events were observed, but only telomere–DSB fusions were induced by radiation, and this in a dose-dependent, linear fashion [10]. Our results demonstrated for the first time that the radiation-sensitive phenotype of *scid* cells is not solely the result of ineffective repair of DSB. Rather, telomere–DSB misjoining provides an additional pathway for misrepair in *scid* cells that does not exist in repair-proficient cells. These novel chromosomal rearrangements, which inappropriately maintain interstitial blocks of telomere sequence, are expected to have unusual properties whose consequences for the cell are not well understood. Interstitial telomere sequences have been shown to be a source of instability [11]. Importantly, telomere–DSB fusion removes just one of the two ends created by a DSB, thereby rendering the remaining broken end capable of driving ongoing chromosomal instability [12]. It is also noteworthy that telomere–DSB fusions only require a single ionizing radiation-induced DSB, a process that will influence the shape of the dose–response curve in unpredictable ways at low doses.

Results and Discussion

Our work supports a link between partial deficiency of DNA-PKcs, impaired telomeric end capping, and the radiogenic breast cancer-prone phenotype of BALB/c mice. Examination of mammary epithelial clones revealed telomere fusion events in a tumorigenic clone. Continued investigation utilizing the BALB/c mouse model has not only confirmed the presence of telomere–telomere fusion, but has also demonstrated a dose response for telomere–DSB fusion in BALB/c mouse mammary cells that rivals and even surpasses dicentric formation. Additionally, we now have evidence suggesting that, following exposure to low doses of γ-rays, telomere fusion events in the BALB/c background of partial DNA-PKcs deficiency contribute to delayed instability in mouse mammary epithelial cells.

To identify chromosomes involved in BALB/c telomere–DSB fusions, as well as to characterize any clonal rearrangements, an essential aspect of demonstrating the oncogenic potential of these novel fusion events, we developed an approach to combine mouse SKY (spectral karyotyping) with telomere CO-FISH (termed

SKYCO-FISH). Preliminary comparisons of side-by-side images revealed a clonal translocation (8:12) possessing a CO-FISH telomere-DSB signal/pattern at the translocation breakpoint. Another approach we are using to determine loci involved in instability and tumorigenesis in mouse mammary cells has been to analyze radiation-altered cells using BAC-CGH array technology. Comparison of BALB/c normal mammary versus mammary tumor DNA revealed an amplification on chromosome 11 (BAC D11MIT253) that corresponds to a region previously identified by DePinho's group as recurring in mouse adenocarcinomas, and additionally has synteny to human 17q 25.1, a region frequently amplified in breast carcinoma [13].

We continue characterization of dysfunctional telomeres in DNA-PKcs deficient backgrounds, including BALB/c, and have additional evidence supporting our model that these uncapped telomeres behave as DSBs, despite the presence of ample telomeric sequence. One particularly revealing approach has been to combine immunofluorescence detection of the damage response factor γ-H2AX with telomere FISH to identify telomere dysfunction foci (TIFs) [14]. In agreement with our molecular cytogenetic analyses, colocalization of γ-H2AX foci and telomere signals in S-phase interphase nuclei demonstrates that telomeres are experiencing end-capping failure following replication and are triggering a γ-H2AX DSB damage response. We have previously demonstrated that the kinase activity of DNA-PKcs is required for effective telomeric end-capping function [15]. Utilizing another specific inhibitor of DNA-PKcs kinase activity in Ligase IV–/– mouse cells, we now confirm that telomere fusion is mediated by NHEJ; that is, they require LigIV. These studies provide new mechanistic insight, but they also suggest that the telomere phenotype of DNA-PK deficiency is underestimated because the pathway responsible for telomere fusion formation is the same one that creates the dysfunction.

Most recently, we have explored the telomeric roles of newly identified DNA-PKcs autophosphorylation sites/clusters. We find that autophosphorylation of Thr-2609, but not Ser-2056, is an important in vivo target for DNA-PKcs end-capping function at mammalian telomeres. Our results fit the proposed reciprocal action of these two autophosphorylation sites, separating function of end-processing versus end-joining [16]. They also suggest a possible mechanism of DNA-PKcs action at telomeres and, therefore, in preserving genomic stability.

Conclusions

Impaired telomere function, as a significant source of spontaneous and radiation-induced chromosomal instability, has the potential to contribute to the cancer-prone phenotype associated with even partial DSB repair deficiency [17]. Beyond their established role in maintaining the lengths of terminal sequences, telomeres have additional critical capping functions that influence both chromosomal radiosensitivity and preservation of genomic stability. Increasing our understanding of previously unrecognized relationships between the radiation/DNA damage response and telomere function will facilitate predicting the carcinogenic risk of exposure to low doses of ionizing radiation.

References

1. Ponnaiya B, Cornforth MN, Ullrich RL (1997) Radiation-induced chromosomal instability in BALB/c and C57BL/6 mice: the difference is as clear as black and white. Radiat Res 147:121–125
2. Yu Y, Okayasu R, Weil MM, et al (2001) Elevated breast cancer risk in irradiated BALB/c mice associates with unique functional polymorphism of the Prkdc (DNA-dependent protein kinase catalytic subunit) gene. Cancer Res 61:1820–1824
3. Okayasu R, Suetomi K, Yu Y, et al (2000) A deficiency in DNA repair and DNA-PKcs expression in the radiosensitive BALB/c mouse. Cancer Res 60:4342–4345
4. de Lange T (2005) Shelterin: the protein complex that shapes and safeguards human telomeres. Genes Dev 19:2100–2110
5. Mitelman F (2000) Recurrent chromosome aberrations in cancer. Mutat Res 462:247–253
6. Bailey SM, Meyne J, Chen DJ, et al (1999) DNA double-strand break repair proteins are required to cap the ends of mammalian chromosomes. Proc Natl Acad Sci U S A 96:14899–14904
7. Bailey SM, Cornforth MN, Kurimasa A, et al (2001) Strand-specific postreplicative processing of mammalian telomeres. Science 293:2462–2465
8. Bailey SM, Cornforth MN, Ullrich RL, et al (2004) Dysfunctional mammalian telomeres join with DNA double-strand breaks. DNA Repair 3:349–357
9. Bailey SM, Goodwin EH, Cornforth MN (2004) Strand-specific fluorescence in situ hybridization: the CO-FISH family. Cytogenet Genome Res 107:14–17
10. Bailey SM, Cornforth MN (2007) Telomeres and DNA double-strand breaks: ever the twain shall meet? Cell Mol Life Sci 64:2956–2964
11. Kilburn AE, Shea MJ, Sargent RG, et al (2001) Insertion of a telomere repeat sequence into a mammalian gene causes chromosome instability. Mol Cell Biol 21:126–135
12. Sabatier L, Ricoul M, Pottier G, et al (2005) The loss of a single telomere can result in instability of multiple chromosomes in a human tumor cell line. Mol Cancer Res 3:139–150
13. DePinho RA, Polyak K (2004) Cancer chromosomes in crisis. Nat Genet 36:932–934
14. Takai H, Smogorzewska A, de Lange T (2003) DNA damage foci at dysfunctional telomeres. Curr Biol 13:1549–1556
15. Bailey SM, Brenneman MA, Halbrook J, et al (2004) The kinase activity of DNA-PK is required to protect mammalian telomeres. DNA Repair 3:225–233
16. Meek K, Douglas P, Cui X, et al (2007) Trans-autophosphorylation at DNA-dependent protein kinase's two major autophosphorylation site clusters facilitates end processing but not end joining, Mol Cell Biol 27:3881–3890
17. Zhang Y, Zhou J, Cao X, et al (2007) Partial deficiency of DNA-PKcs increases ionizing radiation-induced mutagenesis and telomere instability in human cells. Cancer Lett 250:63–73

Secretory Clusterin Is a Marker of Tumor Progression Regulated by IGF-1 and Wnt Signaling Pathways

Yonglong Zou, Eva M. Goetz, Masatoshi Suzuki, and David A. Boothman

Summary. Secretory clusterin (sCLU) is a pro-survival factor that can be induced by cellular stress, including ionizing radiation (IR), many cytotoxic agents, and during cellular replicative or low doses of stress-induced senescence. sCLU expression changes with tumor stage and grade in various types of cancer. Previously our laboratory found that sCLU was induced by IR through activation of the IGF-1R/Src/MEK/Erk/Egr-1 pathway. APC loss in Min–/– mice was also linked to elevated sCLU expression, especially in human colon cancer. We now find that Wnt signaling can cross talk with IGF-1 signaling to regulate sCLU expression. The cross talk between the IGF-1 and Wnt signaling pathways is very complex, not only because they share many components but also because they are delicately regulated by time, dose, and cell type. Both positive and negative feedback regulation loops regulate sCLU expression. Understanding these complicated signaling pathways will be essential for delineating the roles of Wnt, IGF-1, and sCLU expression in tumor progression, aging, and cancer, as well as in heart and Alzheimer's diseases aberrant where sCLU expression has been implicated.

Key words Clusterin · IGF-1 · Wnt · TGF-β_1 · GSK3β · β-catenin · TCF · APC · Egr-1

Introduction

Secretory clusterin (sCLU) is a glycosylated protein found in all bodily fluids. sCLU is also known as apolipoprotein J, the testosterone repressed prostate message-2 (TRPM-2), sulfated glycoprotein-2 (SGP-2), and X-ray-inducible transcript leading to protein-8 (xip8) [1]. sCLU has many important functions noted by its involvement in various physiological processes, such as immune regulation, cell adhesion, morphological transformation, lipid transportation, tissue remodeling, membrane recycling, and cell–cell interactions [2].

Laboratory of Molecular Stress Responses, Program in Cell Stress and Cancer Nanomedicine, Department of Oncology, Simmons Comprehensive Cancer Center, University of Texas Southwestern Medical Center at Dallas, ND 2.210k, TX 75390-8807, USA

sCLU expression is up-regulated after cell injury and stress, including after stroke or heart attack, and in cells and tissues treated with cytotoxic or cytostatic agents [3,4]. sCLU expression has been implicated in cellular senescence, early carcinogenesis, and in later steps of tumor progression [5,6]. Endogenous overexpression of sCLU in human colon, prostate, and breast cancers was linked to increased aggressiveness and metastatic ability [2].

Insulin-like growth factor (IGF)-1 induces sCLU expression through the IGF-1R/Src/Erk/Egr-1 pathway; however, the p53 tumor suppressor can greatly repress sCLU expression [4,7]. One possible mechanism is that IGF-1/Akt signaling enhances Mdm2-mediated ubiquitination and degradation of p53, which could cause upregulation of sCLU [8].

Wnt genes encode a family of secreted proteins that are important in development and maintenance of adult tissues. Abnormalities in Wnt signaling promote both human degenerative diseases and cancer [9]. Since adenomatous polyposis coli (APC/Min) knockout mice have elevated gastrointestinal sCLU expression [10] and APC suppresses Wnt signaling, we hypothesized that Wnt signaling may influence sCLU expression. In this review, we discuss our published and unpublished data in which cross talk between IGF-1 and Wnt pathways plays a major role in the complex regulatory mechanisms that controls sCLU expression.

IGF-1 and Wnt Pathways Share Important Components

Recent data from our laboratory strongly suggest that glycogen synthase kinase 3β (GSK-3β) is not only an important component of the IGF-1 signaling pathway but also plays a key inhibitory role in the Wnt signaling pathway. Treatment of cells with reagents such as insulin/IGF-1 or Wnt causes inactivation of GSK-3β [11,12], although mechanisms of inactivation differ between stimuli. In resting cells, GSK-3β is constitutively active and phosphorylates β-catenin, causing degradation of β-catenin and inhibition of downstream Wnt signaling [12]. GSK-3β also phosphorylates other Wnt components, such as Axin, APC, and T cell factor (TCF) [13,14]. Because these are important factors in downstream Wnt signaling, phosphorylation of these substrates, in turn, prevents transactivation of Wnt target genes. However, after insulin and/or IGF-1 stimulation, the PI3-K/Akt/GSK-3β pathway may not be the sole pathway to mediate lymphoid enhancer-binding factor 1 (LEF1/TCF)-dependent transcription, as the Ras/Raf/MEK1 pathway can also be a redundant pathway playing a role in its signaling [15–17].

Stimulation of the Wnt receptor activates Frizzled receptor signaling, which then triggers Disheveled (Dvl) and Frat activity [18,19], regulating the function of β-catenin. β-Catenin is the key mediator of Wnt signaling, and mutations in β-catenin that prevent its phosphorylation by GSK-3β are common in colon, prostate, liver, and ovarian cancers [20]. GSK-3β often requires a priming kinase to make a substrate more suitable for further phosphorylation [21]. Casein kinase I (CKI) can act as one of the priming kinases, and phosphorylates β-catenin on Ser45, priming it for further phosphorylation on Ser41, -37, and -33 by GSK-3β in a sequential manner, thereby allowing β-catenin to be ubiquitinated for proteasomal degradation [22]. In the presence of Wnt, activated Frizzled receptor initially leads to formation of a complex between Dvl, Frat, Axin, and GSK-3β that results in inactivation of GSK-3β [23,24]. As a consequence, β-catenin is not phosphorylated. As a result, stabilized β-catenin then enters the nucleus to interact with TCFs, leading to transactivation of Wnt downstream genes.

In contrast to Wnt signaling where GSK-3β is sequestered, IGF-1 treatment causes phosphorylation of Ser9 on GSK-3β, which inactivates the enzyme [11]. It has been discovered that Wnt and IGF-1/AKT signaling pathways affect two distinct pools of GSK-3β that, in turn, target different substrates [25]. Thus, IGF-1/AKT signaling alone cannot initiate the Wnt pathway, but it can potentiate Wnt signaling [26,27].

Epithelial-to-Mesenchymal Transition (EMT) Caused by IGF-1 and Wnt Pathways

Tumor metastasis is the most common cause of death in cancer patients. It is a major problem in breast and prostate cancers, where the primary cancers have been controlled by therapy. The first step of metastasis requires epithelial-to-mesenchymal transition (EMT) [28]. Both IGF-1 and Wnt signaling are known to be involved in EMT responses [29]. It is generally accepted that both loss of E-cadherin and increased levels of vimentin are representative markers of EMT responses in most cell types [30]. Although EMT is developmentally important for diverse processes during tissue formation and organogenesis, cancer cells treated with different ligands such as IGF-1, Wnt, and transforming growth factor (TGF)-$β_1$ also undergo EMT [31]. These common ligands usually required for cell growth or differentiation can actually promote EMT responses and tumor metastasis under certain circumstances. Thus, it may be important to suppress these signaling pathways and subsequent EMT responses in tumor cells to prevent tumor metastasis.

Cell–cell junction reorganization is a crucial step in cells undergoing an EMT response [30]. In resting cells, the IGF-1R forms a membrane complex with E-cadherin and β-catenin in coated pits, and this aggregate is quickly internalized in response to IGF-1 stimulation [32]. Consequentially, IGF-1R is either degraded (via Nedd4 and MDM2 ubiquitination) or recycled to the cell surface, but E-cadherin is trapped in organelles surrounding the nucleus and eventually concentrated within the nucleus [33,34]. In contrast, IGF-1 signaling can promote phosphorylation of E-cadherin and β-catenin, which is a main regulatory pathway for association between these two proteins. Induction or activation of IGF-1 signaling can lead to activation of Src, which then phosphorylates β-catenin on tyrosine 654, disrupting the E-cadherin–β-catenin complex on the membrane [35]. Thus, Src activation can promote reshaping of the cells, an important step in EMT.

β-Catenin is not only involved in cell–cell adhesion but also serves as a mediator of Wnt signaling. β-Catenin forms a complex with TCFs to transactivate downstream genes, including vimentin. β-Catenin phosphorylation is not only critical for E-cadherin–β-catenin interaction but is also important for association between TCF and β-catenin transcriptional complex formation. Phosphorylated residues involved in the interaction between TCF and β-catenin are the same as those required for E-cadherin and β-catenin [36]. Thus, IGF-1/Src signaling can induce β-catenin phosphorylation and disrupt the TCF/β–catenin transcriptional complex.

Another downstream signaling molecule of the IGF-1R signaling cascade, Akt, is also involved in the Wnt signaling pathway. The distribution of β-catenin within the plasma membrane, cytoplasm, and nucleus can be regulated by AKT [37]. In epithelial cells, which do not express an exogenously active form of AKT, most of the β-catenin is present at the plasma membrane bound by E-cadherin. In cells expressing an active exogenous form of AKT, β-catenin was localized to the cytoplasm, even though the total amount of β-catenin was lower in cells expressing exogenous AKT than in parental cells [37].

It was recently reported that TGF-$β_1$ treatment promoted the translocation of β-catenin from cytosol to nuclei in a Smad3-dependent manner [38], indicating that there might be some similarities or cross talk between downstream pathways of TGF-$β_1$, IGF-1, and Wnt. Both IGF-1 and Wnt signaling pathways repress E-cadherin, which is required to keep cells in a mesenchymal state. Short-term exposure to IGF-1 induces a slight degradation of extracellular E-cadherin, probably as a result of post-translational regulation of E-cadherin in lysosomes [39]. In contrast, the long-term effect of IGF-1 treatment on E-cadherin expression was evaluated by expressing a constitutively active form of AKT. The constitutively active AKT pathway activated NF-κB to transactivate Snail, a major repressor of E-cadherin, lowering E-cadherin levels [40]. The role of AKT/NF-κB/Snail signaling on E-cadherin loss during EMT was validated by showing that active NF-κB subunit p65 alone was sufficient to cause an EMT response [41]. Opposing NF-κB, GSK-3β is a known endogenous inhibitor of Snail. GSK-3β phosphorylates Snail at two consensus motifs and suppresses Snail function. Inhibition of GSK-3β by AKT results in the upregulation of Snail and downregulation of E-cadherin in vivo [42].

Interestingly, suppression of E-cadherin function leads to retarded cellular proliferation and reduced viability from unknown Akt and mitogen-activated protein kinase (MAPK) inhibition [43], indicating that there could be a feedback loop between IGF-1/AKT signaling and alterations of cell–cell adhesion.

Regulation of sCLU by IGF-1 and Wnt

Our laboratory previously reported that p53 suppressed sCLU [7]. IGF-1 stimulation activates MDM2 (via Akt-dependent phosphorylation of Ser168) and stabilizes MDM2 (by an unknown mechanism) to enhance Mdm2-mediated ubiquitination and degradation of p53 [8]. Taken together, our data suggest that sCLU repression by p53 may be relived by IGF-1 treatment. Furthermore, we reported that Egr-1 was the transcription factor necessary for sCLU expression, and that blocking Egr-1 function abrogated sCLU induction [1]. It was originally thought that Wnt signaling would induce sCLU, as APC/min-deficient mice have higher sCLU expression [10]. However, Wnt signaling has been shown to suppress Egr-1 function in mouse breast epithelial cells [44], suggesting that Wnt signaling pathway may actually suppress sCLU. Our recent studies have shown that blocking any factor in the IGF-1R/Src/MAPK/Egr-1 pathway will decrease basal and inducible expression levels of sCLU, strongly suggesting that sCLU was solely downstream from the IGF-1R signaling pathway [1]. Any alteration of sCLU expression by Wnt is, therefore, likely the result of some unknown interaction between Wnt and IGF-1 signaling pathways. Furthermore, TGF-β_1 was shown to induce rat sCLU expression [45], indicating that there may be cross-talk between IGF-1 and TGF-β_1 signaling pathways. Interestingly, sCLU also bound and inhibited TGF-β_1 receptor I and II, indicating there may be a negative feedback regulation loop for sCLU expression [46].

Taken together, the IGF-1, Wnt, and TGF-β pathways can converge and cross talk to give a steady-state expression of sCLU. Cross talk between IGF-1, Wnt, and TGF-β_1 pathways has been implied in many studies. For example, inhibition of GSK3-β activity by Wnt signaling pathway causes stabilization of Samd3 and increases the cellular sensitivity to TGF-β [47]. Also, TGF-β_1 enhances growth in certain cells by an unknown mechanism of activation of the IGF-1/MAPK pathway [48,49]. The interaction between IGF-1, Wnt, or even TGF-β_1 could systematically regulate sCLU expression dependent on cell type, dose, and time of exposure to a given stimulus, including after IR (Fig. 1).

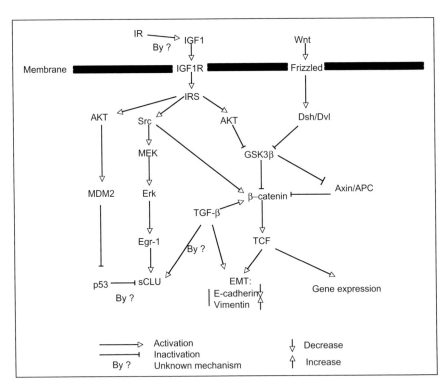

Fig. 1. The cross talk between insulin-like growth factor (IGF)-1, Wnt, and transforming growth factor (TGF)-β_1 pathways

Concluding Remarks

The cross-talk between IGF-1 and Wnt signaling pathways is complex as these pathways share many components that are delicately regulated by time of exposure, dose of stimulus, and context of a given cell type. Furthermore, the downstream signaling pathways stimulated by IGF-1 or Wnt form many positive and/or negative feedback regulation loops. To further study the function of these pathways in cancer cells and during tumor progression, a simple, straightforward endpoint is required. In our laboratory, we have focused on examining the functions of sCLU, which is regulated by IGF-1, TGF-β_1, and, as we recently have shown, Wnt. One of the most important questions we are trying to answer is what is the role of sCLU in EMT responses stimulated by IGF-1, TGF-β_1, or Wnt signaling. Since a prior study showed that the glycosylation inhibitor tunicamycin abolished morphological changes associated with EMT responses induced by TGF-β_1 [50], we hypothesize that sCLU could play a role during the TGF-β_1- or Wnt-induced EMT responses. Indeed, we will soon be reporting the roles of sCLU on tumor metastasis in vivo.

Acknowledgments. This work was supported by Department of Energy (DOE) grant # DE-FG-0221791-16-18 to D.A.B. This is CSCN paper #037.

References

1. Criswell T, Beman M, Araki S, et al (2005) Delayed activation of insulin-like growth factor-1 receptor/Src/MAPK/Egr-1 signaling regulates clusterin expression, a pro-survival factor. J Biol Chem 280:14212–14221
2. Pucci S, Bonanno E, Pichiorri F, et al (2004) Modulation of different clusterin isoforms in human colon tumorigenesis. Oncogene 23:2298–2304
3. Krijnen PAJ, Cillessen SAGM, Manoe R, et al (2005) Clusterin: a protective mediator for ischemic cardiomyocytes? Am J Physiol Heart Circ Physiol 289:H2193–H2202
4. Shannan B, Seifert M, Leskov K, et al (2006) Challenge and promise: roles for clusterin in pathogenesis, progression and therapy of cancer. Cell Death Differ 13:12–19
5. Suzuki1 M, Goetz EC, Venezianoa G, et al (2007) Secretory clusterin (sCLU) is a hallmark sensor of DNA damage, cell stress, and cellular senescence: evidence for similar regulation of sCLU expression after cellular stress and replicative senescence. Radiation Risk Perspectives: Proceedings of the Second Nagasaki Symposium of International Consortium for Medical Care of Hibakusha and Radiation Life Science 1299:150–157
6. Trougakos IP, Pawelec G, Tzavelas C, et al (2006) Clusterin/Apolipoprotein J up-regulation after zinc exposure, replicative senescence or differentiation of human haematopoietic cells. Biogerontology 7:375–382
7. Criswell T, Klokov D, Beman M, et al (2003) Repression of IR-inducible clusterin expression by the p53 tumor suppressor protein. Cancer Biol Ther 2:372–380
8. Ashcroft M, Ludwig RL, Woods DB, et al (2002) Phosphorylation of HDM2 by Akt. Oncogene 21:1955–1962
9. Ishikawa Y (2005) Wnt signaling and orthopedic diseases. Am J Pathol 167:1–3
10. Chen X, Halberg RB, Ehrhardt WM, et al (2003) Clusterin as a biomarker in murine and human intestinal neoplasia. Proc Natl Acad Sci U S A 100:9530–9535

11. van Weeren PC, de Bruyn KM, de Vries-Smits AM, et al (1998) Essential role for protein kinase B (PKB) in insulin-induced glycogen synthase kinase 3 inactivation. Characterization of dominant-negative mutant of PKB. J Biol Chem 273:13150–13156
12. Rubinfeld B, Albert I, Porfiri E, et al (1996) Binding of GSK3β to the APC-β-catenin complex and regulation of complex assembly. Science 272:1023–1026
13. Hart MJ, de los Santos R, Albert IN, et al (1998) Downregulation of β-catenin by human Axin and its association with the APC tumor suppressor, β-catenin and GSK3 β. Curr Biol 8:573–581
14. Lee E, Salic A, Kirschner MW (2001) Physiological regulation of β-catenin stability by TCF3 and CK1epsilon. J Cell Biol 154:983–993
15. Staal FJT, Burgering BT, van de Wetering M, et al (1999) TCF-1 mediated transcription in T lymphocytes: differential role for glycogen synthase kinase-3 in fibroblasts and T cells. Int Immunol 11:312–317
16. Yuan H, Mao J, Li L, et al (1999) Suppression of glycogen synthase kinase activity is not sufficient for leukemia enhancer factor 1 activation. J Biol Chem 274:30419–30423
17. Christèle D, Axelle C, Marie-José B, et al (2001) Insulin and IGF-1 stimulate the bold-catenin pathway through two signalling cascades involving GSK-3β inhibition and Ras activation. Oncogene 20:252–259
18. Li L, Yuan H, Weaver CD, et al (1999) Axin and Frat1 interact with dvl and GSK, bridging Dvl to GSK in Wnt-mediated regulation of LEF-1. EMBO J 18:4233–4240
19. Yost C, Farr G, Pierce SB, et al (1998) GBP, an inhibitor of GSK-3, is implicated in *Xenopus* development and oncogenesis. Cell 93:1031–1041
20. Polakis P (2000) Wnt signaling and cancer. Genes Dev 14:1837–1851
21. Harwood AJ (2001) Regulation of GSK-3 a cellular multiprocessor. Cell 105:821–824
22. Amit S, Hatzubai A, Birman Y, et al (2002) Axin-mediated CKI phosphorylation of β-catenin at Ser 45: a molecular switch for the Wnt pathway. Genes Dev 16:1066–1076
23. Salic A, Lee E, Mayer L, et al (2000) Control of β-catenin stability: reconstitution of the cytoplasmic steps of the wnt pathway in *Xenopus* egg extracts. Mol Cell 5:523–532
24. Farr GH, Ferkey DM, Yost C, et al (2000) Interaction among GSK-3, GBP, axin, and APC in *Xenopus* axis specification. J Cell Biol 148:691–702
25. Ding VW, Chen RH, McCormick F (2000) Differential regulation of glycogen synthase kinase 3β by insulin and Wnt signaling. J Biol Chem 275:32475–32481
26. Chen RH, Ding WV, McCormick F (2000) Wnt signaling to beta-catenin involves two interactive components. Glycogen synthase kinase-3beta inhibition and activation of protein kinase C. J Biol Chem 275:17894–17899
27. Fukumoto S, Hsieh CM, Maemura K, et al (2001) Akt participation in the Wnt signaling pathway through Dishevelled. J Biol Chem 276:17479–17483
28. Fidler IJ (2003) The pathogenesis of cancer metastasis: the "seed and soil" hypothesis revisited. Nat Rev Cancer 3:453–458
29. Leader M, Collins M, Patel J, et al (1987) Vimentin: an evaluation of its role as a tumour marker. Histopathology (Oxf) 11:63–72
30. Thiery JP (2002) Epithelial-mesenchymal transitions in tumour progression. Nat Rev Cancer 2:442–454
31. Shook D, Keller R (2003) Mechanisms, mechanics and function of epithelial-mesenchymal transitions in early development. Mech Dev 120:1351–1383
32. Morali OG, Delmas V, Moore R, et al (2001) IGF-II induces rapid β-catenin relocation to the nucleus during epithelium to mesenchyme transition. Oncogene 20:4942–4950
33. Vecchione A, Marchese A, Henry P, et al (2003) The Grb10/Nedd4 complex regulates ligand-induced ubiquitination and stability of the insulin-like growth factor I receptor. Mol Cell Biol 23:3363–3372
34. Girnita L, Girnita A, Larsson O (2003) Mdm2-dependent ubiquitination and degradation of the insulin-like growth factor 1 receptor. Proc Natl Acad Sci U S A 100:8247–8252
35. Avizienyte E, Wyke AW, Jones RJ, et al (2002) Src-induced de-regulation of E-cadherin in colon cancer cells requires integrin signalling. Nat Cell Biol 4:632–638

36. Graham TA, Weaver C, Mao F, et al (2000) Crystal structure of a β-catenin/TCF complex. Cell 103:885–896
37. Grille SJ, Bellacosa A, Upson J, et al (2003) The protein kinase Akt induces epithelial mesenchymal transition and promotes enhanced motility and invasiveness of squamous cell carcinoma lines. Cancer Res 63:2172–2178
38. Jian H, Shen X, Liu I, et al (2006) Smad3-dependent nuclear translocation of β-catenin is required for TGF-$β_1$-induced proliferation of bone marrow-derived adult human mesenchymal stem cells. Genes Dev 20:666–674
39. Palacios F, Tushir JS, Fujita Y, et al (2005) Lysosomal targeting of E-cadherin: a unique mechanism for the down-regulation of cell-cell adhesion during epithelial to mesenchymal transitions. Mol Cell Biol 25:389–402
40. Julien S, Puig I, Caretti E, et al (2007) Activation of NF-kappaB by Akt upregulates Snail expression and induces epithelium mesenchyme transition. Oncogene 26:7445–7456
41. Chua HL, Bhat-Nakshatri P, Clare SE, et al (2007) NF-kappaB represses E-cadherin expression and enhances epithelial to mesenchymal transition of mammary epithelial cells: potential involvement of ZEB-1 and ZEB-2. Oncogene 26:711–724
42. Bachelder RE, Yoon SO, Franci C, et al (2005) Glycogen synthase kinase-3 is an endogenous inhibitor of Snail transcription: implications for the epithelial-mesenchymal transition. J Cell Biol 168:29–33
43. Reddy P, Liu L, Ren C, et al (2005) Formation of E-cadherin-mediated cell-cell adhesion activates AKT and mitogen activated protein kinase via phosphatidylinositol 3 kinase and ligand-independent activation of epidermal growth factor receptor in ovarian cancer cells. Mol Endocrinol 19:2564–2578
44. Tice DA, Soloviev I, Polakis P (2002) Activation of the Wnt pathway interferes with serum response element-driven transcription of immediate early genes. J Biol Chem 277:6118–6123
45. Jin G, Howe HP (1997) Regulation of clusterin gene expression by transforming growth factor β. J Biol Chem 272:26620–26626
46. Reddy KB, Karode MC, Harmony AK, et al (1996) Interaction of transforming growth factor β receptors with apolipoprotein J/clusterin. Biochemistry 35:309–314
47. Guo X, Ramirez A, Waddell DS, et al (2008) Axin and GSK3-β control Smad3 protein stability and modulate TGF-signaling. Genes Dev 22:106–120
48. Marcopoulou CE, Vavouraki HN, Dereka XE, et al (2003) Proliferative effect of growth factors TGF-$β_1$, PDGF-BB and rhBMP-2 on human gingival fibroblasts and periodontal ligament cells. J Int Acad Periodontol 5:63–70
49. Yan Z, Deng X, Friedman E (2001) Oncogenic Ki-ras confers a more aggressive colon cancer phenotype through modification of transforming growth factor-β receptor III. J Biol Chem 276:1555–1563
50. Wegrowski Y, Perreau C, Martiny L, et al (1997) Transforming growth factor β-1 up-regulates clusterin synthesis in thyroid epithelial cells. Exp Cell Res 247:475–483

Target of Radiation Carcinogenesis Is Protein: Becoming Triploid Is Proximate Cause of Cell Transformation

Masami Watanabe and Hanako Yoshii

Summary. Although numerical chromosome aberration is closely related to expression of malignant transformation, it is not clear how a change of chromosome number occurs. Here we propose that aneuploidy, which is ubiquitous in cancer and inevitably unbalances thousands of synergistic genes, destabilizes the structure of chromosomes. We obtained primary cells from embryos of the p53 wild-type and p53 knockout (KO) mouse and cultured the cells by 5T10 culture protocol. Both types of cells were easily immortalized, and immortalized p53 wild-type cells became a tetraploid population and immortalized p53 KO cells became a triploid population. In addition, only immortalized p53 KO cells showed tumorigenicity at around 30 passages, but p53 wild-type cells did not do so, even at more than 100 passages. These results strongly suggest that aneuploidy is the cause rather than a consequence of carcinogenesis. Loss of p53 function promotes derivation of aneuploidy closely.

Key words Aneuploidy · Triploidy · Tetraploidy · p53 function · Radiation carcinogenesis

Introduction

It has been believed that the first target of radiation carcinogenesis is DNA. However, this hypothesis is not yet proved for carcinogenesis from low-dose radiation directly. We analyzed our results of research on malignant cell transformation by low-dose radiation during the past 30 years and came to strongly believe that a radiation cancer-causing primary target was not DNA itself. One piece of evidence that supports our thought is that transformation frequency in Syrian hamster embryo (SHE) cells irradiated with a low dose of X-rays is 500–1000 times higher than that of somatic mutation [1,2]. This observation contradicts "the multistage mutation theory" by which carcinogenesis is produced from the accumulation of three

---

Laboratory of Radiation Biology, Department of Radiation Life Science, Research Reactor Institute, Kyoto University, 2-1010 Asashiro-nishi, Sennan-gun, Osaka 590-0494, Japan

to five independent mutations. Transformation frequency, theoretically, should be smaller than independent mutation frequency.

Recently, several reports including our own reports suggested that nontarget effects, such as bystander effect and delayed effect, modify cell transformation frequency [3,4]. From these results, we speculate that nongenetic damage plays an important role in the initial process of cellular malignant transformation. However, another important finding is that this process is strictly inhibited in a human cell in vitro [5]. Therefore, in this study, we were searching for an intracellular target related to carcinogenesis in SHE cells and human embryo cells.

Materials and Methods

Mouse embryonic fibroblast (MEF) cells were derived from 13-day-old embryos of p53 wild-type and p53 knockout C57BL mice. Cells were cultured in Eagle's MEM containing 10% fetal bovine serum by 5T10 culture protocol using a P75 culture flask in a 5% CO_2 incubator. During cultivation, we examined cell growth ability, chromosome aberration, intracellular oxidation level, centrosome structural aberration, and subsequent tumorigenicity. Chromosome aberrations were measured by multicolor fluorescence in situ hybridization (FISH).

Results and Discussion

We found that the degree of intracellular oxidation, such as reactive oxidative radicals and long-lived radicals, was elevated by high-density culture and radiation exposure in both SHE cells and HE cells. These radicals attack several proteins, such as telomere-related protein and centrosome, and destroy their structure [6,7]. Telomere destabilization induces telomere fusion and makes a dicentric chromosome. In fact, the dicentric chromosome is the dominant aberration induced by low-dose radiation [8]. Telomere destabilization causes chromosomal instability by the bridge-fusion-breakage cycle. However, it is very likely that this route is accompanied by chromosomal breakage, produces genetic deficiency, and causes cell death. On the other hand, centrosome destabilization induces nondisjunction and raises the frequency of aneuploidy. Our results suggested that, in the early process of cell transformation, structural aberration of chromosomes does not occur but aneuploidy is seen with high frequency. Because aneuploidy is not accompanied by genome loss, aneuploid cells easily survive. Our results suggested that aneuploidy preceded malignant transformation, but that tetraploidy did not.

These results suggest a possibility that a main target of radiation carcinogenesis is not DNA, but the centromere and centrosome, which are the proteins that constitute the chromosomal homeostasis maintenance mechanism. If our results are correct, the "mutation theory" of carcinogenesis is wrong. We suggest a new

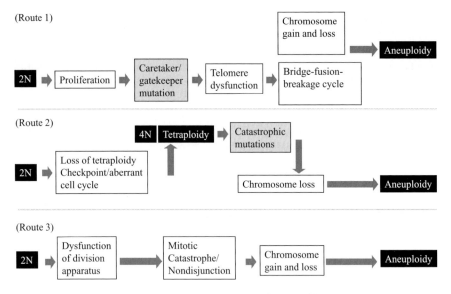

Fig. 1. Three potential mechanisms for the generation of aneuploid cells

hypothesis about radiation carcinogenesis, which we named the "protein-target hypothesis," or, alternatively, the "aneuploidy-cancer hypothesis." As a conclusion of this study, in Fig. 1, we show three potential routes to generate aneuploid cells. Storchova and Pellman [9] suggested that the two upper routes (routes 1 and 2) introduce aneuploidy. In route 1, telomere destabilization promotes telomere fusion and increases the frequency of a dicentric chromosome. It is well known that a dicentric chromosome is lethal. It is likely that aneuploidy is induced by route 2. However, in both routes 1 and 2, mutation is the key event to the process. Using route 1 and 2, therefore, we cannot explain the results that aneuploidy (cell transformation) is generated in higher frequency than mutation. Therefore, we newly add the third route (route 3 in Fig. 1), indicating that the generation of aneuploidy should be the main route for radiation carcinogenesis.

References

1. Watanabe M, Horikawa M, Nikaido O (1984) Induction of oncogenic transformation by low doses of X-rays and dose-rate effect. Radiat Res 98:274–283
2. Watanabe M, Suzuki K (1991) Expression dynamics of transforming phenotypes in X-irradiated Syrian hamster embryo cells. Mutat Res 249:71–80
3. Suzuki K, Yasuda N, Suzuki F, et al (1989) Trisomy of chromosome 9q: specific chromosome change associated with tumorigenicity during the progress of X-ray-induced neoplastic transformation in golden hamster embryo cells. Int J Cancer 44:1057–1061

4. Watanabe M, Suzuki K, Kodama S (1990) Karyotypic changes with neoplastic conversion in morphologically transformed golden hamster embryo cells induced by X-rays. Cancer Res 50:760–765
5. Kodama S, Mori I, Roy K, et al (2001) Culture condition-dependent senescence-like growth arrest and immortalization in rodent embryo cells. Radiat Res 155:254–262
6. Urushibara A, Kodama S, Suzuki K, et al (2004) Involvement of telomere dysfunction in the induction of genomic instability by radiation in scid mouse cells. Biochem Biophys Res Commun 313:1037–1043
7. Undarmaa B, Kodama S, Suzuki K, et al (2004) X-ray-induced telomeric instability in *Atm*-deficient mouse cells. Biochem Biophys Res Commun 315:51–58
8. Roy K, Kodama S, Suzuki K, et al (2000) Hypoxia relieves X-ray-induced delayed effect in normal human embryo cells. Radiat Res 154:659–666
9. Storchova Z, Pellman D (2004) From polyploidy to aneuploidy, genome instability and cancer. Nat Rev Mol Cell Biol 5:45–54

Adult Stem Cells, the Barker Hypothesis, Epigenetic Events, and Low-Level Radiation Effects

James E. Trosko[1] and Keiji Suzuki[2]

Summary. The convergence of new experimental findings, such as human adult stem cells as potential target cells for cancer and the epigenetic effects of oxidative stress-inducing agents, and of old concepts, such as the multi-stage, multi-mechanism process of carcinogenesis and the stem cell theory of cancer, has called into question the linear, no-threshold hypothesis of radiation-induced health effects. Specifically, the integration of the multistage, multiple mechanism concept of carcinogenesis, the stem cell theory of cancer, the Barker effect on prenatal/postnatal development, which affects disease risks later in life, and epigenetic effects induced by low-level exposure to oxidative stress-inducing agents, such as ionizing radiation, the effect of intercellular communication on modifying the effects of ionizing radiation in tissues, and the effect of caloric restriction on reducing risks to chronic diseases, should be all considered in interpreting the risk to exposure to low-level ionizing radiation. All these concepts might help to explain radiation-induced observations of the adaptive response, bystander effects, genomic instability, and the Barker hypothesis.

Key words Stem cells · Radiation-induced epigenetic signaling · Barker hypothesis · Caloric restriction · Oxidative stress · Bystander effect

Introduction: Challenge to the Paradigm of Radiation-Induced Genotoxicity at Low-Level Ionizing Radiation

Until recently, because of the paucity of actual experimental or epidemiological data at low-level ionizing radiation exposure, extrapolation from available experimental in vitro and in vivo animal data and epidemiological data, derived from

---

[1]Department of Pediatrics and Human Development, College of Human Medicine, Michigan State University, East Lansing, MI 48824, USA
[2]Course of Life Science and Radiation Research, Graduate School of Biomedical Sciences, Nagasaki University, Nagasaki, Japan

high-level exposures, involved the use of the genotoxicity paradigm to explain potential health effects that might be the result of such exposures. However, because of theoretical predictions of the suspected genotoxic mechanisms of action of ionizing radiation (e.g., DNA strand breakage, gene and chromosome mutations), as well as many new conceptual ideas of the mechanisms of radiation-induced long-term health effects, such as the carcinogenic process, the current view seems to call into question the linear, no-threshold (LNT) model of low-level radiation [1]. In addition, new insights have been developed as to how past, and many current, in vitro model systems might generate misleading mechanistic interpretations for potential risk extrapolations to human in vivo health effects, such as cancer [2]. Equally important, new insights have been reported related to the factors that might influence the mechanisms of low-level radiation effects on the specific cells which lead to the pathogenesis of the carcinogenic process [3]. This short review offers an alternative interpretation of acute and chronic low-level radiation effects on one potential health consequence by examining (a) the role of adult stem cells as the potential target cells of carcinogenesis [4]; (b) the role of epigenetic signaling on adult stem cells and on the multi-stage, multi-mechanism concept of carcinogenesis [5]; (c) limitations of past two-dimensional in vitro models, using abnormal rodent and human cells grown at abnormal non-in-vivo conditions [6,7]; and (d) the potential roles of environmental and dietary factors in modulating the risk from low-level radiation [5]. We consider how modulation of adult stem cells during prenatal and early postnatal development, that is, the Barker hypothesis [8], might influence low-level radiation health effects.

In addition, the isolation of adult human stem cells and their ability to be neoplastically transformed in vitro [9], together with the discovery of "cancer stem cells" [10], and reported evidence of the derivation of the cancer stem cell from the normal adult stem cell [11], suggest in vitro mechanistic studies on nonstem cells in vitro might have little relevance to in vivo radiation-induced health effects, particularly at low doses.

The convergence of the limitations of nonmeasurable experimental or epidemiologically determined health endpoints related to low-level radiation effects and the many theoretical and experimental findings related to shared molecular mechanisms of radiation and chemical exposures, such as oxidative stress-induced intracellular signaling and epigenetic changes, force a reexamination of the paradigms related to radiation-induced cancer.

Although the prevailing paradigm in radiation carcinogenesis has assumed that radiation-induced DNA damage in cells, measured at high doses, can induce both gene and chromosome mutations (usually non-point mutations, but also chromosome deletions and rearrangements), as well as cell death by either apoptosis or necrosis, the one-"hit" idea of an acute exposure to ionizing radiation (low or high dose) does not fit the current knowledge that carcinogenesis consists of multiple steps and multiple mechanisms.

Although apoptosis is the major mode of cell death in some types of tissue, such as hematopoietic tissue and thymic tissue, most of the mesenchymal and epithelial cells do not induce apoptosis in response to a low dose of ionizing radiation. Also, necrosis is more apparent when cells received higher doses, for example, 10 Gy [12]. Moreover, the ability of ionizing radiation to induce premature senescence has been noted in vitro when human fibroblasts are exposed to high doses of ionizing radiation. Considering what might be the consequence of either cell death by necrosis, apoptosis, or premature senescence in an irradiated tissue, one could see multiple effects on the surviving cells at low or high doses. At low doses in tissues with a few stem cells, many progenitor or transit cells, and terminally differentiated cells, probably little necrosis occurs with any of these three cell types.

At high doses, necrosis and possible induced premature senescence could occur differentially between the cell types. The release of various inflammatory factors from the dead cells could trigger "compensatory hyperplasia" in the surviving adult stem cells and transit cells. On the other hand, communication via a number of signaling mechanisms and molecules from senescent fibroblasts has been shown to promote the growth of epithelial cells [13,14]. At lower nonnecrotic doses, induction of apoptosis and premature senescence could produce a very different scenario. Post irradiation, the stromal–epithelial interaction between normal cells will have been altered such that this new stromal–epithelial interaction might be between premature aged stromal cells and new progenitor and adult stem cells. The potential long-term altered signaling between surviving stromal and epithelial cells might lead to long-term health effects that might not be predicted or interpreted correctly [15]. The long-term effects that might be induced by acute low-level exposures would be hard to explain using the one-hit, genotoxic paradigm, but more easily explained by stable epigenetic effects, not on a single targeted cell but by the general alteration of many cells of a tissue. This speculation, however, must be rigorously tested in new model systems, particularly in vitro, using three-dimensional organoids, generated with various human stem cells, to mimic some aspects of in vivo tissues.

In addition, even if DNA damage were the primary event leading to mutations, the existence of DNA repair mechanisms in cells introduces a step that would complicate a one-hit hypothesis.

Several concepts derived from radiation studies during the past few decades have shown that there exists an "adaptive response," a "bystander effect," or "genomic instability," in irradiated cells [16], ionizing radiation-induced oxidative stress-induced cell signaling [3], a differential response to radiation-induced cell killing when cells are irradiated in sparse, two-dimensional log-phase conditions compared to two-dimensional stationary-phase in vitro condition or in a three-dimensional condition [17]. Moreover, the demonstration of differential responses to ionizing radiation-induced cell killing of adult stem cells in small versus large intestinal tissues [18] suggests that no one in vitro cell system, particularly even when human adult stem cells might be used, can be a model system for universal extrapolation to in vivo radiation responses.

New Concepts to Be Considered in Interpreting Potential Health Effects of Low-Level Ionizing Radiation

The very first assumption that must be considered in interpreting radiation health effects is that all health effects noted after radiation exposure must have an underlying molecular/biological mechanism. However, not all measurable molecular/biochemical effects after low-level radiation exposure lead, necessarily, to a detrimental health effect.

In brief, it is speculated that (a) any cancer, correlated with the exposure to an acute low-level radiation exposure, must conform to the multi-step, multi-mechanism model of carcinogenesis; (b) adult stem cells in most, if not all, human organs are the "targets" for radiation-induced cancer, that is, the stem cell theory [19–21] versus the de-differentiation theory of carcinogenesis [22]; (c) the "Barker hypothesis" can influence the consequences of low level radiation effects; (d) both secreted and gap junctional-mediated cell communication mechanisms can contribute to the health consequences of radiation [5]; (e) low-level radiation-induced oxidative stress can lead to epigenetic, not mutagenic, effects that might or might not lead to a health consequence [3]; and (f) there is a potential role of caloric restriction on modifying the ionizing radiation health response [3,5].

Factors Influencing the Multi-Stage/Multi-Mechanism Carcinogenesis Process

Most investigators accept the interpretation that cancers are the result of multiple distinct phases ("initiation" of a single cell; the "promotion" or clonal expansion of that single initiated cell and conversion or "progression" of that initiated cell to an invasive and metastatic cell) and that each phase can consist of multiple molecular mechanisms [23]. The old "one-hit" hypothesis of radiation-induced cancer simply cannot be consistent with this accepted concept of the process of carcinogenesis. It has been *assumed*, because (a) "initiation" is an irreversible process, (b) mutagenesis or genotoxicity leads to an irreversible process, and (c) ionizing radiation can generate free radicals, capable of generating DNA lesions that could lead to gene/chromosomal mutations and cell death by either necrosis or apoptosis, or (d) by inducing premature senescence, that low-level ionizing radiation is responsible for the initiation phase of carcinogenesis by a mutagenic process.

Furthermore, two extreme hypotheses exist for the "target cell" for initiating the carcinogenic process, namely, the adult stem cell [19–21] or any progenitor or differentiated cell [22]. The recent discovery of adult normal human stem cells and of the "cancer stem cells" tends to support the stem cell theory of carcinogenesis and that the adult stem cell is the "target cell" for initiation [4]. The observation that these cancer stem cells seem to exhibit ionizing radiation resistance has major implications for the therapeutic eradication of these cells from a tumor [24].

A relatively old idea has been reintroduced, namely, the "Barker" hypothesis [8]. In brief, it postulates that many adult diseases, such as cancer, can be linked to prenatal and early postnatal developmental events. With the emerging information about stem cells as being the target cells for initiating the carcinogenic process, not only having an initiating event happening in a adult stem cell early in embryonic/fetal development, but the modulation of the stem cell pool during these periods in utero, could, all other things during life being equal, also affect the risk to ultimately getting cancer. This scenario would occur if the pregnant woman were exposed to prenatal dietary or exogenous agents that might increase or decrease the stem cell pool in any organ [25]. The case of pregnant rats exposed to bisphenol A or bisphenol A plus a soy diet, which could either increase or decrease, respectively, the risk of prostate cancers in male offspring who were never exposed to these agents after birth, would be a classic example of the Barker hypothesis [26]. More recently, it has been shown that there is a correlation of umbilical cord blood hematopoietic stem cells with birth weight and its implications for a prenatal influence on cancer risk [25].

One of the factors that is rarely considered in interpreting the cancer frequencies in the survivors of the atomic bombs in Hiroshima and Nagasaki is caloric restriction. In experimental animal dietary restriction studies, the frequencies of many chronic diseases are reduced and lifespan is extended [27,28], and it is known that the general Japanese population of pre-atomic bomb events was significantly calorically restricted [29]. Understandably, caloric restriction results in animals might lead to the wrong conclusions when extrapolated to human beings. Reduction of calories can occur with reduction of nutrients, vital elementary metals, and other factors, as was the case with the victims of Auschwitz, or it could be done with a diet of antioxidant-containing foods and sufficient protein, as was done during the Second World War in Japan, where tea, soy products (tofu, natto), vegetables, and raw fish were available. In the former example, caloric restriction could lead to a more disease-prone state and increased morbidity and mortality, whereas in the latter case, lifespan expansion and reduction of disease risk of chronic diseases might be expected.

In addition, Japanese women consumed significant amounts of soy products for generations before the bombs were dropped. This, then, raises a legitimate question whether both the Barker hypothesis and caloric restriction might have contributed to the frequency of attributed radiation-induced breast cancers in the women survivors of the atomic bombs [5]. What makes this hypothesis even more interesting is the observation that normal human adult breast stem cells have been shown to be induced to differentiate when exposed to genistein, a component of soy products [30]. With a reduced number of breast stem cells in female offspring of mothers who eat significant amounts of soy products, these women would have less breast tissue after puberty and fewer breast stem cells as targets for the initiation process. Furthermore, these women would also be calorically restricted after any initiation or exposure to the atomic bomb radiation, which would probably negatively affect the promotion of any initiated breast stem cell.

Although many experimental animal studies have been linked to anticancer effects, in studies of human health the results seem to be mixed. However, in some studies, the effects of green tea have been suspected to contribute to the lowering of the incidence of cigarette-smoking induced lung cancers [31], and soy isoflavone, or genistein, has been linked to the prevention of prostate cancers [32]. The result of the combination of both these modifying factors, the "Barker effect" and caloric restriction, would be expected to be a reduced risk of cancer in the atomic bomb survivors.

Obviously, postnatal and adult exposure to dietary and exogenous agents, such as smoking, could also increase the risk to the initiated stem cells through increasing the promotion phase.

Modifying Factors of Low-Level Epigenetic Signaling in Adult Stem Cells

In addition, the induction of redox intracellular signaling, caused by the generation of free radicals either as a direct consequence of radiation or by chemicals at nonmutagenic and noncytotoxic necrotic doses/concentration, implies that low-level radiation could alter gene expression in an adult stem cell so that it could die by apoptosis, proliferate, differentiate, or, if already differentiated, adaptively respond. Little is known about low-level induction of intracellular signaling on altered gene expression in the target cells of cancer, namely, the adult stem cells. Only the study of the differential apoptotic response of stem cells after ionizing radiation of the small and large intestine of rodents has demonstrated that there might be specific organ stem cell differential responses to ionizing radiation [18].

It is assumed that low-level exposure to ionizing radiation does not induce initiation of a single adult stem cell by inducing either a point or chromosome mutation. Rather, dietary and environmental factors during embryonic/fetal development could increase or decrease the number of adult stem cells in specific organs, thereby increasing or decreasing the risk to the initiation event [5,33]. In addition, it can be hypothesized that initiation at low-level exposures is not induced by the radiation but by "errors in replication" of the stem cells. This event also would be influenced by a Barker effect and caloric restriction. In other words, diets or environmental toxins/toxicants could stimulate or retard the proliferation of stem cells. In turn, each time a stem cell's DNA replicates, there is a finite chance that an error of replication in any gene could occur. One such example could be taken from the results of the study of the mutation spectra of mutated oncogenes in lung tumors of smokers and nonsmokers [34]. Given that Thilly [34] found that the mutation spectra for these two classes of tumors were essentially identical, it appears smoking acted more as a promoter of preexisting "spontaneously" existing initiated cells whose oncogenes might have been mutated simply by an error in replication [2]. Since all organs have initiated cells, when exposed to low- or high-level ionizing radiation, any tumor that could arise later might have been the result of the radiation acting as a promoter [35].

Little is known how this "promoting effect" might occur at low doses, but at high doses where ionizing radiation-induced cell killing would occur, the death of cells could act as an indirect tumor promoter by some compensatory hyperplasia of a surviving spontaneously initiated cell. On the other hand, because apoptosis, not necrosis, is caused by an epigenetic event, low-level radiation might eliminate spontaneously induced initiated stem cells, thereby leading to a reduction of cancers, rather than an increase. Ionizing radiation, by having some of its effects mediated by the "bystander effect" to nonirradiated cells/tissues, could bring about "epigenetic" effects. Epigenetic effects would involve alterations in gene expression. Depending on the cell type affected by these nontargeted radiation effects, molecular changes, such as DNA methylation or histone modification, could lead to altered cell behavior (proliferation, differentiation, or apoptosis) [36].

Even more significantly, epigenetic effects on adult stem cells exposed in utero to dietary or environmental agents might trigger altered gene expression in adult stem cells, which might modulate the quantity or quality of stem cells, such that the risk to cancers later in life might be increased or decreased, that is, the Barker hypothesis [5,8]. The past demonstration of bystander effects from complex gap junction intercellular communication [37], secreted factors, complex extracellular matrix and stromal–epithelial interactions, adaptive responses, induced radiosensitivity and radioresistance, and genomic instability [16] will have to be incorporated in any explanation of in vivo effects based on in vitro models of questionable validity.

The recent demonstration that a bystander effect, induced by microbeam irradiation, of increased levels of apoptosis, of micronuclei formation, loss of nuclear DNA methylation, and of an increased fraction of senescent cells in an in vitro human three-dimensional model, illustrates that this more realistic model of irradiating cells could help to resolve potential health effects of low-level ionizing radiation exposure [38]. With observations such as these, for example, ionizing radiation induction of fibroblast senescence, and the altered signaling between senescent stromal cells and epithelial cells, studies to determine the lowest level of ionizing radiation that might bring about senescence in a three-dimensional model of a human tissue, in which the adult epithelial stem cell could be monitored (i.e., with the Oct-4 gene) for either cell proliferation, differentiation, or apoptosis, would seem to be a strategy to test the biological effects of low-level radiation.

Looking back at some uses of ionizing radiated human fibroblasts, it has been shown that normal human kidney adult stem cells (which expressed Oct-4A gene and did not have functional gap junctional intercellular communication), but not the progenitor or terminally differentiated cells, could grow on the radiation-induced senesced fibroblast monolayer [39]. In addition, many human carcinoma cells also grew on these radiation-induced senesced human fibroblasts. This finding implies that the senesced fibroblasts produced some growth-stimulating factor which allowed both the normal adult stem cells and cancer stem cells to proliferate but that the normal progenitor and differentiated cells could not grow. While the fibroblasts were irradiated, separately, at very high doses from the normal kidney epithelial cells, the stage is set for identifying the lowest dose that could reproduce this effect. In addition, with use of both normal and immortalized, but not tumorigenic, adult human stem cells to produce three-dimensional "organoids," co-culturing these "organoids" after exposure to low-level ionizing radiation with induced senescent cells might be shown to act as a tumor promoter.

Of course, many in vitro studies have contributed to mechanistic understanding of many biological effects. However, intrinsically, no in vitro assay can accurately represent how any given cell type would behave in vivo, given the absence of physiological events (episodic circadian rhythm effects, dietary surges, immunological system effects, cell matrix–stromal–epithelial interactions, in vivo stem cell niche interactions with progenitor and differentiated daughter cells, oxygen tension effects, etc.) (Fig.1). Therefore, in vitro results of any biological endpoints, such as cell death, mutations, mitogenesis, apoptosis, differentiation, or in vitro neoplastic transformation, cannot be accurately extrapolated in vivo.

Specifically, the in vitro assays for "genotoxicity" are all afflicted by some limitations or artifacts [2], especially those for chemicals that have been classified as mutagens/carcinogens. One example is the 6-thioguanine system. Agents are classified as being "genotoxic" if a treated population of 6-thioguanine-positive cells gives rise to some 6-thioguanine-negative colonies (cells that do not have

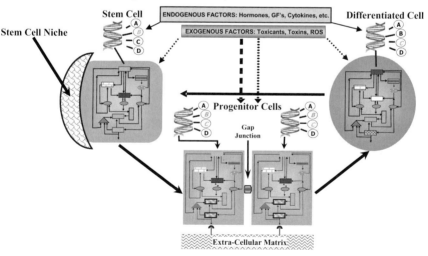

Fig. 1. Diagrammatic representation of the adult stem cell, progenitor, and terminally differentiated daughter cells within a tissue. Each cell type expresses different genes and is differentially affected by endogenous and exogenous signaling molecules that trigger various cross-talking intracellular signals, which in turn affects the transcription of different genes in each cell type, causing differential alterations in cell proliferation, differentiation, apoptosis, and adaptive responses

functional hypoxanthine-guanine phosphoribosyltransferase enzyme to metabolize the 6-thioguanine agent into a lethal metabolite). However, if the agent can point-mutate or delete this gene, the cell is truly a mutant cell and the agent is a genotoxicant. However, if the agent induces transcription suppression of the gene (epigenetic toxicant), the cell has no enzyme activity to metabolize the drug and is phenotypically indistinguishable from the true mutation. In addition, if the agent was selected from the population of preexisting spontaneously mutated cells, it too would be misclassified as a "genotoxicant."

Finally, clearly, the task of understanding the complex normal biological processes that help to maintain homeostatic control of cell proliferation, differentiation, and apoptosis of adult stem cells, their progenitors, and the differentiated lineage n-stage cells must be accomplished with realistic in vitro and in vivo model systems. The traditional two-dimensional in vitro systems, particularly normal or abnormal rodent cell systems, while possibly providing insights to mechanisms, cannot be used for extrapolation to three-dimensional in vivo human tissue. The future development of three-dimensional normal human tissue-specific systems with markers for monitoring adult stem cells before and after low-level ionizing radiation seems to be the best alternative to studying millions of survivors of low-level ionizing irradiation. In the case of human responses to either acute or chronic low-level radiation, the roles of diet and environmental and pharmaceutical chemicals during embryonic and fetal development must be considered in the risk assessment. That consideration implies the necessity for the study of environmental and dietary factors that might affect organ-specific adult stem cells during prenatal and early postnatal development, factors to which an irradiated population or person might have been exposed before being irradiated.

References

1. NCRP (2001) Evaluation of the linear-nonthreshold dose-response model for ionizing radiation. Report 136. National Council on Radiation Protection and Measurements, Bethesda, MD
2. Trosko JE, Upham BL (2005) The emperor wears no clothes in the field of carcinogen risk assessment: ignored concepts in cancer risk assessment. Mutagenesis 20:81–92
3. Upham BL, Trosko JE (2005) A paradigm shift in the understanding of oxidative stress and its implications to exposures of low level ionizing radiation. Acta Med Nagasaki 50:63–68
4. Trosko JE, Tai MH (2006) Adult stem cell theory of the multi-stage, multi-mechanism theory of carcinogenesis: role of inflammation on the promotion of initiated stem cells. In: Dittmar T, Zaenkar KS, Schmidt A (eds) Infection and inflammation: impacts on oncogenesis. Contributions to microbiology. Vol.13, Karger, Basel, pp 45–65
5. Trosko JE (2007) Concepts needed to understand potential health effects of chronic low-level radiation exposures: role of adult stem cells and modulated cell-cell communication. Int Congr Ser 1299:101–113
6. Pampaloni F, Reynaud EG, Stelzer EHK (2007) The third dimension bridges the gap between cell culture and live tissue. Nat Rev/Mol Cell Biol 8:839–845
7. Smalley KS, Lioni M, Herlyn M (2006) Life isn't flat: cancer biology to the next dimension. In Vitro Cell Dev Biol-Anim 42:242–247

8. Barker DJP (ed) (1998) Mothers, babies, and health in later life, 2nd edn. Churchill Livingstone, New York
9. Kang KS, Sun W, Nomata K, et al (1998) Involvement of tyrosine phosphorylation of p185 C-erbB2/neu in tumorigenicity induced by X-rays and the neu oncogene in human breast epithelial cells. Mol Carcinog 21:225–233
10. Hajj MA, Wicha MS, Benito-Hernandez A (2003) Prospective identification of tumorigenic breast cancer cells. Proc Natl Acad Sci U S A 100:3983–3988
11. Tai MH, Chang CC, Kiupel M, et al (2005) Oct-4 expression in adult stem cells: evidence in support of the stem cell theory of carcinogenesis. Carcinogenesis (Oxf) 26:495–502
12. Suzuki K, Mori I, Nakayama Y, et al (2001) Radiation-induced senescence-like growth arrest requires TP53 function but not telomere shortening. Radiat Res 155:(1 pt 2):248–253
13. Krtolica A, Parrinello S, Lockett S, et al (2001) Senescent fibroblasts promote epithelial cell growth and tumorigenesis: a link between cancer and aging. Proc Natl Acad Sci U S A 98:12072–12077
14. Coppe JP, Kauser K, Campisi J, et al (2006) Secretion of vascular endothelial growth factor by primary human fibroblasts at senescence. J Biol Chem 281:29568–29574
15. Barcellos-Hoff MH, Park C, Wright EG (2005) Radiation and the microenvironment: tumorigenesis and therapy. Nat Rev Cancer 5:867–875
16. Schollnberger H, Mitchel RJ, Redpath JL, et al (2007) Detrimental and protective effects: a model approach. Radiat Res 168:614–626
17. Santini MT, Rainaldi G, Indovina PL (1999) Multicellular tumor spheroid in radiation biology. Int J Radiat Biol 75:787–799
18. Potten CS (1989) The role of stem cells in the regeneration of intestinal crypts after cytotoxic exposure. In: Butterworth BE, Slaga TJ, Farland W, McClain M (eds) Chemically induced cell proliferation: implications for risk assessment. Wiley-Liss, New York, pp 155–171
19. Pierce GB (1974) Neoplasms, differentiation and mutations. Am J Pathol 77:103–118
20. Markert C (1968) Neoplasia: a disease of differentiation. Cancer Res 28:1908–1914
21. Potter VR (1978) Phenotypic diversity in experimental hepatomas: the concept of partially-blocked ontogeny. Br J Cancer 38:1–23
22. Sell S (1993) Cellular origin of cancer: differentiation or stem cell maturation arrest? Environ Health Perspect 101:15–26
23. Weinstein IB, Cattoni-Celli S, Kirschmeier P, et al (1984) Multistage carcinogenesis involves multiple genes and multiple mechanisms. J Cell Physiol 3:127–137
24. Rich JN (2007) Cancer stem cells in radiation response. Cancer Res 67:8980–8984
25. Strohsnitter WC, Savarese TM, Low HP, et al (2008) Correlation of umbilical cord blood haematopoietic stem and progenitor cell levels with birth weight: implications for a prenatal influence on cancer risk. Br J Cancer 98:660–663
26. Ho SM, Tang WY, de Frausto JB, et al (2006) Developmental exposures to estradiol and bisphenol A increases susceptibility to prostate carcinogenesis and epigenetically regulates phosphodiesterase type 4 variant 4. Cancer Res 66:5624–5632
27. Ross MH, Bras G (1971) Lasting influence of early caloric restriction on prevalence of neoplasms in the rat. J Natl Cancer Inst 47:1095–1113
28. Tannenbaum A, Silverstone H (1953) Effect of limited food intake on survival of mice bearing spontaneous mammary carcinoma and on the incidence of lung metastases. Cancer Res 13:532–536
29. Willcox BJ, Willcox DC, Dodoriki H, et al (2007) Caloric restriction, the traditional Okinawan diet, and healthy aging: the diet of the world's longest-lived people and its potential impact on morbidity and life span. Ann N Y Acad Sci 1114:434–455
30. Hsieh CY, Chang CC (1999) Stem cell differentiation and reduction as a potential mechanism for chemoprevention of breast cancer. Chinese Pharm J 51:15–30
31. Stellman SD, Takezaki T, Wang L, et al (2001) Smoking and lung cancer risk in American and Japanese men: an international case-control study. Cancer Epidemiol Biomark Prev 10:193–1199

32. Perabo FGE, Von Low EC, Ellinger J, et al (2008) Soy flavone genistein in prevention and treatment of prostate cancer. Prostate Cancer Prostat Dis 11:6–12
33. Trosko J, Chang CC, Upham B, et al (2004) Ignored hallmarks of carcinogenesis: stem cells and cell-cell communication. Ann N Y Acad Sci 1028:192–201
34. Thilly WG (2003) Have environmental mutagens caused oncomutations in people? Nat Genet 3:255–259
35. Trosko JE (1998) Radiation, signal transduction, and modulation of intercellular communication. In: Peterson LE, Abrahamson S (eds) Effects of ionizing radiation. John Henry Press, Washington, DC, pp 177–192
36. Kovalchuk O, Baulch JE (2008) Epigenetic changes and nontargeted radiation effects: is there a link? Environ Mol Mutagen 49:16–25
37. Trosko JE, Chang CC (2003) Hallmarks of radiation carcinogenesis: ignored concepts. In: Shibata Y, Yamashita S, Watanabe M, Tomonaga M (eds) Radiation and Humankind. Int Congr Ser 1258. Elsevier B.V., Amsterdam, The Netherlands, pp. 31–36
38. Sedelnikova OA, Nakamura A, Kovalchuk O, et al (2008) DNA double-strand breaks form in bystander cells after microbeam irradiation of three dimensional human tissue models. Cancer Res 67:4295–4302
39. Chang CC, Trosko JE, El Fouly MH, et al (1987) Contact sensitivity of a subpopulation of normal human fetal kidney epithelial cells and of human carcinoma cell lines. Cancer Res 47:1634–1645

Combined Effect of Ionizing Radiation and *N*-Ethyl-*N*-Nitrosourea on Mutation Induction and Lymphoma Development

Kazumi Yamauchi, Shizuko Kakinuma, Akifumi Nakata, Tatsuhiko Imaoka, Takashi Takabatake, Mayumi Nishimura, and Yoshiya Shimada

Summary. Carcinogenesis in humans is thought to result from exposure to numerous environmental factors. Little is known, however, about how these different factors work in combination to cause cancer. Mouse thymic lymphoma is a good model for research on radiation and chemical carcinogenesis. We examined here the occurrence of thymic lymphoma and mutation induction following exposure to both X-rays and *N*-ethyl-*N*-nitrosourea (ENU) in B6C3F1 mice. Mice were exposed weekly to whole-body X-irradiation (0.2 or 1.0 Gy per each exposure) for 4 consecutive weeks, ENU (200 ppm) in the drinking water for 4 weeks, or X-irradiation followed by ENU treatment. The incidence of lymphoma after 0.2 and 1.0 Gy were 0% and 10%, respectively. ENU treatment induced lymphoma in 20% of exposed mice. When ENU was combined with 1.0 Gy, lymphoma incidence increased up to 94%, showing a synergistic effect. In contrast, combination of ENU with 0.2 Gy resulted in a decrease in lymphoma incidence, that is, an antagonistic effect. Mutant frequency of the reporter transgene *gpt* after ENU exposure alone increased by tenfold compared to untreated controls. Combined exposure of ENU with 0.2 Gy X-rays dramatically decreased mutant frequency. In contrast, 1.0 Gy X-rays combined with ENU further enhanced mutant frequency and accelerated clonal expansion of mutated cells. In conclusion, the mutagenic and carcinogenic effect of combined exposure of X-rays with ENU is dose dependent.

Key words Thymic lymphoma · Combined genotoxic effect · *N*-Ethyl-*N*-nitrosourea · Radiation · Clonal expansion

Introduction

Human beings are exposed to numerous natural and man-made agents that are potentially carcinogenic. Therefore, cancer risk by ionizing radiation should be assessed as a result of combined exposures with other agents, including tobacco,

---

Experimental Radiobiology for Children's Health Research Group, National Institute of Radiological Sciences, 4-9-1 Anagawa, Inage-ku, Chiba 263-8555, Japan

genotoxic and nongenotoxic chemicals, hormones, viruses, and metals. Alkylating agents are found in plants, food, cigarette smoke, fuel combustion products, and commonly used industrial solvents. Some alkylating agents are also used for cancer therapy in combination with ionizing radiation. However, available data on the combined effect are relatively few, especially on its mechanism. In the present study, we report the dose dependence of the mode of combined effect of radiation with *N*-ethyl-*N*-nitrosourea on mutation induction and lymphoma development.

Materials and Methods

Female B6C3F1 mice were exposed to whole-body X-irradiation at a weekly dose of 0.2 or 1.0 Gy for 4 consecutive weeks or to *N*-ethyl-*N*-nitrosourea (ENU) at 200 ppm in drinking water. The mice were also exposed to X-rays followed by ENU (Fig. 1). X-ray irradiation was performed at a dose rate of 0.7 Gy/min. The mice, which had symptoms of thymic lymphoma 2 to 4 months after exposure, were killed under anesthesia and autopsied. The B6C3F1 *gpt*-delta mice were similarly treated with both X-rays and ENU. After the 4th week of exposure, the thymus was analyzed for the frequency and spectrum of *gpt* mutation as described previously [1]. Recurrent mutations derived from the tissue of a single animal could be the result of clonal expansion that occurred early after mutagen treatment.

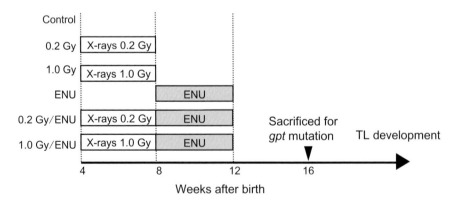

Fig. 1. Experimental design for thymic lymphomagenesis (TL) and *gpt* mutation analysis in mice treated with X-ray irradiation, *N*-ethyl-*N*-nitrosourea (ENU), or a combination of the two. Mice were exposed to X-rays weekly. ENU was administered at a concentration of 200 ppm in drinking water

Results

Combined Effect of X-Rays and ENU on Thymic Lymphomagenesis

Repeated exposure to X-rays at 1.0 Gy per exposure (4.0 Gy in total) increased the incidence of thymic lymphomas to 10%, whereas X-rays at 0.2 Gy did not induce lymphomas at all. ENU at 200 ppm induced lymphomas at an incidence of 20%. Combined exposure of ENU with 1.0 Gy X-rays resulted in a dramatic increase in lymphoma incidence at 94%, indicating a synergy. When ENU was combined with low-dose X-rays (0.2 Gy), the incidence was significantly reduced compared to that of ENU treatment alone, suggesting a protective role of low-dose X-rays for ENU-induced lymphomagenesis.

Induction of Gpt Mutation after Combined Exposure

DNA mutations play a central role in carcinogenesis. The frequency and type of mutations that result from combined treatment may shed light on the molecular mechanism(s) underlying the carcinogenic effects of combined exposure to ENU and radiation. To delineate such mechanisms, we have examined the occurrence of mutations in thymic cells of B6C3F1 (*gpt+/−*) mice after combined exposure [2]. It was found that ENU increased mutant frequency by ten-fold relative to untreated controls (Fig. 2). The mutant frequency in mice exposed to 0.2 Gy or 1.0 Gy X-rays alone was, surprisingly, reduced compared to the control ($P < 0.05$). Exposure to high-dose X-rays (1.0 Gy) followed by ENU increased mutant frequency by three-fold relative to ENU alone and facilitated clonal expansion of mutated cells. When low-dose X-ray (0.2 Gy) was combined with ENU, mutant frequency was, unexpectedly, reduced, which was primarily the result of a decrease in G:C to A:T and

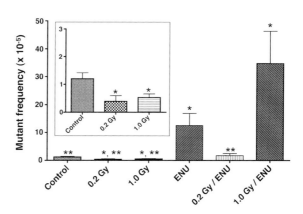

Fig. 2. Mutant frequency analysis of *gpt* recovered from thymus DNA from control, irradiated (0.2 Gy or 1.0 Gy), ENU-treated, and irradiated/ENU-treated mice. The *inset* shows an expanded scale for mutant frequency for the first three conditions. *$P < 0.05$, significantly different from control; **$P < 0.05$, significantly different from ENU. *Bars* represent mean ± SD

A:T to T:A mutations. In addition, clonality was drastically reduced compared with ENU alone (24.6% vs. 82.2%). The mode and mechanism of combined exposure clearly differs between low and high doses of radiation.

Discussion

We report here the dose dependency of the mode of thymic lymphomagenesis and mutagenesis after combined exposure to X-rays and ENU. It was shown that low-dose X-rays suppressed lymphoma induction by ENU whereas high-dose X-rays enhanced induction. In accord with this, low-dose X-rays reduced ENU-induced mutant frequency and clonal expansion of mutated cells and high-dose X-rays promoted both.

It is reported that preirradiation of X-rays decreases the incidence of brain tumors in rats exposed in utero [3]. This protective effect of preirradiation appears to correspond to the inductive effect of ionizing irradiation on O^6-alkylguanine alkyltransferase (ATase), which protects cells from G to A mutation. Induction of ATase by irradiation has been frequently observed in several tissues both in vitro and in vivo [4,5]. Our results, showing that 0.2 Gy X-rays combined with ENU decreased the G to A transition, suggest increased activity of ATase by radiation.

On the other hand, high-dose radiation can kill the target cells, thereby providing an environment for the surviving cells to expand. Irradiation of thymic epithelial cells enhances interleukin (IL)-7 production, and thymocytes at the preleukemic stage proliferate more vigorously in response to IL-7 [6,7]. We previously found frequent mutations of *Ikaros* in X-ray- and ENU-induced thymic lymphomas [8–10]. T cells with reduced or dominant-negative Ikaros activity, which may result from either a lack of or a point mutation in the zinc finger responsible for DNA binding, exhibit a greater proliferative response to IL-2 [11]. Taken together, these results suggest that high-dose radiation provides a thymic microenvironment ripe for the occurrence of prelymphoma cells, which harbor growth-advantageous mutations following ENU treatment.

In conclusion, low-dose (0.2 Gy) X-rays reduce not only the frequency of spontaneously occurring but also ENU-induced mutations, suggestive of an adaptive response. Low-dose X-rays also reduce the clonal expansion of cells following ENU treatment, whereas 1.0 Gy X-rays accelerate cell expansion. Thus, low- and high-dose radiation plays different roles in lymphomagenesis when combined with ENU exposure.

Conclusion

Combined exposure of carcinogens is a characteristic of ordinary human life. The dose of radiation is a critical factor to determine the mode of combined effect of radiation and ENU.

Acknowledgments. We thank Ms. Y. Amasaki, Ms. U. Enzaka, Ms. M. Okabe, Mr. J. Nagai, Ms. S. Hirano, and Ms. Y. Miyayama and the staff in the Animal Facility of our institute for their assistance with laboratory analysis and mouse husbandry. This work was supported in part by a grant from the Long-range Research Initiative (LRI) of the Japan Chemical Industry Association (JCIA), a grant from the 'Ground-based Research Announcement for Space Utilization' promoted by the Japan Space Forum, a grant from the Ministry of Health, Labour and Welfare, Japan, and a Grant-in-Aid from the Ministry of Education, Culture, Sports, Science, and Technology of Japan.

References

1. Nohmi T, Katoh M, Suzuki H, et al (1996) A new transgenic mouse mutagenesis test system using Spi- and 6-thioguanine selections. Environ Mol Mutagen 28:465–470
2. Yamauchi K, Kakinuma S, Sudo S, et al (2007) Differential effects of low- and high-dose X-rays on *N*-ethyl-*N*-nitrosourea-induced mutagenesis in thymocytes of B6C3F1 *gpt*-delta mice. Mutat Res 640:27–37
3. Stammberger I, Schmahl W, Nice L (1990) The effects of X-irradiation, *N*-ethyl-*N*-nitrosourea or combined treatment on O^6-alkylguanine-DNA alkyltransferase activity in fetal rat brain and liver and the induction of CNS tumours. Carcinogenesis (Oxf) 11:219–222
4. Chan CL, Wu Z, Eastman A, et al (1992) Irradiation-induced expression of O^6-methylguanine-DNA methyltransferase in mammalian cells. Cancer Res 52:1804–1809
5. Wilson RE, Hoey B, Margison GP (1993) Ionizing radiation induces O^6-alkylguanine-DNA-alkyltransferase mRNA and activity in mouse tissues. Carcinogenesis (Oxf) 14:679–683
6. Nishimura M, Kakinuma S, Yamamoto D et al (2004) Elevated interleukin-9 receptor expression and response to interleukins-9 and -7 in thymocytes during radiation-induced T-cell lymphomagenesis in B6C3F1 mice. J Cell Physiol 198:82–90
7. Toki J, Adachi Y, Jin T, et al (2003) Enhancement of IL-7 following irradiation of fetal thymus. Immunobiology 207:247–258
8. Shimada Y, Nishimura M, Kakinuma S, et al (2000) Radiation-associated loss of heterozygosity at the *Znfn1a1* (*Ikaros*) locus on chromosome 11 in murine thymic lymphomas. Radiat Res 154:293–300
9. Kakinuma S, Nishimura M, Sasanuma S, et al (2002) Spectrum of *Znfn1a1* (*Ikaros*) inactivation and its association with loss of heterozygosity in radiogenic T-cell lymphomas in susceptible B6C3F1 mice. Radiat Res 157:331–340
10. Kakinuma S, Nishimura M, Kubo A, et al (2005) Frequent retention of heterozygosity for point mutations in *p53* and *Ikaros* in *N*-ethyl-*N*-nitrosourea-induced mouse thymic lymphomas. Mutat Res 572:132–14
11. Avitahl N, Winandy S, Friedrich C, et al (1999) Ikaros sets thresholds for T cell activation and regulates chromosome propagation. Immunity 10:333–343

γ-Ray-Induced Mouse Thymic Lymphomas: Bcl11b Inactivation and Prelymphoma Cells

Ryo Kominami, Hiroyuki Ohi, Kenya Kamimura, Masaki Maruyama,
Takashi Yamamoto, Ken-ichi Takaku, Shin-ichi Morita, Rieka Go, and
Yukio Mishima

Summary. Bcl11b+/− heterozygous mice and Bcl11b+/−p53+/− doubly heterozygous mice showed more susceptibility to γ-ray-induced thymic lymphomas than Bcl11b wild-type mice and p53+/− mice, respectively. Most of the thymic lymphomas developed in irradiated Bcl11b+/−p53+/− mice retained the Bcl11b wild-type allele, indicating that Bcl11b is a haploinsufficient tumor suppressor gene. Of interest is the high retention of the wild-type Bcl11b allele in those radiation-induced tumors, and this leads to the implication that the main contribution of irradiation in the Bcl11b+/−p53+/− mice is not to tumor initiation, by inducing allelic losses, but to the promotion of thymic lymphoma development. Although the reason for this unexpected high retention is unclear, an explanation might be the apoptosis given by loss of Bcl11b in the Jurkat T-cell line, because apoptosis appears to contradict the predicted property of tumor suppressors. Our chapter also shows the presence of clonally growing large thymocytes in atrophic thymuses at 40 days after irradiation. Those cells are probably prelymphoma cells because of the genetic alteration detected. However, the cell number was low, and therefore abrogation of the hindrance in cell proliferation through additional genetic and/or epigenetic changes may be a prerequisite for lymphoma development.

Key words γ-Radiation · Bcl11b/Rit1 · Mouse thymic lymphoma · Prelymphoma

Introduction

Gamma (γ) radiation induces DNA double-strand breaks (DSBs), and some of them result in allelic losses of chromosomes after DNA recombination and repair [1]. Therefore, allelic losses at tumor suppressor loci found in radiogenic tumors are thought to be mostly a consequence of γ-irradiation. We performed genome-wide analysis of allelic losses in γ-ray-induced mouse thymic lymphomas [2,3] and

---

Department of Molecular Genetics, Graduate School of Medical and Dental Sciences, and Transdisciplinary Research Center, Niigata University, Asahimachi 1-757, Niigata 951-8510, Japan

localized candidate chromosomal regions harboring tumor suppressor genes. Subsequent sequence analysis allowed us to identify Ikaros on mouse chromosome 11 [4] and to clone a novel gene, Bcl11b/Rit1, on mouse chromosome 12 [5,6]. The Bcl11b/Rit1 (also called CTIP2) gene encodes zinc-finger proteins and plays a key role in $\alpha\beta$ T-cell development [5], whereas Ikaros also encoding zinc-finger proteins controls the development of lymphoid tissues [7]. One of the consequences given by Ikaros inactivation is to prevent apoptosis, one of the six hallmarks of cancer cells proposed by Hanahan and Weinberg [8]. On the other hand, Bcl11b inactivation leads to apoptosis in mouse thymocytes in vivo [5]. Hence, Ikaros and Bcl11b probably differ in the manner of contribution to lymphomagenesis.

In this chapter, we report haploinsufficiency of Bcl11b for tumor suppression and effects given by Bcl11b inactivation in Jurkat human T cells. We also show the detection of probable prelymphoma cells that develop in atrophic thymuses 40 days after irradiation. Finally, we claim that the contribution of γ-irradiation is to the promotion of thymic lymphoma development rather than its initiation.

Materials and Methods

Mice and Lymphoma Development

Bcl11b+/− BALB/c mice and p53+/− MSM mice used in this study were maintained under specific pathogen-free conditions in the animal colony of Niigata University. Mice were exposed to a single dose of 3 Gy γ-ray radiation at 4 weeks of age. Development of thymic lymphoma was diagnosed by observation of labored breathing and palpable induration of thymic tumor. All animal experiments comply with the guidelines by the animal ethics committee for animal experimentation of Niigata University.

DNA Isolation and PCR Analysis of Allelic Differences

DNA was isolated from brain and lymphomas using the DNeasy Tissue Kit (Qiagen, Hilden, Germany). Genotyping of Bcl11b and p53 were carried out with polymerase chain reaction (PCR) as described previously [4–6]. Loss of the wild-type allele and allelic loss at Bcl11b were analyzed using the D12 Mit181 marker in the vicinity of Bcl11b, and allelic loss at Ikaros was analyzed using the D11 Mit62 marker.

Flow Cytometry

Thymocytes were analyzed by a FACSAria flow cytometer (Becton-Dickinson, San Jose, CA, USA). Data were analyzed with the Flow-Jo software (Tree-Star, Inc, Ashland, OR, USA).

Results

Haploinsufficiency of Bcl11b for Tumor Suppression

Recent studies have indicated that the human Bcl11b locus is recurrently involved in chromosomal aberrations in hematopoietic malignancies, mostly of T-cell origin [9–11]. However, the majority of T-ALL expresses Bcl11b from an undisrupted allele, and therefore it was not concluded whether Bcl11b acts as a tumor suppressor gene or an oncogene. We thus examined whether Bcl11b+/− heterozygous mice show susceptibility to tumors. A total of 49 F_1 hybrids between Bcl11b+/− BALB/c and MSM mice were produced and subjected to γ-irradiation. Figure 1A displays the cumulative tumor incidence of mice of Bcl11b+/− and Bcl11b+/+ genotypes. Bcl11b+/− mice developed tumors at a higher incidence and a shorter latency than those of Bcl11b+/+ ($P = 0.0037$ in Mantel–Cox test). Allelic loss analysis using the D12Mit181 marker in the vicinity of Bcl11b showed that 14 (54%) of the 26 thymic lymphomas lost the wild-type allele. These results are consistent with Knudson's two-hit model [12] and clearly indicate the tumor suppressive property of Bcl11b/Rit1. However, the frequency (54%) of loss of the wild-type allele in the lymphomas was lower than expected, because the frequency of loss of the wild-type p53 allele was as high as 86% in irradiated p53+/− mouse thymic lymphomas [2]. Therefore, we further analyzed thymic lymphomas induced in mice doubly heterozygous for Bcl11b and p53. These mice spontaneously developed thymic lymphomas, and the frequency of loss of the wild-type Bcl11b allele was as low as 2 of the 14 lymphomas (14%). We then subjected the Bcl11b+/−p53+/− mice to γ-irradiation and obtained 27 thymic lymphomas. The loss frequency of the wild-type allele was also low, 6 of the 27 lymphomas (22%). These results, that most lymphomas retained the wild-type alleles, suggest that Bcl11b is haploinsufficient for tumor suppression, a situation

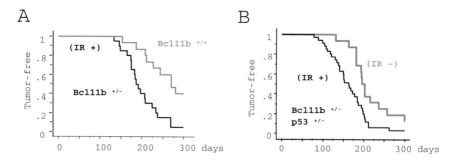

Fig. 1. Kaplan–Meier analysis of tumors developed in irradiated (IR+) Bcl11b+/− (*black line*) and wild-type (*gray line*) mice (**A**), and irradiated (*black line*) and unirradiated (*gray line*) mice of Bcl11b+/−p53+/− genotype (**B**)

in which functional loss of only one allele confers a selective advantage for tumor growth [13,14]. Accordingly, loss-of-function alterations of one Bcl11b allele may contribute to the development of human T-cell lymphoma and leukemia. Of note was a prominent difference in the latency, the mean latency being 203 days in unirradiated Bcl11b+/−p53+/− mice whereas 159 days in irradiated Bcl11b+/−p53+/− mice ($P = 0.0079$) (Fig. 1B). Namely, irradiation enhanced the lymphoma development but did not markedly increase the frequency in loss of the wild-type Bcl11b allele.

Inactivation of Bcl11b Results in Apoptosis

Thymocytes of Bcl11b−/− mice exhibit apoptosis when the cells enter the DN3 developmental stage during thymocyte differentiation [5,15]. At the DN3 stage, thymocytes start to proliferate rapidly to produce CD4-CD8 double-positive cells. We produced Bcl11b-knockdown (KD) Jurkat T-cell leukemia cells by introducing the plasmid DNA expressing Bcl11b siRNA. The KD cells were viable but not healthy. The level of apoptosis increased in KD cells after the elevation of serum concentration from 5% to 10%, and the increase was prominent at the S phase of the cell division cycle. This effect was accompanied with concomitant decreases in a cell-cycle inhibitor, p27, and an antiapoptotic protein, Bcl-xL. The decreases were regulated at the transcriptional level because their RNA expression decreased promptly after growth stimuli. The mechanism for this transcriptional repression was not known, but it was a likely consequence of the impairment of Sirt1, a NAD-dependent deacetylase associating with Bcl11b [16]. Other changes in KD cells were cleavage of the mediator protein, Claspin, and inhibition of phosphorylation of cell-cycle checkpoint kinase 1 (Chk1). Chk1 was phosphorylated in Jurkat cells when UV-irradiated but KD cells and Bcl11b−/− thymocytes failed to phosphorylate Chk1. Because Claspin and Chk1 play a central role in sensing and responding to incomplete replication, increased DNA replication stress in Bcl11b-lacking cells may be a cause of apoptosis.

Existence of Prelymphoma Cells in Radiation-Induced Atrophic Thymus

Whole-body irradiation to mice causes thymic atrophy and two-thirds of them eventually develop thymic lymphomas within 300 days. Thus, the atrophic thymus may be a microenvironment that allows damaged thymocytes to develop precancerous cells. If a subpopulation of clonally growing cells exists in the atrophic thymus, clonal expansion of thymocytes may be detectable. We thus isolated atrophic thymuses at 40 days after irradiation from apparently healthy mice. The cell

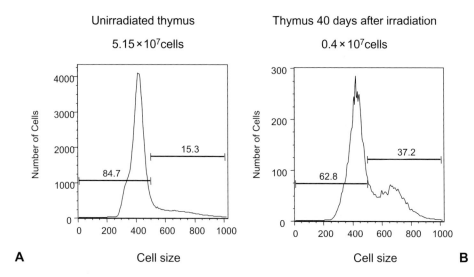

Fig. 2. Flow cytometric analysis of thymocytes from a mouse at 40 days after 3 Gy γ-irradiation (**A**). Analysis of thymocytes from an unirradiated mouse is also shown as a control (**B**). The percentage of cells in the large-sized cell fraction is shown above the *right line in the boxes*

number in most of them ranged from 3×10^6 to 10^7 cells, lower than $3-6 \times 10^7$ cells in unirradiated thymus. Figure 2 displays an example of flow cytometric analysis of an atrophic thymus, showing the presence of a population of large-sized thymocytes. This phenotype is interesting because the overt thymic lymphoma cells are nearly diploid but large in size. The percentage of this large-sized cell fraction tended to increase in irradiated atrophic thymuses. One-third of the thymuses contained the large-sized cells at more than 25%, although unirradiated thymuses contained them at approximately 15%. We thus studied the relationship between the large-sized thymocytes and clonal growth or clonal expansion. The clonality of thymocytes was examined with a conventional protocol using PCR [17,18] that determines D-J recombination of the TCRβ gene. Three sets of primers were used, one set for recombination between the Dβ1 and Jβ1 locus, one for the Dβ2 and Jβ2 locus, and the remaining one for the Dβ1 and Jβ2 locus. DNA from brain provided no signals for rearrangement whereas DNA from normal thymus showed six bands reflecting rearrangements at six sites between different Dβ and Jβ positions. In contrast, DNA from thymic lymphomas of monoclonal origin showed only one or two prominent bands. Analysis of 21 thymuses revealed that 12 of them showed one or two prominent bands, similar to thymic lymphomas but not to normal thymus. These results suggest a clonally growing population(s) present in atrophic thymuses at a high frequency that may comprise prelymphoma cells.

Genetic Changes Occur at Bcl11b Earlier Than at Ikaros During Thymic Lymphoma Development

Existence of a clonally growing cell population(s) in atrophic thymuses raised a possibility that these thymocytes have already progressed to a premalignant stage with genetic changes of some tumor suppressor genes. Hence, we examined allelic loss at Bcl11b and Ikaros loci in thymic lymphomas and the atrophic thymuses that showed clonal expansion at 40 days after irradiation. This analysis was done using MIT microsatellite markers that detected differences between BALB/c and MSM alleles. Allelic loss frequency at Bcl11b was 89% (31/35) in thymic lymphomas and 42% (5/12) in atrophic thymuses. This finding indicated a gradual increase in the frequency during thymic lymphoma development. On the other hand, the frequency at Ikaros was 43% (15/35) in thymic lymphomas and no change at Ikaros in atrophic thymuses. Although this study did not examine mutation of remaining alleles of the two genes, frequent inactivation (50%) of the remaining Ikaros allele has been reported [19]. The result indicated that the allelic loss frequency at Ikaros markedly differed between thymic lymphomas and atrophic thymuses. Taken together, these results suggest that genetic changes occur at Bcl11b locus earlier than at Ikaros locus during thymic lymphoma development.

Discussion

This study shows the effects of Bcl11b inactivation on the development of mouse thymic lymphomas and has analyzed genetic changes at Bcl11b and Ikaros in thymic lymphomas and atrophic thymuses at 40 days after irradiation. Bcl11b+/− heterozygous mice showed more susceptibility than Bcl11b wild-type mice, indicating that Bcl11b is a tumor suppressor gene. Of interest is that most of the thymic lymphomas that developed in irradiated Bcl11b+/−p53 +/− mice retained the Bcl11b wild-type allele. This finding suggests that the Bcl11b heterozygous state can contribute to lymphomagenesis without further loss of the wild-type allele [20]. However it remains open how this haploinsufficiency contributes to lymphomagenesis.

Apoptosis is a major phenotype seen in thymocytes of Bcl11b knockout mice [5,15]. The phenotype seems to contradict Bcl11b as a tumor suppressor because apoptosis has been considered as a mechanism to eliminate deleterious cells with DNA damage. We thus examined the relationship between Bcl11b inactivation and apoptosis using Bcl11b-KD T-cell lines. When exposed to growth stimuli, the KD cells exhibited extensive apoptosis with concomitant decrease in Bcl-xL antiapoptotic protein. The result is consistent with the start of in vivo apoptosis at the DN3 developmental stage where thymocytes proliferate rapidly. This finding implicates Bcl11b in the remedy for DNA replication stress and maintenance of genomic integrity. One possible explanation for contribution of the apoptotic phenotype to lymphomagenesis is that it reflects accumulation of DNA damages or a deregulated elevation in cell-cycle progression in those cells. Indeed, hyperplastic or dysplastic cells often exhibit apoptotic phenotype together with high mitotic index [21,22]. Such precancerous cells probably develop a rapidly progressive tumor phenotype when they acquire the ability to escape apoptosis.

We showed the clonally growing large thymocytes in atrophic thymuses at 40 days after irradiation. Those cells are probably prelymphoma cells because of clonal growth and genetic alteration. Consistently, it was reported that prelymphoma cells, which can form a tumor in transplanted thymus, exist in one-fourth of the atrophic thymuses within 40 days after irradiation [23]. However, the cell number was low in the atrophic thymuses and showed hindrance in cell proliferation. Therefore, abrogation of this hindrance through additional genetic and/or epigenetic changes may be a prerequisite for lymphoma development.

It is well accepted that radiation contributes to carcinogenesis through induction of allelic losses resulting from DSBs and subsequent DNA recombination [1]. In this study, however, we showed high retention of the wild-type Bcl11b allele in thymic lymphomas developed in irradiated Bcl11b+/−p53+/− doubly heterozygous mice, and the frequency was similar to that in unirradiated doubly heterozygous mice. The high retention is probably related to the doubly heterozygous mice used in this study and might be ascribed to the apoptotic phenotype given by Bcl11b inactivation, which is distinct from the antiapoptotic phenotype by inactivation of other haploinsufficient tumor suppressor genes including Pten. In contrast to the Bcl11b+/− or p53+/− singly heterozygous mice, the doubly heterozygous mice spontaneously develop thymic lymphomas at a high frequency, and hence the Bcl11b+/−p53+/− genotype may have potential to initiate the development of thymic lymphomas. Such synergistic effect has been reported in various genes such as Pten and p53 [24–26], although it remains open what mechanism governs the synergistic cooperativity. Cells losing the wild-type allele probably develop in irradiated thymus, but those cells acquire a relatively weak selective advantage in the doubly heterozygous mice [11–13]. The high retention of wild-type alleles even in radiation-induced tumors suggests that the main contribution of irradiation in the Bcl11b+/−p53+/− mice is not tumor initiation by inducing DSBs. Rather, irradiation contributes to the promotion of thymic lymphoma development, possibly by changing the normal thymic microenvironment into an impaired one that founds prelymphoma cells [3].

References

1. Little JB (2000) Radiation carcinogenesis. Carcinogenesis (Oxf) 21:397–404
2. Matsumoto Y, Kosugi S, Shinbo T, et al (1998) Allelic loss analysis of gamma-ray-induced mouse thymic lymphomas: two candidate tumor suppressor gene loci on chromosomes 12 and 16. Oncogene 16:2747–2754
3. Kominami R, Niwa O (2006) Radiation carcinogenesis in mouse thymic lymphomas. Cancer Sci 97:575–581
4. Okano H, Saito Y, Miyazawa T, et al (1996) Homozygous deletions and point mutations of the Ikaros gene in γ-ray-induced mouse thymic lymphomas. Oncogene 18:6677–6683

5. Wakabayashi Y, Watanabe H, Inoue J, et al (2003) Bcl11b is required for differentiation and survival of αβ T lymphocytes. Nat Immunol 4:533–539
6. Wakabayashi Y, Inoue J, Takahashi Y, et al (2003) Homozygous deletions and point mutations of the Rit1/Bcl11b gene in γ-ray induced mouse thymic lymphomas. Biochem Biophy Res Commun 301:598–603
7. Georgopoulos K, Moore DD, Derfler B (1992) Ikaros, an early lymphoid-specific transcription factor and a putative mediator for T cell commitment. Science 258:808–812
8. Hanahan D, Weinberg RA (2000) The hallmarks of cancer. Cell 100:57–70
9. MacLeod RA, Nagel S, Kaufmann M, et al (2003) Activation of HOX11L2 by juxtaposition with 3'-BCL11B in an acute lymphoblastic leukemia cell line (HPB-ALL) with t(5;14)(q35;q32.2). Genes Chromosomes Cancer 37:84–91
10. Nagel S, Kaufmann M, Drexler HG, et al (2003) The cardiac homeobox gene NKX2-5 is deregulated by juxtaposition with BCL11B in pediatric T-ALL cell lines via a novel t(5;14)(q35.1;q32.2). Cancer Res 63:5329–5334
11. Przybylski GK, Dik WA, Wanzeck J, et al (2005) Disruption of the BCL11B gene through inv(14)(q11.2q32.31) results in the expression of BCL11B-TRDC fusion transcripts and is associated with the absence of wild-type BCL11B transcripts in T-ALL. Leukemia 19:201–208
12. Sherr CJ (2004) Principles of tumor suppression. Cell 116:235–246
13. Cook WD, McCaw BJ (2000) Accommodating haploinsufficient tumour suppressor genes in Knudson's model. Oncogene 19:3434–3438
14. Quon KC, Berns A (2000) Haplo-insufficiency? Let me count the ways. Genes Dev 15:2917–2921
15. Inoue J, Kanefuji T, Okazuka K, et al (2006) Expression of TCRαβ partly rescues developmental arrest and apoptosis of αβT cells in Bcl11b–/– mice. J Immunol 176:5871–5879
16. Cismasiu VB, Adamo K, Gecewicz J, et al (2005) BCL11B functionally associates with the NuRD complex in T lymphocytes to repress targeted promoter. Oncogene 24:6753–6764
17. Kawamoto H, Ohmura K, Fujimoto S, et al (2003) Extensive proliferation of T cell lineage-restricted progenitors in the thymus: an essential process for clonal expression of diverse T cell receptor beta chains. Eur J Immunol 33:606–615
18. Ohi H, Mishima Y, Kamimura K, et al (2007) Multi-step lymphomagenesis deduced from DNA changes in thymic lymphomas and atrophic thymuses at various times after γ-irradiation. Oncogene 26:5280–5289
19. Kakinuma S, Nishimura M, Sasanuma S, et al (2002) Spectrum of Znfn1a1 (Ikaros) inactivation and its association with loss of heterozygosity in radiogenic T-cell lymphomas in susceptible B6C3F1 mice. Radiat Res 157:331–340
20. Kamimura K, Ohi H, Kubota T, et al (2007) Haploinsufficiency of Bcl11b for suppression of lymphomagenesis and thymocyte development. Biochem Biophys Res Commun 355:538–542
21. Bartkova J, Horejsi Z, Koed K, et al (2005) DNA damage response as a candidate anti-cancer barrier in early human tumorigenesis. Nature (Lond) 434:864–870
22. Gorgoulis VG, Vassiliou LV, Karakaidos P, et al (2005) Activation of the DNA damage checkpoint and genomic instability in human precancerous lesions. Nature (Lond) 434: 907–913
23. Sado T, Kamisaku H, Kubo E (1991) Bone marrow-thymus interactions during thymic lymphomagenesis induced by fractionated radiation exposure in B10 mice: analysis using bone marrow transplantation between Thy 1 congenic mice. J Radiat Res 32:168–180
24. Mao JH, Wu D, Perez-Losada J, et al (2003) Genetic interactions between Pten and p53 in radiation-induced lymphoma development. Oncogene 22:8379–8385
25. Celeste A, Difilippantonio S, Difilippantonio MJ, et al (2003) H2AX haploinsufficiency modifies genomic stability and tumor susceptibility. Cell 114:371–383
26. Freeman DJ, Li AG, Wei G, et al (2003) PTEN tumor suppressor regulates p53 protein levels and activity through phosphatase-dependent and -independent mechanisms. Cancer Cell 3:117–130

Radiation Risk Management

Framework of Radiation Safety Management in Japan: Laws, Administrative Agencies, and Supporting Associations

Naoki Matsuda, Masahiro Yoshida, Hideaki Takao, and Miwa Miura

Summary. Radiation safety management in Japan stands upon a global framework. The concerted activities of international organizations including the International Commission on Radiological Protection (ICRP), United Nations Scientific Committee on the Effects of Atomic Radiation (UNSCEAR), International Atomic Energy Agency (IAEA), and World Health Organization (WHO) form the baseline of radiation safety in Japan by incorporation of their recommendations and guidelines into laws and regulations such as the law concerning Prevention of Radiation Hazards Due to Radioisotopes, etc., and the law for Regulations of Nuclear Source Material, Nuclear Fuel Material and Reactors. To support radiation safety management, the Japan Health Physics Society (JHPS), the Japan Radioisotope Association (JRIS), and the Japanese Society of Radiation Safety Management (JRSM) play their roles by providing seminars, meetings, and publications of updated information on radiation regulations and also for technical transfer. In each radiation facility, a "radiation protection supervisor," entitled by national examination, is required to not only supervise but also promote radiation safety management including radiation monitoring inside/outside control areas and the estimation of external/internal exposure, education, and training of radiation workers. The goal of radiation safety management is, of course, to reduce the radiation health risk of the public as well as that of radiation workers. The expansion of radiation safety-risk control from legal demand to the daily life of the public, including medical exposure and emergency preparedness, through dosimetry, protection, and education is definitely important.

Key words Radiation safety management · International organizations · Supporting associations · Radiation protection supervisor

---

Division of Radiation Biology and Protection, Center for Frontier Life Sciences, Nagasaki University, 1-12-4 Sakamoto, Nagasaki 852-8523, Japan

Introduction: Overview of the Radiation Safety Framework

Radiation safety management in Japan stands upon a global framework, that is, the International Commission on Radiological Protection (ICRP), United Nations Scientific Committee on the Effects of Atomic Radiation (UNSCEAR), International Atomic Energy Agency (IAEA), and World Health Organization (WHO). The ICRP was founded in 1928 to advance the science of radiological protection for public benefit, in particular by providing recommendations and guidance on all aspects of protection against ionizing radiation. The report on biological effects of ionizing radiation issued by UNSCEAR supports the scientific background of those recommendations, and the IAEA publishes a variety of documents regarding basic safety standards (BSS) for radiation protection. WHO, within its sustainable development and healthy environments cluster, operates the radiation and environmental health program to evaluate health risks and public health issues related to environmental and occupational radiation exposure.

These concerted activities of international organizations form the baseline of radiation safety in Japan by means of incorporation of their guidelines into laws and regulations. The latest amendment, for example, to the Japanese law concerning Prevention of Radiation Hazards Due to Radioisotopes, etc., was made in 2004, when the new standard for exemption limit of radionuclides described in safety series No. 115, "International Basic Safety Standards (BSS) for protection against ionizing radiation and for the safety of radiation sources" by IAEA in 1996, was incorporated. As the exemption limit for some nuclides, such as tritium, is more than 100 times higher than the previous limit in Japan, most of the biochemical work using a small amount of tritium as a tracer can be done legally outside a control area. This drastic change after the strict Japanese regulation on the use of radioisotopes for many years has caused confusion in the context of how to manage radiation safety outside control areas. Another example includes the incorporation of the previous ICRP recommendation in 1990, which proposed the change of the effective limit from 50 mSv/year to 100 mSv/5 years into Japanese law in 2000. The new ICRP recommendation was published at the end of 2007 and is supposed to be a reflection of an amendment of the laws, through the new guidelines by IAEA, in 10 years. In the new recommendation, dose limit-related issues are not changed; however, radiation weighting factors and tissue weighting factors are modified so that changes in dose calculations and control level of releasable radioactivity from radiation facilities are able to be amended.

Japanese Laws and Regulations

The Atomic Energy Basic Law, established in 1955, is the basis of radiation-related regulations in Japan and gave birth to two major laws, the law concerning Prevention of Radiation Hazards Due to Radioisotopes, etc. and the law for Regulations of Nuclear Source Material, Nuclear Fuel Material and Reactors, according to Article

20, "Protective Measures of Radiation Hazards," and Article 12, "Regulation Concerning Nuclear Fuel Materials," respectively. The former regulates the use, sale, lease, disposal, and other handling of radioisotopes, the use of radiation-generating equipment, and the disposal and other handling of articles contaminated by radioisotopes to prevent radiation hazards, whereas the latter enforces the necessary regulations on manufacture, processing, storage, reprocessing, and disposal activities of nuclear source materials, fuel materials, and nuclear reactors. When we think about radioisotopes, most of them, except for thorium, uranium, and plutonium, are regulated by the law concerning Prevention of Radiation Hazards Due to Radioisotopes. Besides these laws, the Industrial Safety and Health Law and the Medical Service Law also contain radiation safety issues. Therefore, the radiation facility in Japan is managed under the regulation of two or three different laws. As the detailed requirements for control of radiation health risk are not identical in these different laws, the dual or triple regulations sometimes cause confusion in radiation safety practice. For example, a medical checkup for radiation workers is required every 6 months by the Industrial Safety and Health Law whereas the law concerning Prevention of Radiation Hazards Due to Radioisotopes requires this every 12 months.

Handling of radiation and radioisotopes is strictly regulated by these laws. As of the end of 2007, approximately 4600 facilities are approved to handle radioisotopes. In each facility, radiation can be used only in the designated control area equipped with radiation shielding walls and ventilation systems. Radioactive wastes should be stored inside the control area until they are taken away by the Japan Radioisotope Association (JRIS), which takes care of radiation waste management in Japan. Radiation workers are subject to medical checkups, education/training, and dosimetry of internal/external exposure to secure the radiation safety of each individual. The dosimetry of external exposure for radiation workers from April 2005 to March 2006 by the radiophotoluminescence technology distributed by Chiyoda Technol Corporation resulted in 39 681.6 mSv as a population (222 343 workers) dose and 0.17 mSv as an average dose per worker (Table 1). The workers

Table 1. Annual effective dose in Japan (external exposure, April 2005–March 2006)

Dose (mSv)	Medical	Educational	Nondestructive examination	Industrial	Total
Population dose	35 839.30	1 018.70	875.60	8 851	39 681.60
Average dose	0.25	0.02	0.37	0.05	0.17
ND	103 610	45 091	1 722	32 673	183 096
	(74.76)	(96.28)	(74.10)	(94.43)	(82.35)
–0.10	1 948.00	947	124	583	902
	(6.39)	(2.02)	(5.34)	(1.69)	(2.61)
0.11–1.00	16 637	562	277	10 505	18 378
	(12.00)	(1.20)	(11.92)	(4.72)	(8.27)
1.01–5.00	8 418	188	170	364	9 140
	(6.07)	(0.40)	(7.31)	(1.05)	(4.11)

(continued)

Table 1. (continued)

Dose (mSv)	Medical	Educational	Nondestructive examination	Industrial	Total
5.01–10.00	981	43	28	70	1 122
	(0.71)	(0.09)	(1.21)	(0.20)	(0.50)
10.01–50.00	91	0	2	7	100
	(0.06)	(0.00)	(0.08)	(0.02)	(0.02)
50.00–	1	0	1	0	2
	(<0.01)	(0.00)	(0.04)	(0.00)	(0.00)
Total	138 589	46 831	2 324	34 599	222 343
	(100.00)	(100.00)	(100.00)	(100.00)	(100.00)

Monitored by Radio-photo Luminescence technology (Glass Budge™, Chiyoda Technology Corporation, Tokyo, Japan)

involved in nondestructive examination using X-rays or γ-rays demonstrated the highest level of average dose at 0.37 mSv, while the lowest was found in educational workers at 0.02 mSv. Two workers, one who is a medical and the other a nondestructive examination worker, exhibited doses higher than 50 mSv.

Specialists of Radiation Safety Management and Supporting Associations

Because radiation safety management procedures need basic knowledge and understanding of radiation physics, chemistry, biology, technology, psychology, and education as well as laws and regulations, the number of specialists in radiation safety is limited. Under the law concerning Prevention of Radiation Hazards, a specialist entitled a "radiation protection supervisor" by national examination should be assigned in each radiation facility. At present, more than 4600 radiation protection supervisors are playing roles in radiation safety management including radiation monitoring inside/outside control areas, estimation of external/internal exposure, and education and training of radiation workers. Although the legal responsibilities of radiation protection supervisors are only those named within the law, expansion of their activities to widespread radiation safety includes training for radiation emergency preparedness and safety operation in radiation accidents. Collaborative efforts with radiologists, radiological technologists, and medical physicists are also necessary to contribute to regional safety, such as radiation emergency preparedness and risk communications (Fig. 1).

From academic societies to the committee of radiation protection supervisors, there are several nonprofit organizations to promote radiation safety management in Japan. The Japan Health Physics Society (JHPS) is the official member of the International Radiation Protection Association (IRPA) and therefore acts as a scientific organization to reflect their activities to the society and the practices of

Fig. 1. Personnel and specialties required for radiation safety/risk management

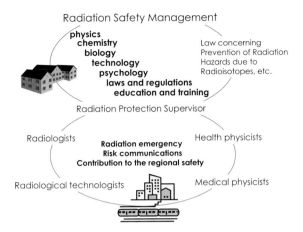

radiation protection. JRIS, working for wider application of knowledge and technology, maintains a complete system from supply to disposal of radioisotopes for the sake of promotion of utilization of radioisotopes in Japan. The radiation protection supervisor's committee of JRIS organizes the radiation safety staff of registered radiation facilities to maintain all the radiation facilities with the latest information on radiation safety regulations and guidelines. To put a wide variety of radiation safety management procedures together in a scientific research field, the Japanese Society of Radiation Safety Management (JRSM), which was founded in 2001, covers basic, applied, and practical research not only in natural sciences but also in the social sciences. Collaborative actions of these organizations, such as a scientific meeting, is also performed, depending on the topic.

Conclusion: Radiation Health Risk Management in the Framework

The goal of radiation safety management is, of course, to reduce radiation health risk in the world. However, it could be possible that accurate estimation of radiation health risk, including estimation of exposed dose, has been performed for radiation workers only because of legal requirements. The expansion of radiation safety-risk control from legal demand to the daily life of the public, including medical exposure and emergency preparedness, through dosimetry, protection, and education, is definitely important.

Background Radiation Dose to the Population Around the Kudankulam Nuclear Power Plant

Subramaniyan Selvasekarapandian, Jeyapandian Malathi, Gopalganapathi M. Brahmanandhan, and David Khanna

Summary. In Kudankulam (a small village near Cape Comerin, the southernmost tip of the Indian subcontinent), two nuclear power reactors of 1000 MWe each are now under construction. To create baseline data regarding natural background radiation, systematic measurements of the radiation levels in soil, sand, air, and indoors have been performed. Five taluks situated in three different districts lying within a 30-km radius have been chosen as the study area for the present measurements. Primordial radionuclide concentration in sand and soil samples has been measured, and sparse distribution of monazite has been discovered in some places along the coastal areas of Kanyakumari district. The annual effective dose from the three primordial radionuclides in soil samples to the population living around the Kudankulam nuclear power plant is 0.149 mSv/year. The average annual effective dose from primordial radionuclides in sand samples is found to be 0.994 mSv/year. The annual effective dose from indoor gamma radiation has been calculated as 1.18 mSv/year. The effective dose rate from radon, thoron, and their progeny varied from 0.05 to 22.23 mSv/year, with a geometric mean value of 0.62 mSv/year. The overall dissolved radon concentration in drinking water samples was found to vary between background level (<26 mBq/l) and 9939 ± 247 mBq/l.

Key words Nuclear power plant · Gamma radiation · Radon · Thoron

Introduction

The sources of natural background radiation are three primordial radionuclides (potassium-40, thorium-232, and uranium-238) found in soil and sand. People living in dwellings also acquire radiation exposure from building materials along with background radiation from the soil. Radon (^{222}Rn) and thoron (^{220}Rn) are radioactive gases that are released during decay of uranium and thorium series, respectively, which are found in homes and can contribute to internal exposure by

---

Solid State and Radiation Physics Laboratory, Department of Physics, Bharathiar University, Coimbatore 641–046, India

inhalation. The radon that is released from rocks can easily dissolve in water and give an internal dose by ingestion when this water is used. This chapter considers these issues in detail.

The Indian government is pursuing an ambitious programme of generating 20 000 MWe of power through nuclear energy alone by 2020 A.D. To realize this dream, efforts are being carried out in all fronts of nuclear science and technology. The Nuclear Power Corporation of India Limited under the aegis of the Department of Atomic Energy has signed up for collaboration with Atomstroyexport of the Russian Federation to set up two 1000 MWe nuclear reactors of advanced light water type in Kudankulam. Before the commencement of any nuclear power stations or industry, it is mandatory to carry out measurement of existing natural background radiation levels around the power project site. Baseline data around the Kudankulam Nuclear Power Plant site have been created by these methods:

1. Estimation of primordial radionuclides in sand samples collected along the beaches and measurement of external gamma radiation
2. Estimation of primordial radionuclides in soil samples collected from all the five taluks and the associated gamma background dose
3. Indoor gamma radiation measurement using thermoluminescent dosimeters (TLDs) in different types of dwellings throughout the five taluks
4. Measurement of the concentration of indoor radon, thoron, and their progeny in different types of dwellings spread throughout the five taluks using solid state nuclear track detectors (SSNTD)-based passive detector technique
5. Measurements of dissolved radon in drinking water

The results of these measurements are presented in this chapter. Figure 1 shows the study area map.

Materials and Methods

Gamma-ray spectrometry offers a convenient, direct, and nondestructive method for the measurement of the activity of different radionuclides in environmental samples from their characteristic gamma line in the spectrum. A detector consisting of NaI(Tl) crystals 3 in. × 3 in. was used in the present investigation. Standard soil sample collection and processing methods have been adopted [1]. The gamma-ray spectrometer has been characterized using standard gamma sources [1]. To measure indoor gamma radiation, the thermoluminescence technique has been adopted. A TLD is a piece of thermoluminescent phosphor material kept in a small brass capsule 1 mm thick and 5 mm long. $CaSO_4$:Dy, prepared in the laboratory by the acid evaporation technique [2], was used as the phosphor material. The radon-thoron mixed-field dosimeter designed by the Bhabha Atomic Research Centre and employed for the present measurements consists of a twin chamber system, and LR115 type (type II, strippable) film was used [3]. All the indoor gamma radiation

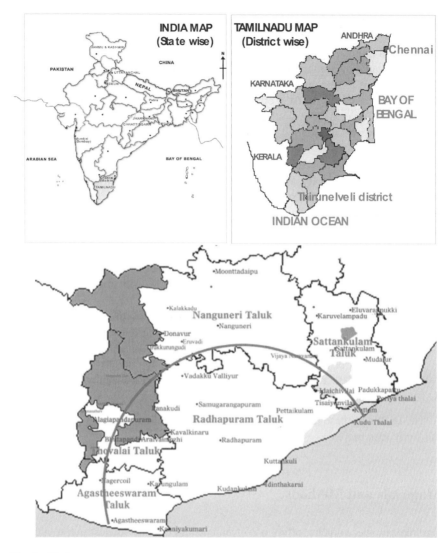

Fig. 1. Study area map

and indoor radon-thoron measurements have been performed on a quarterly basis (90 days) covering a year. Radon in drinking water samples was measured using the standard scintillation cell method utilizing radon bubblers [4]. Throughout the study area, different types of drinking water sources have been collected. Chromosomal study has been carried out where the indoor gamma radiation is high. Human peripheral blood leukocyte cultures have been used for chromosomal analysis using G-banding technique in the present study.

Results

Radioactivity in Soil and Sand Samples

Soil. We collected 470 soil samples around the Kudankulam Nuclear Power Project plant site, and activity levels of primordial radionuclides (^{232}Th, ^{238}U, and ^{40}K) have been measured using a NaI(Tl) gamma-ray spectrometer. In soil samples, ^{232}Th activity varied between 18.4 and 2181.6 Bq/kg with a geometric mean of 148.1 Bq/kg; the variation of ^{238}U and ^{40}K was calculated as background level (8.5Bq/kg) – 453.7 Bq/kg and 13.25 – 1713.2 Bq/kg, with a geometric mean of 29.9 Bq/kg and 238.8 Bq/kg, respectively. Using the United Nations Scientific Committee on the Effects of Atomic Radiation (UNSCEAR) conversion factors [5], the estimated total dose from these three radionuclides was calculated; the results varied between 14.3 and 1552.8 nGy/h. The activity level of ^{232}Th was found to be higher within a 5- to 10-km region, that is, the Teri region situated around Thillaivalanthoppu. The structured soil in the Teri region has a high abundance of natural radionuclides compared to other soil types existing in the Kudankulam environment. The annual effective dose from the three primordial radionuclides to the population living around the Kudankulam nuclear power plant is estimated to be 149 µSv/year.

Sand. We collected 78 sand samples around the seashore of the Kudankulam nuclear power plant site. The activity level of ^{232}Th was found to be 24.3 times higher than that of the world average (30 Bq/kg) reported in UNSCEAR (2000) [5]. The activity level of ^{238}U series was 2.8 times higher than the world average (35 Bq/kg). The estimated average annual effective dose is found to be 993.5 µSv/year. A clear upward trend is observed in the ^{232}Th concentration if one moves east from the Kanyakumari (Cape Comorin). The ^{232}Th concentration remained at a high level up to Kudankulam, after which it decreased towards the Thoothukudi district. Hence it is observed that the monazite deposition, which is responsible for the high activity of ^{232}Th, is present only in the Kanyakumari to Kudankulam shore.

Indoor Gamma Dose

Throughout the surrounding areas of Kudankulam, 341 houses have been surveyed for indoor gamma radiation estimation. CaSO$_4$:Dy phosphor has been used in the present measurements. Indoor gamma radiation has been monitored on a quarterly basis covering all the seasons of the year. Geometric mean values of indoor gamma radiation were estimated as 278.2, 255.2, 217.2, and 202.1 nGy/h in summer, autumn, winter, and spring seasons, respectively. Higher values of indoor gamma radiation have been recorded in the seashore villages where the activity level of primordial radionuclides was found to be high. High values of indoor gamma radiation have also been observed in summer because of the very high temperature prevalent around the Kudankulam environment. The annual effective dose from indoor gamma radiation has been estimated as 1.18 mSv/year around the Kudankulam Nuclear Power Plant site.

Radon, Thoron, and Their Progeny

We randomly selected 250 houses for measuring radon, thoron, and their progeny concentrations around the Kudankulam Nuclear Power Project site. The ^{222}Rn gas level was found to vary from background level to 110.9 Bq/m^3 in all seasons, with a geometric mean of 26 Bq/m^3. The ^{220}Rn gas level was found to vary from background level to 116 Bq/m^3 with a geometric mean of 17.6 Bq/m^3. The ^{222}Rn progeny level estimated varied from background level to 21.2 mWL with a geometric mean (GM) value of 3.3 mWL (working level). The ^{220}Rn progeny level was found to vary from background level to 165.2 mWL with a geometric mean of 9.8 mWL. The equilibrium factor for ^{222}Rn and its progeny varied from 0.01 to 0.71; that for ^{220}Rn varied from 0.001 to 0.39. The estimated effective dose rate from these radionuclides using UNSCEAR (2000) conversion factors varied from 0.05 to 22.2 mSv/year with a GM of 0.62 mSv/year, based on an indoor occupancy factor of 0.8 for ^{222}Rn and 0.03 for ^{220}Rn.

Dissolved Radon in Drinking Water

We collected 118 drinking water samples from different sources of water such as open wells, borewells, ponds, rivers, and taps around the Kudankulam Nuclear Power Project site. The overall dissolved ^{222}Rn level estimated varied from background level (<26 mBq/l) to 9939 mBq/l (excluding one abnormal value). In general, drinking water samples collected from borewell water sources demonstrated significantly higher levels of dissolved ^{222}Rn as compared to that from other sources. The overall highest concentration of ^{222}Rn was found in a borewell sample collected in Dharmapuram in the Agastheeswaram taluk. Only this drinking water sample was found to have a higher dissolved ^{222}Rn concentration (13.47 Bq/l) than that of the maximum contaminant level (11 Bq/l) proposed by the U.S. Environmental Protection Agency (EPA).

Discussion

The baseline study carried out for natural background radiation around the upcoming Kudankulam Nuclear Power Plant, Tirunelveli District, Tamil Nadu, India has been presented in this chapter. Primordial radionuclide levels in sand and soil samples have been measured, and a sparse distribution of monazite was discovered in some places along the coastal areas of Kanyakumari district. The annual effective dose from three primordial radionuclides in soil samples to the population living around the Kudankulam nuclear power plant was calculated as 0.15 mSv/year. The average annual effective dose from primordial radionuclides in sand samples is estimated to be 1.0 mSv/year. The annual effective dose from indoor gamma radiation has been calculated as 1.18 mSv/year. The estimated effective dose rate from indoor ^{222}Rn, ^{220}Rn, and their progeny in dwellings varied from 0.05 to 22.2 mSv/year with a geometric mean value of 0.62 mSv/year. The overall dissolved ^{222}Rn levels in drinking water samples varied from background level (<26 mBq/l) to 9939 mBq/l.

References

1. Malathi J, Selvasekarapandian S, Brahmanandhan GM, et al (2005) Study of radionuclide distribution around Kudankulam nuclear power plant site (Agastheeswaram taluk of Kanyakumari district, India). Radiat Prot Dosim 113:415–420
2. Malathi J, Selvasekarapandian S, Brahmanandhan GM, et al (2008) Gamma dose measurement in dwellings of Agastheeswaram taluk of Kanyakumari district, lying 30 km radius from Kudankulam nuclear power plant site. Environ Monit Assess 137:163–168
3. Eappen KP, Mayya YS (2004) Calibration factors for LR-115 (Type-II) based radon thoron discriminating dosimeter. Radiat Meas 38:5–17
4. Selvasekarapandian S, Sivakumar R, Muguntha Manikandan N, et al (2002) A study on the radon concentration in water in Coonoor, India. J Radioanal Nucl Chem 252:345–347
5. UNSCEAR (2000) Report on sources and effects of ionizing radiation of general assembly with scientific annexes. United Nations, New York

International Cooperation in Radiation Emergency Medical Preparedness: Establishment of a Medical Network in Asia

Makoto Akashi

Summary. Although accidents of radiation exposure fortunately occur only rarely, potential sources for exposure accidents can be found anywhere. When persons are accidentally exposed to ionizing radiation, physicians in medical practice may be involved in their immediate assessment and care; of course, their early diagnosis and dose assessment are crucial. Ionizing radiation cannot be seen by the human eye, nor smelled, heard, or otherwise detected by our normal senses, nor do symptoms/signs appear soon after radiation exposure. Moreover, these symptoms/signs are not specific for the exposure. Thus, radiation exposure is a highly emotional subject, causing widespread public concern, and the psychological aspects of radiation accidents also require attention. On the other hand, the experience gained in the medical care of recent radiation accident patients has enabled us to develop new assessment and treatment modalities and has provided more information about complications and the numerous problems yet to be solved. The knowledge of triage, assessment, initial diagnostic methods, and general treatment protocols has to be shared among medical professionals throughout the world. Human error and inadequate control or regulation of radiation sources can result in significant exposure among workers and the general public. However, one of the problems is that there are few chances to obtain this knowledge, especially in the Asian region, and not every country has developed capabilities for responding to radiation emergencies. Moreover, new concerns regarding emergency response against the threat of malicious acts require international/regional networks. As the practice of medicine is based on science as well as past experiences, a system for exchanging and sharing information on radiation accidents needs to be established for a smooth medical response anywhere in the Asian region. The National Institute of Radiological Sciences (NIRS) has introduced international training courses for medical professionals in Asia, on the basis that previous efforts have proved that international cooperation is effective.

Key words Radiation · Accidents · Network · Asia · Medical response

Center for Radiation Emergency Medicine, National Institute of Radiological Sciences (NIRS), 4-9-1 Anagawa, Inage-ku, Chiba-city, Chiba 263-8555, Japan

Introduction

A radiation accident is defined as an unintentional exposure to ionizing radiation or contamination with radionuclides, resulting in possible deleterious effects for the exposed and/or contaminated individuals [1]. Since the discovery of X-rays in 1885 by Roentgen and of radioactivity by Becquerel in 1886, radiation exposure accidents have occurred in society. As early as in 1887, Becquerel observed an erythema on his abdomen, and ascribed it to radioactive materials. Today, on the other hand, devices or locations whereby an individual could be exposed to radioactive materials are not rare. These potential sources of exposure accidents include industrial radiography, therapeutic devices, sterilizers, transportation accidents, and nuclear power plants; devices used for industrial radiography and accelerators are frequent sources of external exposure accidents.

Radiation accidents requiring treatment are rare. Medical response to a radiological emergency means providing first-aid-treatment and taking appropriate actions to protect yourself and others from radiation [2]. However, there are few medical professionals who have the experience of taking care of patients involved in radiation accidents, for the simple reason that such occurrences are not common. Nonetheless, it is on the basis of past experiences that medical care by medical professionals and first response by ambulance and police staff are carried out. These professionals are called upon at the time of radiation accidents. To respond to radiation accidents, knowledge of radiation and lessons learned from past accidents are essential [3,4]. Thus, it is important to share and exchange information of accidents internationally, especially because the information is limited [5–7]. In this chapter, I introduce our international cooperation on radiation emergency medical preparedness at the National Institute of Radiological Sciences (NIRS) and propose the establishment of a medical network in Asia.

Training and Drills

Ionizing radiation can only be detected by radiation detection instruments. This characteristic makes radiation emergencies different from other types of emergencies such as earthquakes and explosions. To prepare effectively for radiation emergencies, it is necessary to understand what radiation is, what types of events can cause a radiological emergency, and what harmful effects could result from such an event. NIRS has three domestic training courses for medical professionals. "The Seminar on Radiation Emergencies: A Pre-hospital Course" covers the principles of radiation protection against patients contaminated with radionuclides for first responders such as ambulance staff, firefighters, and policemen. "The Seminar on Radiation Emergencies: A Hospital Course" provides a general introduction to radiological protection for doctors, nurses, and radiation technologists, and also covers medical care for contaminated and/or heavily exposed patients. In "The Seminar on Radiation Measurement for Emergencies," radiation detection/measurement and also use of a whole-body counter (WBC) for the dose assessment of internal exposure are introduced to radiation technologists. Occasionally, we have invited medical leaders in radiation emergency medical preparedness from Asian countries to these courses, and introduced these courses as seminars for trainers.

We have also introduced several courses on radiation emergency medical preparedness for medical professionals in the Asian region at NIRS. IAEA (International Atomic Energy Agency)/RCA (Regional Co-operative Agreement for Research) training courses on radiation emergency for medical doctors were held in 2001 and 2004. On request, we planned four seminars for Asian medical doctors; these seminars were held for Korean and also Taiwanese doctors in 2005 and 2007. Moreover, a seminar for trainers on radiation emergency medicine in the Asian region was introduced for doctors from seven Asian countries in 2007. In these seminars, basics of radiation and radiation detection/measurement were covered, and treatment for acute radiation syndrome (ARS) and internal contamination, management of contaminated victims with radionuclides, and lessons learned from our experiences of a criticality accident, which occurred in 1999, were introduced [8–11]. Furthermore, the response to the general public was emphasized, and several past accidents were reviewed. Participants from various countries presented their systems of medical response to radiation emergency in their respective countries. Thus, knowledge and information were shared and exchanged at these seminars.

Meetings and Workshops

NIRS also planned meetings and workshops on radiation emergency medical preparedness for Asian countries. In cooperation with WHO, the "WHO-REMPAN (Radiation Emergency Medical Preparedness and Assistance) Regional Workshop on Radiation Emergency Medical Preparedness and Response in the Eastern Asia" was held in 2006. In the workshop, a medical network system in the Asian region was discussed, and the participants reached an agreement that the network is important and its establishment is required. In the same year, the "International Workshop on Radiation Emergency Medical Preparedness Within the Framework of the Asian Nuclear Safety Network (ANSN)" was held in cooperation with IAEA. In this workshop, the network system in Latin America was introduced, and establishment of the network in Asia was discussed. Although there are many problems to be resolved, medical professionals are in agreement regarding the importance of establishment of the network in the Asian region. Figure 1 shows a map of the facilities of the participants in the training courses and/or workshops/meetings of Asia at NIRS.

Radiation Emergency Medical Preparedness Network in Asia 257

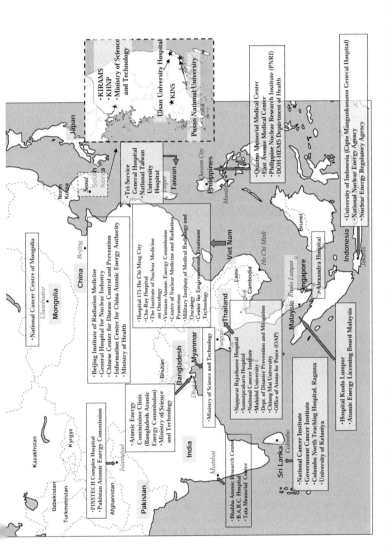

Fig. 1. Map of the facilities of the participants in training courses or workshops/meetings in Asia at the National Institute of Radiological Sciences (NIRS). For Korea: KIRAMS, KHNP, Ministry of Science and Technology, Seoul National University Hospital, Gachon Medical School, Ajou University Hospital, Chungnam National University Hospital, Chonnam National University Hospital, Kyungpook National University Hospital, Halla General Hospital, Gyeongsang National University Hospital, Chungbuk National University Hospital, Kijang Hospital, Chonbuk National University Hospital, Yeong Gwang General Hospital, Dongguk University Gyongju Hospital, Yeong Gwang Christian Hospital, Uljin Medical Center, Chungbuk National University Hospital, Gachon University Gil Medical Hospital, Ulsan University Hospital, and Pusan National University are included. For Taiwan: Tri-Service General Hospital, National Cheng Kung University, Department of Health, Executive Yuan, Taipei Veterans General Hospital, Far Eastern Memorial Hospital, National Taiwan University Hospital, Taichung Veterans General Hospital, Chung-Ho Memorial Hospital, Kaohsiung Medical University, Kaohsiung Veterans General Hospital, and Chang-Gung Memorial Hospital are included

International Response to Accidents

In 2000, a radiation source accident occurred in Thailand. In response to a request from IAEA, NIRS sent an expert to the country. In 2001, about 20 patients were exposed to high-dose radiation as a consequence of a dosage miscalculation at the department of radiation/oncology in a hospital in Panama. According to a request from IAEA, a medical expert in radiation from NIRS was sent to Panama. In 2006, the Health Protection Agency (HPA) of the United Kingdom informed us that several Japanese people might be involved in contamination with polonium-210 (^{210}Po) in London. We advised these Japanese to undergo testing of ^{210}Po levels in 24-h urine. Some of them had urine examinations at NIRS; no increases in levels of ^{210}Po were detected when compared to those of healthy volunteers.

Discussion

In spite of the fact that radiation accidents requiring treatment rarely occur, medical preparedness for such accidents is vital, because radiation is essential in modern life. Accidents of external exposure are different from radiation contamination; exposed patients do not carry radioactive materials after the radioactive materials have been removed. However, there are many misunderstandings concerning radiation exposure and its effects, as even medical professionals have few opportunities to learn about radiation. The system for the annual exchange and sharing of information on radiation accidents should result in a smooth medical response. In this respect, NIRS has introduced training courses and meetings for medical professionals in Asia. We believe that efforts should be made toward the establishment of a medical network for radiation emergencies in the Asian region.

References

1. Guskova AK (2001) Radiation sickness classification. In: Gusev IA, Guskova AK, Mettler FA Jr (eds) Medical management of radiation accidents. CRC Press, Boca Raton, pp 23–30
2. REAC/TS: Managing Radiation Emergencies: Guidance for Hospital Medical Management, Oakridge, TN. http://www.orau.gov/reacts/syndrome.htm
3. Fliedner TM, Friesecke I, Beyrer K (eds) (2001) Medical management of radiation accident: manual on the acute radiation syndrome. METREPOL (European Commission Concerted Action), British Institute of Radiology, Oxford
4. Friesecke I, Beyrer K, Fliedner TM, et al (2001) Medical treatment protocols for radiation accident victims as a basis for a computerised guidance system. How to cope with radiation accidents: the medical management. Br J Radiol 74:121–122
5. Gorin NC, Fliedner TM, Gourmelon P, et al (2006) Apperley: consensus conference on European preparedness for haematological and other medical management of mass radiation accidents. Ann Hematol 85:671–679

6. Weisdorf D, Chao N, Waselenko JK, et al (2006) Acute radiation injury: contingency planning for triage, supportive care, and transplantation. Biol Blood Marrow Transplant 12:672–682
7. Meineke V, Fliedner TM (2005) Radiation-induced multi-organ involvement and failure: a challenge for pathogenetic, diagnostic and therapeutic approaches and research. Br J Radiol 27:S196–S200
8. Hirama T, Akashi M (2005) Multi-organ involvement in the patient who survived the Tokai-mura criticality accident. Br J Radiol 27:S17–S20
9. Akashi M (2005) Role of infection and bleeding in multiple organ involvement and failure. Br J Radiol 27:S69–S74
10. Maekawa K (2002) Overview of medical care for highly exposed victims. In: Ricks RC, Berger ME, O'Hare FM Jr (eds) The medical basis for radiation-accident preparedness: the clinical care of victims. Proceedings of the fourth international REAC/TS conference on the medical basis for radiation-accident preparedness, March 2001, Orlando, Florida. Parthenon, New York, pp 313–318
11. Akashi M, Hirama T, Tanosaki S, et al (2001) Initial symptoms of acute radiation syndrome in the JCO criticality accident in Tokai-mura. J Radiat Res 42:S157–S166

Disaster and Mental Health

Long-Term Biopsychosocial Consequences of Disaster: Focus on Atomic Bomb Survivors

Naotaka Shinfuku

Summary. All disasters have biopsychosocial consequences including short-term and long-term impacts. Reviews of the mental health consequences of atomic bomb survivors of Hiroshima and Nagasaki have revealed that a variety of psychological problems were observed among survivors after the disaster and that these problems persisted after 50 years. Included were somatic complaints, anxiety, fatigue feelings, and other psychosomatic symptoms. A radiation disaster poses special mental health problems because the stressors are invisible.

Key words Radiation disaster · Biopsychosocial consequences · Nagasaki · Atomic bomb

Introduction

More than 60 years have passed since the tragedy of the atomic bombs in Hiroshima and Nagasaki in August 1945. More than 110000 people in Hiroshima and more than 70000 people in Nagasaki were killed by atomic bombs. Survivors suffered for many years from health problems caused by radiation. Immediate survivors succumbed to leukemia and radiation-related diseases one by one.

Survivors experienced the loss of loved family members, houses, and belongings. They witnessed the terrible scenes after the disaster. Naturally, they endured traumatic experiences and they showed many signs of psychological distress. However, for decades people did not pay much attention to the psychological distress of survivors of the atomic bombs. It was only in the 1980s that the mental health aspects of the disaster victims received due attention. In the United States, posttraumatic stress disorder (PTSD) appeared to describe the psychological consequences among Viet Nam veterans, and the mental health problems of disaster victims gradually gained recognition.

Department of Social Welfare, School of Human Sciences, Seinan Gakuin University, 6-2-92 Nishijin, Sawara-ku, Fukuoka 814-8511, Japan

The Chernobyl atomic power plant exploded in April 1986, killing people and spreading radioactive substance for more than 300 km. This radiation accident in Chernobyl caused panic, fear, anxiety, and other specific psychological problems in nearby countries because the stressors were invisible. In Japan, the Great Hanshin Awaji Earthquake in January 1995 provided the opportunity for medical professionals to pay attention to the psychological dimension of disaster victims.

A series of surveys on atomic bomb survivors by psychiatrists at Nagasaki University revealed that a considerable number of survivors were still suffering from psychological distress after 50 years. This chapter provides an overview of psychological consequences of disaster in general and the specific features of psychological problems caused by radiation disasters.

Subjects and Methods

This chapter is an overview of disaster mental health based on my personal observation of the long-term health consequences of the Hanshin Awaji Earthquake victims from 1995 to present [1]. The author lived in Kobe in 1995 and experienced the Hanshin Awaji Earthquake. Since then, he has been engaged in activities for the psychological care of disaster victims as well as epidemiological research on the mental health of disaster victims [2].

Included is a literature review of health problems related to radiation disasters, among them several reports on the psychological consequences of Hiroshima and Nagasaki atomic bomb victims (*Hibakusha*) by Japanese researchers, as well as reports by Russian experts on the Chernobyl nuclear plant disaster. The author served on several occasions as a member of a committee and research team of the Ministry of Health and Welfare to study mental health impacts of disaster victims of the Hanshin Awaji Earthquake, the Tokai Nuclear Plant accident, and Nagasaki atomic bomb survivors.

Results

Biopsychosocial Consequences of Disasters in General

All disasters have biopsychosocial consequences, including short-term and long-term impacts. In the case of the Hanshin Awaji Earthquake, biological consequences included death, injuries, and stress-related health problems such as peptic ulcers and hypertension. Psychological problems included anxiety, depression, and PTSD. Social impacts included poverty, isolation and emigration. It appears that at times psychological and social impacts of disasters were not accorded sufficient attention [2].

The foregoing biopsychosocial consequences are considered to be general reactions to any kind of disaster, either small or large, by the victims. Disasters differ greatly in their nature and the amount of damage. However, there are some commonalities among the psychological impacts. As well, the psychological impact on the victims changes over time. A worsening of general health conditions continues for decades or more for a sizable number of the victims of disasters. Man-made disasters pose more severe and long-lasting psychological damage than do natural disasters. Certain population groups are more vulnerable than other groups. Women are more vulnerable than men to the disaster, and younger people and children are more vulnerable than adults. Panic reaction, psychosomatic problems, neurotic symptoms and depression are psychiatric problems commonly seen after a disaster. Insomnia and fear are commonly seen soon after a disaster. A depressive reaction is common for those who have lost family members, homes and their belongings. Some victims develop personality problems and alcohol and substance abuse as they have lost their will to live in a constructive manner. PTSD may be considered a part of a wider range of neurotic and depressive symptoms. Such psychological dimensions are sometimes overlooked by policy makers. Human care for the victims could greatly relieve psychological suffering of victims in the long run. Thus, it is important to provide comprehensive and long-term care to the victims of disasters. The victims of a disaster become survivors of the disaster and potential helpers to other disaster victims through their valuable experiences [3].

Psychological Problems of Atomic Bomb Survivors

The atomic bombs in Hiroshima and Nagasaki in August 1945 killed more than 110 000 persons in Hiroshima and more than 70 000 in Nagasaki. The survivors are very old now, and many of them are still suffering from a variety of physical, mental and social difficulties. Studies on the psychological aspects of the victims are scarce compared with those on their physical problems.

Nonetheless, there were a few reports on the psychological aspects of the victims of the atomic bombs. There was no scientific report on the mental health of atomic bomb survivors immediately after the disaster. All medical facilities in Hiroshima and Nagasaki were destroyed by the atomic bombs. The hospitals of affected areas were destroyed. Medical resources, if they existed, were mobilized for the physical care of the survivors. Psychiatrists Okumura and Hikita from Kyusyu University, Fukuoka, visited the National Omura Hospital near Nagasaki in November 1945 and interviewed survivors 4 months after the atomic bombing of Nagasaki. They reported cases of general neurotic complaints, panic attack with stupor, and a few cases of neurosis and psychosis [4]. In 1953, Konuma reported the psychological problems of atomic bomb victims in Hiroshima. He observed that about 25% of the respondents were suffering from a variety of problems that would be diagnosed as PTSD today; these were, among others, an increase in the sensitivity to light and sound, nightmares, intrusive thoughts about the scene soon after the bombing, and avoidance of the event, place and person recalling the scene [5]. Konuma also reported the persistence of smelling bad smells (olfactory hallucination) among survivors. Many survivors experienced terrible odors from the decay of human bodies after the atomic bomb disaster. In 1961, Nishikawa also reported the results of a survey of atomic bomb survivors in Nagasaki. He was then professor and chairman of the Department of Psychiatry at Nagasaki University. Nishikawa reported a high prevalence of psychosomatic and neurotic symptoms among the survivors. Nervous system disturbances, feelings of bodily fatigue, forgetfulness and headaches were mentioned as common psychological problems of the survivors [6]. At that time, the term neuro-asthenia was used among Japanese psychiatrists to describe a wide range of psychological distresses. Many of them may be termed as somatoform disorder or PTSD in modern classification systems based on the *Diagnostic and Statistical Manual of Mental Disorders (DSM)* and the International Classification of Diseases (ICD).

Mental Health Surveys of Atomic Bomb Survivors After 50 Years

In March 1957, 11 years after the atomic bomb disaster, the Japanese government formulated a law to provide free medical checkups and free medical care to the survivors of the atomic bombs in Hiroshima and Nagasaki. The law specified the population who could benefit from these services to be the residents of certain designated geographical areas. Since then, a series of legal measures were promulgated to provide medical and humanitarian services to the population certified as *Hibakusha* (atomic bomb victims) by central and local governments. However, the mental health aspects of survivors were not accorded due attention for many years; leukemia and other malignancies resulting from atomic bomb radiation receiving the majority of medical attention. Nakane and his colleagues at the Department of Psychiatry, Nagasaki University, undertook a series of surveys of the mental health aspects of survivors in the 1990s. In 1994, Nakane and his colleagues in Nagasaki carried out a survey of the psychological consequences among atomic bomb survivors in Nagasaki after 50 years [7]. Nakane used the cases registered at the Atomic Bomb Survivors Regular Health Check. Of 38 827 registered cases, 7 600 survivors participated in the first screening survey and received a test using the simple version of the General Health Questionnaire (GHQ). Residents close to the center of the bombing scored high. Then, 226 survivors participated in the second survey and were interviewed by specialists using the structured interview schedule. Interviews by psychiatrists reported 83 cases (36.7%) as clinical cases. Among them, survivors with mood disorders constituted 33 cases, survivors suffering from neurotic disorders, stress disorder, and somatoform disorders comprised 36 cases, and 10 survivors showed behavioral problems related to physical and somatic factors such as insomnia and eating disorders. Also, 4 survivors had substance abuse disorders such as alcohol dependency. These figures showed that among all atomic bomb survivors, 14.6% could be given psychiatric diagnoses. Nakane observed the high rates of somatic complaints, anxiety, and somatoform disorders among survivors. Their Quality of Life (QOL) and GHQ scores were poor compared to the general population. Nakane et al. found that closely similar psychological symptoms to those described by Konuma and Nishikawa persisted after 50 years among atomic bomb victims (*Hibakusha*) [7].

Nakane also conducted a mental health survey on 8700 residents who lived within 12 km from the center of the atomic bombing and who were still living in the same designated area. He used the Clinician-Administered PTSD Scale (CAPS) and was able to obtain valid data from 312 respondents. He found 20 cases (6.4%) of complete PTSD and 57 cases (18.3 %) of incomplete PTSD [8].

There were strong requests from the residents outside of the designated area to enlarge the geographical area that could benefit from the law enacted in 1957. Many residents outside of the designated area complained of physical and mental health distress resulting from the atomic bomb. In 1999, Ohta et al. carried out a survey on "atomic bomb experience and psychological trauma" for residents outside the designated area of the city of Nagasaki and reported that a considerable number of survivors outside of the designated area were also suffering from long-lasting psychological trauma [9]. The work by Nakane and his colleagues contributed greatly to raise the awareness of long-term psychological distress suffered by *Hibakusha* [10]. Their work has influenced the Atomic Bomb Health Law and contributed to enlarging the coverage of the designated area, enabling the residents to access free medical care [11].

Radiation Disaster and Specific Mental Health Problems

Radiation disasters have the following aspects as unique features: (1) invisible stressor; (2) difficulty in knowing the degree and extent of the damage by radiation; (3) possible serious side effects at a later stage; (4) difficulty in identifying hidden side effects and genetic damage; and (5) contaminated soils and buildings as possible source for further damage.

Radiation is commonly used in medical practices for diagnoses and treatment. X-ray filming, computer tomography, and radiation therapy are important parts of modern medicine. Radiation poses specific psychological consequences to the patients. They are fearful of genetic influences, harm to the reproductive system, cancer caused by radiation, and countless unforeseen side effects. Soejima, a Japanese radiologist, reported that about one-fourth of patients receiving radiation therapy for cancer in Japan were afraid of the side effects of radiation [12]. Soejima pointed out that the high rate of anxiety among these patients might be a consequence of the unique experience of atomic bombing. However, fear of radiation therapy is worldwide. Informed consent based on education is necessary to reduce the fear of radiation therapy.

In March 1979, a nuclear plant accident took place at Three Mile Island, north of New York City, on the east coast of the United States. About 14 000 inhabitants within 10 miles of the nuclear plant were evacuated. Although the actual damage to human life was minimal, the fear and anxiety of the nearby inhabitants lasted for a long time. Pregnant women and women with young children showed continuing psychological distress. According to a survey by the National Institute of Mental Health (NIMH) 1 year after the accident, mothers with young children reported scores more than twice as high for depression, anxiety, hostility, and somatoform complaints. The Three Mile nuclear accident showed the massive psychological implications of a radiation accident even though the actual damage to physical health was not great.

In April 1986, the Chernobyl atomic power plant in the northern part of the Ukraine Republic exploded, spreading radioactive material for more than 10 days. The accident caused serious radiation disturbances to more than 200 people, killed 32 people immediately, and caused the evacuation of more than 100000 people within a 30 km radius. The Chernobyl accident was the biggest nuclear plant accident ever recorded. A survey in 1989, 3 years after the accident, detected a considerable amount of radioactive material at areas more than 300 km from the explosion site. It is well known that a variety of radiation-induced health problems appeared in contaminated areas near Chernobyl. In some areas, the incidence of thyroid tumors among children was more than 100 times higher than for children of nonaffected areas.

Russian psychiatrists carried out mental health surveys among the affected population in Chernobyl soon after the accident [13]. The survey of 1572 persons who were near Chernobyl 2 to 10 days after the accident showed very high rates of acute stress reactions, neurosis, and psychotic symptoms; 75% of respondents had some form of acute stress symptoms. Acute stress reactions included anxiety, recklessness, psychomotor agitation, inability to think and act properly, disturbance of speech, headache, thirst, loss of appetite, abnormal sense of body, anticipation of death, and depression. These symptoms fluctuated greatly and changed with time; 13% of respondents were diagnosed with neurosis ranging from strong anxiety and panic attack to somatoform disorders, and 3.8% were judged by Russian psychiatrists as having psychotic disorders. Confusion and delusional states were included in this category, although this category disappeared based on a survey 6 months later. The forgoing survey has several flaws in sampling and diagnostic reliability. However, this study showed that a wide range of mental health problems were observed among victims of the Chernobyl nuclear disaster. At 3.5 years after the disaster, the International Atomic Energy Agency (IAEA) conducted a survey of the population of the affected area and compared the data with those of a nonaffected area: 44.5% of the population in the affected area attributed their ill health to radiation and more than 70% of the population had a desire to emigrate.

Several studies on the psychological aspects among the survivors of Chernobyl showed that survivors suffered a wide range of mental problems and that these problems were of a long-lasting nature. One could argue that survivors of the atomic bomb in Nagasaki and survivors of the atomic plant explosion of Chernobyl showed similar long-lasting psychological distress.

In September 1999, an accident at the nuclear plant at Tokai, Ibaraki Prefecture, north of the Tokyo area, killed two people and injured a few employees. This accident, although small in scale, caused panic to the nearby population. Vegetables from this area were refused by markets. The nearby population had to be evacuated. School children from this area were stigmatized.

Mrs. Kyoko Hayashi, a famous writer who experienced the atomic bomb in Nagasaki, wrote a story about a young Japanese girl in Nagasaki who would not accept a marriage proposal from the man she loved because she was *Hibakusha*. She stigmatized herself as incompetent to live a normal life because of possible ill health and the bad consequences for her offspring. This story clearly shows the long-lasting psychological trauma of radiation disasters.

Discussion

My personal experience as a victim of the Hanshin Awaji Earthquake and a review of psychological consequences of disaster victims demonstrates that a whole range of biopsychosocial problems appear with time after the disaster. Any disaster has biopsychosocial impacts on the victims and affects the population, while the psychological trauma and social stigma of the victims is long lasting. Radiation disasters pose specific mental health problems as the stressors are invisible. Also, it is hard to identify the hidden side effects and genetic damage. The survivors who experienced the atomic bombings still suffer from various psychosomatic problems 60 years after the disasters. They rate low in GHQ and QOL scores. Long-term support is necessary and valuable to reduce the negative consequences of disasters.

Finally, the author would like to highlight the following measures as important to reduce the psychological problems of disaster victims: (1) dissemination of accurate scientific data; (2) complete disclosure of the data; (3) regular check of victims' physical and mental condition; (4) antistigma education; (5) support for their accommodation and life; and (6) a comprehensive health support and care system.

Acknowledgments. The author is grateful to Prof. Yoshibumi Nakane, former professor and chairman of the Department of Psychiatry, Nagasaki University. His work has formed the basis for studies on mental health aspects of atomic bomb survivors in Japan.

References

1. Shinfuku N (1999) To be a victim and a survivor of the great Hanshin-Awaji earthquake. J Psychosom Res 46:541–548
2. Shinfuku N (2005) The experience of the Kobe earthquake. In: Lopez-Ibor JJ, Christodoulou G, Maj M (eds) Disasters and mental health. World Psychiatric Association, Wiley, West Sussex, pp 127–136

3. Shinfuku N (2002) Disaster mental health-lessons learned from the Hanshin-Awaji earthquake. World Psychiatry 1:158–159
4. Okumura N, Hikita H (1949) Neuro-psychiatric findings of victims of atomic bomb (in Japanese). Kyusyu Neuro-Psychiatric Journal 1:50–52
5. Konuma M, Furuya M, Kubo S (1999) Diencephalic syndromes as atomic bomb consequences. Japan Medical News (Nihoniji-shinpou) 1547:4853–4860
6. Nishikawa T, Chikujyo S (1961) Psychiatric survey on atomic bomb victims (in Japanese). Nagasaki Medical Journal 36:717–722
7. Nakane Y, Honda S, Mine M, et al (1996) The mental health of atomic bomb survivors. In: Nagataki S, Yamashita S (eds) Nagasaki Symposium on Radiation and Human Health. Elsevier, Amsterdam, pp 239–246
8. Nakane Y, Takada K, Imamura Y, et al (1998) Mental health among atomic bomb survivors in Nagasaki. Hiroshima International Council for Health Care of the Radiation-Exposed (HICARE) & World Health Organization (eds) Proceedings of the WHO/HICARE Symposium on Radiation Accidents and Environmental Epidemiology: a decade after the Chernobyl accident. WHO, Geneva, Switzerland, pp 93–105
9. Ohta Y, Mine M, Wakasugi M, et al (2000) Psychological effect of Nagasaki atomic bombing on survivors after half a century. Psychiatry Clin Neurosci 54:97–103
10. Honda S, Shibata Y, Nakane Y, et al (2002) Mental health conditions among atomic bomb survivors in Nagasaki. Psychiatry Clin Neurosci 56:575–583
11. Nakane Y (2006) The long path to psychological disorder authorization in atomic bomb being bombed (in Japanese). Clinical Psychiatry 48:273–285
12. Kokai M, Soejima T, Wang XD, et al (2001) Psychological disturbances at radiation disasters (in Japanese). Japanese Journal of Psychiatric Treatment 16:387–394
13. Spivak LI (1992) Psychiatric aspects of the accident at Chernobyl nuclear power station. Eur J Psychiatry 6:207–212

Health Status of Children Exposed to the Chernobyl Accident In Utero: Observations in 1989–2003 and the Implications for Prioritizing Prophylactic Programs

Nataliya A. Korol[1] and Yoshisada Shibata[2]

Summary. To elucidate the health effects of exposure in utero to the Chernobyl accident, we compared the health status of 406 children (201 boys and 205 girls) born from women pregnant at the time of the accident (exposed group), and 406 children matched for gender and year of birth (control group) born from mothers who had been living in the same district of Kiev as mothers of the exposed group since before the accident, on the basis of biennial checkup results from 1989 through 2003. Prevalence was significantly higher in the exposed group than in the control group in bronchitis, liver system disorders, and stomach disorders observed in 1995–2003 and in vegetative nervous system disorder and cardiovascular disorders observed in 1997–2003. The prevalence of neurotic disorders was significantly higher in the exposed group than in the control group in 1989–1997; it increased dramatically until 1993, then decreased dramatically in 1995–1997, and the difference diminished in effect in 1999–2003. The results of the present study suggest the effectiveness of the massive psychosocial support programs launched in 1993 by national and international nongovernmental organizations (NGOs) for those exposed in utero as a "social target group." People exposed in utero are still in need of prophylactic intervention with the emphasis on bronchitis, stomach disorders, liver system disorders, cardiovascular disorders, and vegetative nervous system disorder.

Key words Chernobyl accident · Exposed in utero · Somatic diseases · Neurotic disorders · Prophylactic programs

Introduction

At 1:23 A.M. on April 26, 1986, two successive explosions took place at unit IV of the Chernobyl nuclear power plant (NPP) during a test of the electrical system. By 7 A.M. on April 27, 1986, radiation exposure reached 180–600 mR/h in some

---

[1]Laboratory for Chernobyl Children Population Health, Research Center for Radiation Medicine, Academy of Medical Sciences of Ukraine, Melnikov str. 53, Kiev, Ukraine
[2]Atomic Bomb Disease Institute, Nagasaki University Graduate School of Biomedical Sciences, Nagasaki, Japan

districts of Pripyat, the town where Chernobyl NPP staff members and their families were living. Evacuation from Pripyat started at 2 P.M. on April 27, more than 36 h after the disaster, and finished at 7 P.M. on the same day.

Approximately 45 000 people who were evacuated from Pripyat received permanent accommodation in Kiev. The main purpose in locating evacuated families to Kiev was to enforce serving Chernobyl NPP and cleanup work on qualified specialists.

The chaotic and poorly organized evacuation undoubtedly brought evacuees many chronic stress factors, such as confusion about dose of radiation exposure received, lost homes and property, changes in lifestyle, and future health outcome.

Among evacuees, women who were pregnant at the time of the disaster and their children exposed in utero are at the highest risk. The objective of the present study was to evaluate health status dynamics in children exposed in utero for developing prophylactic strategies.

Materials and Methods

The subjects of the present study were 406 children (201 boys and 205 girls) exposed in utero (called exposed group hereafter) and 406 gender- and year of birth-matched children (called control group hereafter) born from mothers who had been living in the same district of Kiev as mothers of exposed group since before the accident. The children of both groups have received biennial checkups at the Research Center for Radiation Medicine in Kiev since 1989. The standard checkup included physical examination, biochemical and hematological analysis, and ultrasound of thyroid gland and abdomen. If necessary, they were hospitalized and underwent, according to a physician's prescription, deep medical examinations, such as electroencephalography, hormone and immune analysis, and other specific medical examinations.

Diagnoses were coded according to ICD-9. We compared the two groups with respect to the prevalence of several groups of diseases: bronchitis (ICD-9, 490), vegetative nervous system disorders (ICD-9, 373.9), liver system disorders (ICD-9, 570–577), stomach disorders (ICD-9, 531–537), cardiovascular diseases (ICD-9, 425–427), neurotic disorders (ICD-9, 300–315), thyroid disorders (ICD-9, 240–246), and diabetes (ICD-9, 250).

Results

During the entire observation period, the prevalence of bronchitis steadily increased in the exposed group, while it has decreased since 1997 in the control group (Fig. 1A). The relative risk (RR), comparing the prevalence of the disease in the exposed

Fig. 1. Prevalence of diseases observed in exposed group and control group at biennial checkup (**A–F**) and the corresponding relative risk (**A′–F′**). **A, A′** Bronchitis (ICD-9, 490); **B, B′** vegetative nervous system disorder (ICD-9, 373.9); **C, C′** liver disorders (ICD-9, 570–577); **D, D′** stomach disorders (ICD-9, 531–537); **E, E′** cardiovascular disorders (ICD-9, 425–427); **F, F′** neurotic disorders (ICD-9, 300–315). *UCL*, upper confidence limit; *LCL*, lower confidence limit

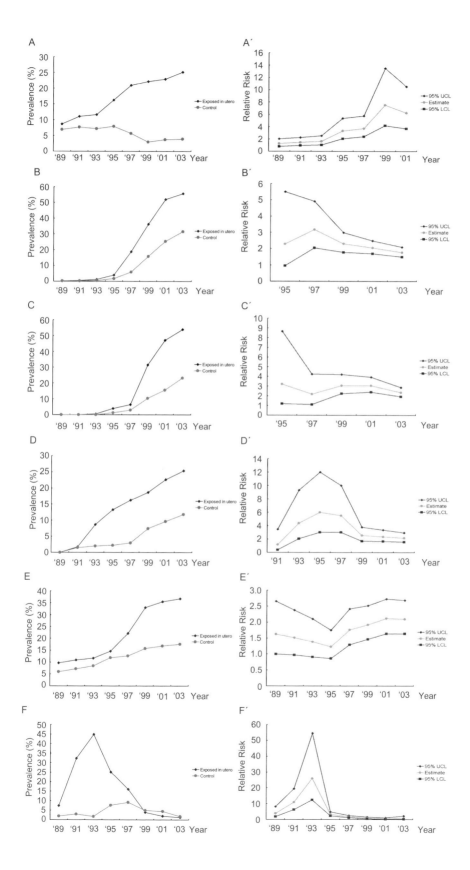

group to that in the control group, was 1.6 [95% confidence interval (CI), 1.04–2.53] in 1993; 3.3 (95% CI, 2.04–5.34) in 1995; 3.7 (95% CI, 2.38–5.74) in 1997; 7.5 (95% CI, 4.17–13.5) in 1999; 6.2 (95% CI, 3.65–10.5) in 2001; and 25.5 (95% CI, 9.48–68.6) in 2003 (Fig. 1A′).

During the entire observation period, the prevalence of vegetative nervous system disease steadily increased in both groups and was significantly higher in the exposed group than in the control group from 1997 through 2003, with a steady decrease (Fig. 1B). RR reached, in 1997, the peak of 3.2 (95% CI, 2.04–4.91), then gradually decreased: RR was 2.3 (95% CI, 1.77–2.98) in 1999; 2.0 (95% CI, 1.69–2.49) in 2001; and 1.8 (95% CI, 1.49–2.09) in 2003 (Fig. 1B′).

Liver disorders were not diagnosed in 1989 or 1991 in the exposed group or in 1989, 1991, or 1993 in the control group (Fig. 1C). The prevalence of these disorders has steadily increased since 1995 in both groups, and was significantly higher in the exposed group than in the control group since then: RR was 3.2 (95% CI, 1.83–8.66) in 1995; 2.2 (95% CI, 1.10–4.24) in 1997; 3.0 (95% CI, 2.21–4.20) in 1999; 3.0 (95% CI, 2.37–3.91) in 2001; and 2.3 (95% CI, 1.90–2.85) in 2003 (Fig. 1C′).

The stomach disorders were not diagnosed in the two groups in 1989, but the prevalence of these disorders has steadily increased since 1991 in both groups (Fig. 1D), and was significantly higher in the exposed group than in the control group since 1993, with the relative risk reaching the maximum in 1995: RR was 4.4 (95% CI, 2.05–9.32) in 1993; 6.0 (95% CI, 3.00–12.0) in 1995; 5.5 (95% CI, 3.02–10.1) in 1997; 2.5 (95% CI, 1.69–3.78) in 1999; 2.4 (95% CI, 1.66–3.35) in 2001; and 2.1 (95% CI, 1.56–2.94) in 2003 (Fig. 1D′).

The prevalence of cardiovascular disorders steadily increased in both groups during the entire period, but a significantly higher prevalence of cardiovascular disorders in the exposed group compared to the control group was observed after 1997 (Fig. 1E): RR was 1.8 (95% CI, 1.28–2.42) in 1997; 1.9 (95% CI, 1.46–2.52) in 1999; 2.1 (95% CI, 1.64–2.73) in 2001; and 2.1 (95% CI, 1.63–2.69) in 2003 (Fig. 1E′).

The prevalence of neurotic disorders observed in the entire observation period showed specific features. The prevalence of these disorders was relatively stable in the control group, whereas it began to increase rapidly in the exposed group after 1989, reaching a peak in 1993, then rapidly decreased to the level comparable to that in the control group in 1999 (Fig. 1F). RR was 3.8 (95% CI, 1.74–8.08) in 1989 and dramatically increased in 1991 (RR, 10.9; 95% CI, 6.14–19.4) and 1993 (RR, 26.0; 95% CI, 12.3–54.7). Then, RR decreased more than eightfold times in 1995 (RR, 3.3; 95% CI, 2.25–4.81); RR was 1.8 (95% CI, 1.20–2.57) in 1997. No significant difference was observed between the two groups in the prevalence of neurotic disorders in 1999–2003 (Fig. 1F′).

No significant difference was observed between the two groups in the prevalence of thyroid disorders or diabetes in 1989–2003.

Discussion

Scientists from Ukraine, Belarus, and Russia claim that somatic diseases dramatically increased in children after the Chernobyl accident [1,2]. The results of the present study showed concordance with their claims. Similar results, that is, health deterioration and an increase in the prevalence of somatic diseases, were observed by Ukrainian scientists in children born to the women who had lived during pregnancy in the zone of strict radiation control as well as in children born to pregnant evacuees from Pripyat [3]. One of the most important international researches was conducted in the framework of the "Brain Damage In Utero" project (IPHECA). The study indicated that incidence of mental retardation (the lowest degree), behavioral disorders, and changes in the emotional problems were higher in children exposed in utero compared to the control group [4]. However, the international community recognized only thyroid cancer among children as radiation-induced outcomes, attributing such an increase in somatic diseases mainly to psychological and social impact [5].

In 1993, national and international nongovernmental organizations (NGOs) recognized children exposed to the Chernobyl accident in utero as a "social target group" and launched massive psychosocial support programs for children exposed in utero to promote their mental health and intellectual and spiritual status. The most important practical program was developed by the "Chernobyl children" NGO, which targeted individually the children exposed in utero. This program included (1) psychological counseling for mothers, especially single mothers or those from an unstable family; (2) lectures for parents about child psychology and physiology, and about the results of national and international research on radiation medicine; (3) developing, publishing, and distributing literature for parents and children about the nature of ionizing radiation with its health effects, especially hereditary effects; (4) psychological counseling for children with emphasis on developing professional skills, self-esteem, tolerance, personal aims, and targeting; (5) group support; 6) organizing holidays and treatment abroad; and (7) humanitarian donations of books, vitamins, clothing, etc.

The results of the present study suggest the effectiveness of these programs for decreasing neurotic disorders in children exposed in utero. However, a significantly high prevalence of somatic disorders in children exposed in utero shown in the present study might reflect that implemented psychosocial support programs were not effective for promoting their somatic health in childhood. Medical monitoring of those exposed in utero, who are now young adults aged 21 years, should be continued and should include investigation of somatic health and of psychological and social issues.

People exposed in utero are still in need of prophylactic intervention with emphasis on bronchitis, stomach disorders, liver system disorders, cardiovascular disorders, and vegetative nervous system disorders. The same scheme of international and national prophylactic programs must be applied to other groups of Chernobyl children, for example, those living in contaminated areas, those born to evacuees and cleanup workers, for promoting their psychological and social situation.

References

1. Romanenko AYe, Nyagu AI, Loganovsky RN (2000) Radiation medicine in an assessment of the consequences of the Chernobyl disaster. Int J Radiat Med 1:3–25
2. Korenev NM, Popov NN, Borisko GA, et al (2003) Some aspects of somatic health forming of descendants of Chernobyl NPP accident liquidators. Int J Radiat Med 5:86–91
3. Stepanova E, Kondrashova V, Galichanskaya T, et al (2003) Effects in children in utero. In: Vozianov A, Bebeshko V, Bazuka D (eds) Health effects of Chernobyl accident. DIA, Kiev, pp 396–404
4. V.5 Mental health of the children irradiated in utero (1996). In: Souchkevitch GN, Tsyb AF (eds) Health consequences of the Chernobyl accident: results of the IPHECA pilot projects and related national programmes. World Health Organization, Geneva, pp 391–394
5. Chernobyl's legacy: health, environmental and socio-economic impacts and recommendations to the governments of Belarus, the Russian Federation and Ukraine. The Chernobyl Forum: 2003–2005, 2nd revised version. IAEA, Vienna, 2006. Available from IAEA (http://www.iaea.org/Publications/Booklets/Chernobyl/chernobyl.pdf)

Psychological Consequences More Than Half a Century After the Nagasaki Atomic Bombing

Yuriko Suzuki[1], Atsuro Tsutsumi[1], Takashi Izutsu[2], and Yoshiharu Kim[1]

Summary. A radioactive disaster can affect people in both their physical and mental health. Previous research has suggested that people who experienced atomic bombing directly showed poor mental health. However, even residents in the areas not designated as an atomic bombing-afflicted area by the government reportedly have poor mental health. Further investigation is warranted to examine whether people who experienced the Nagasaki atomic bomb without direct physical exposure to radiation suffer worse mental health even after 50 years, and to identify risk factors, including social experiences related to the bombing. To examine the psychological consequences of the atomic bombing in the Nagasaki area, we have set the following aims of investigation: (1) whether the people with exposure experience in the non-designated area had fear of exposure, and to what extent and what sort; (2) whether they still remain in poorer mental health than the comparison group; and (3) what sort of demographic and social experiences are related to their poor mental health. This study included subjects who lived in the area non-designated as the atomic bombing-afflicted area, with a comparison group who moved into the area after the war. Using the General Health Questionnaire 28 items (GHQ-28) as a primary indicator, we assessed the mental health status of the participants, along with knowledge of the nature and the effect of the atomic bomb and distressing and humiliating experiences related to the atomic bombing. The results of this study will be published elsewhere.

Key words Mental health · Atomic bombing · Perceived mental health · GHQ-28 · Fear of exposure

---

[1]Department of Adult Mental Health, National Center of Neurology and Psychiatry, National Institute of Mental Health, 4-1-1 Ogawa-Higashi, Kodaira, Tokyo 187-8553, Japan
[2]Department of Forensic Psychiatry, National Center of Neurology and Psychiatry, National Institute of Mental Health, Tokyo, Japan

Introduction

A radioactive disaster could affect people in their physical and mental health. Mental health effects of the Nagasaki radioactive disaster yielded various forms of agony such as injury or disability caused by the disaster, particularly by radioactivity, traumatic memories of the incident, fear of being exposed to invisible radioactivity, and a psychological burden caused by socioeconomic difficulties, including stigma.

Although limited in amount of research, previous studies revealed mental health consequences after a radioactive disaster; for example, in the Chernobyl nuclear power plant accident in 1986, a high prevalence of mental disorders was reported, especially of mood and anxiety disorders among inhabitants in the region severely affected by the accident [1]. The rate of suicide, one of the most serious manifestations of poor mental health consequences, was elevated among the residents and personnel who were engaged in its restoration, and this is deemed to be a result of the mental health consequences already listed [2–6].

Among horrendous historical tragedies of radioactive disasters, the atomic bombs dropped on Hiroshima and Nagasaki in Japan killed approximately 140,000 and 70,000 people, respectively, and these bombings also devastated the people's mental health. However, only a few studies have been conducted to examine the adverse impacts in mental health among survivors of an atomic bombing. A small study 3 months after the bombing reported that less than 10% of the people who were exposed to radiation physically had mental disorders [7]. Approximately 10 years after the event, about 10% of people with radiation exposure reportedly suffered from mental disturbances [8]. A study conducted 50 years after the event demonstrated that 8.4% of those physically exposed to the atomic bomb in Nagasaki had mental health problems, but also aging, loss of family members because of the disaster, and acute symptoms after the event contributed to their deteriorating mental health status [9].

In such cases, proximate distance from the hypocenter was related to adverse mental health status of the atomic bomb survivors with physical radiation exposure [10]. However, the other type of exposure, indirect exposure, which caused fear of radioactive disasters, may also have worsened the mental health of the people. One such example was reported in many survivors' testimonials conducted by the Nagasaki City government. The researchers published a report on the deteriorated mental health condition including post traumatic stress disorder (PTSD) among the people who reside in the peripheral area of the city, where the Japanese government has contended that there is no substantial evidence for radioactivity contamination. The survivors in the area appealed for the needs of financial and medical support from the government based on the city report.

The history of these negotiations goes back to the time of the atomic bombing. After the fall of the atomic bomb in 1945, the Japanese government officially designated the central area of Nagasaki City, where the hypocenter of the bombing was, as the "exposed area," and residents in the area qualified to receive medical and financial support by the government. Yet, the decision on how to define the designated area remained controversial. The towns on the east and north edge of Nagasaki City within several kilometers from the hypocenter were not included in the official designated area, while the towns in the southern area, 10 kilometers (km) away, were designated as the official area, based on the rationale that the wind was blowing from north to south at the time of the bombing and that windborne radiation could not have reached beyond the mountains on the east side of the city of Nagasaki. In 1974 and 1976, as a result of the repeated appeals by the people in the "non-designated area" of Nagasaki City and Nagasaki Prefecture, some districts in the "non-designated area" came to be officially designated as the "partially exposed area." From April 1999 to March 2000, Nagasaki City conducted a wide mail survey to examine the general health condition of the "atomic bomb sufferers" in the "non-designated area" [11]. The response rate was nearly 80%, which reflected the keen concern of the residents in the area. The report concluded that most subjects complained of having various physical illnesses, results that were worse than the results of the preceding National Health Survey. When examined, the testimonials for the open question on the atomic bomb experience, 312 people were recognized to be at high risk for severe mental distress. Using the Clinician-Administered PTSD Scale (CAPS), a structured diagnostic interview procedure, 77 of the interviewees were diagnosed as past PTSD (20, full; 57, partial) as a consequence of the atomic bombing exposure. However, the study did not have a comparison group, and thus it was difficult to determine whether people's current worsened mental condition was a consequence of the atomic bombing more than 50 years ago.

Regardless of the previous investigations that concluded there could not be any substantial contamination with radioactive substances in the non-designated area, the fear of radioactivity exposure may have been presented as the residents' anxiety or traumatic fear from the atomic bombing. Although previous studies focused on assessing the mental health status of people who were physically exposed to the radiation, those who were not physically exposed to radiation but had experienced the intense light, enormous sound, and heat sensations of the atomic bomb may also have caused mental health disturbances; moreover, the bombing caused long-term consequences such as traumatic symptoms and other anxiety-mood disorders given the invisible nature of the radioactive rays. Thus, the subjective experience of being exposed to atomic bombing also warrants future investigation to clarify the degree of mental health status and related experiences regarding atomic bombing—how the people perceived the experience and fear at the time of, and after, the atomic bombing. No previous report, to the author's knowledge, had addressed the fear of exposure in the subjects who have suffered for more than half a century.

Therefore, we have set the following aims of this investigation: to examine (1) whether the people with exposure experience in the non-designated area had fear of exposure, and to what extent and what sort; (2) whether they still remain in poorer mental health than the comparison group; and (3) what sort of demographic and social experiences other than the atomic bombing experience are related to their poor mental health.

Subjects and Methods

Subjects

As subjects for this study, we targeted to sample 400 of the 9,800 residents with exposure experience from the non-designated area as the atomic bombing-afflicted area since the time of the atomic bombing. We defined the "exposure experience" by the degree of perception of the light, sound, and heat, as well as their location at the time of the bombing such as inside/outside a house or in the shelter, etc., without physical exposure to radioactivity, according to the decision of the government. Additionally, their radiation-related symptoms such as dental bleeding, spots on the skin, and epilation, behavior after the bombing, such as reports that they walked into the severely affected area or took care of the fatally wounded victims, and the experience of the atomic bombing by other family members were recorded. The interviews of these "exposure experiences" were later cross-checked by other family members.

To have a demographically representative sample, 30 cells were developed by age, sex, and five degrees of exposure level. In each district of the area, the subjects were selected from each cell corresponding to the distribution pattern. To have a comparison group, residents who moved into the area between 1950 and 1960, which is well after the bombing, were selected with matching by age and sex.

In the end, we approached 405 old residents in the non-designated area as a subject group, of whom 342 completed the interview, and approached 571 new residents who moved into the area after the bombing as a comparison group, yielding 330 people who completed the interview. In the analysis, we examine the data from 342 of the subject group and 288 of the comparison group.

Measurement

The dependent variable was current mental and physical well-being using the General Health Questionnaire-28 (GHQ-28) [12,13]. The GHQ-28 is one of the most widely utilized instruments for assessing general mental health status. It includes 28 items with four grade response sets each, with a higher score indicating worse general mental health status. The cutoff point of the Japanese version of GHQ-28 has been set at 6/7 [14]. The validity and reliability of the Japanese version of GHQ-28 have been confirmed [15]. In addition to total score, GHQ-28 consists of four subdomains, that is, social, physical, depressive, and anxious, each of which can be scored, and its cutoff has been set.

The independent variables were (1) basic sociodemographic characteristics such as age and sex, (2) health-related measures including perceived health status, which were assessed by six degrees from very good to very bad, and the self-report checklist of 20 diseases and treatment received within 6 months, and (3) knowledge of the nature and the effect of the atomic bomb. To detect possible reporting bias resulting from deliberate exaggeration of complaints, the K-Scale of Minnesota Multiphasic Personality Inventory (MMPI) was also administered. Lower score means the subjects tend to have self-reproach and a higher score means they tend to shuffle the responsibility onto an external matter.

With regard to the experience group, experiences related to the atomic bombing were addressed in detail to determine their experience of distress and feeling stigmatized, as well as support experienced in relationship to the atomic bombing. The interviewees were asked about their atomic bombing experiences such as resulting loss of family members. Also, their perception of adversity after the experience, and formal and informal support to care for the atomic bomb experience consequences, were evaluated.

This study was conducted during 12–30 March, 2001, after the study protocol was approved by the ethical committee of the National Center of Neurology and Psychiatry, Japan.

Results

The results of this study will be published elsewhere.

Discussion

Even after more than 50 years have passed from the time the atomic bomb was dropped on Nagasaki, people apparently have adverse mental health status as a consequence of exposure to the atomic bombing. The psychological effects of indirect exposure, namely, fear of the exposure, have been argued; however, the question has not been investigated in a scientifically rigorous manner. Administrative decision should be made based on scientific evidence, balanced with the experience of those who have been suffered for more than half a century.

References

1. Havenaar JM, van den Brink W, van den Bout J, et al (1996) Mental health problems in the Gomel region (Belarus): an analysis of risk factors in an area affected by the Chernobyl disaster. Psychol Med 26:845–855
2. Rich V (1988) Legasov's indictment of Chernobyl management. Nature (Lond) 333:285
3. Smucker P (1993) Suicide following the Chernobyl disaster (in Norwegian). J Sykepleien 16:20
4. Kamarli Z, Abdulina A (1996) Health conditions among workers who participated in the cleanup of the Chernobyl accident. World Health Stat Q 49:29–31

5. Vanchieri C (1997) Chernobyl "liquidators" show increased risk of suicide, not cancer. J Natl Cancer Inst 89:1750–1752
6. Dickson D (1998) Chernobyl claims another victim. Science 240:1402
7. Okumura N, Hikita H (1949) Results of psycho-neurological study on atomic bomb survivors (in Japanese). Kyushu Neuropsychiatry 1:50–52
8. Nishikawa T, Tuiki S (1961) The long-term psychological sequelae of atomic bomb survivors in Hiroshima and Nagasaki (in Japanese). Nagasaki Med J 36:717–722
9. Honda S, Shibata Y, Mine M, et al (2002) Mental health conditions among atomic bomb survivors in Nagasaki. Psychiatry Clin Neurosci 56:575–583
10. Yamada M, Kodama K, Wong FL (1991) The long-term psychological sequelae of atomic bomb survivors in Hiroshima and Nagasaki. In: Hubner KF, Fry SA (eds) The medical basis for radiation accident preparedness. Elsevier, New York, pp 155–163
11. Nagasaki City (2000) Kiitekudasai, watasitachi no kokoronoitade, genshiryokubakudanhibaku-mishiteitiiki syougen-chosa houkokusyo. [Listen to us, our heartbreak: report of the testimonials of people in the non-designated area as atomic bombing afflicted area (in Japanese)]
12. Goldberg DP (1972) The detection of psychiatric illness by questionnaire. Oxford University Press, London
13. Goldberg DP, Hilliler VF (1979) A scaled version of the General Health Questionnaire. Psychol Med 9:139–145
14. Fukunishi I (1990) The assessment of cut-off point of the General Health Questionnaire (GHQ) in the Japanese version (in Japanese). Shinri Rinshou. 3:235–242
15. Nakagawa Y, Daibo I (1985) Japanese version of General Health Questionnarire-28. Nihonbunkakagakusha, Tokyo

Radiation and Cancer

Significance of Oncogene Amplifications in Breast Cancer in Atomic Bomb Survivors: Associations with Radiation Exposure and Histological Grade

Shiro Miura[1], Masahiro Nakashima[2], Hisayoshi Kondo[3], Masahiro Ito[4], Serik Meirmanov[2], Tomayoshi Hayashi[5], Midori Soda[6], and Ichiro Sekine[1,2]

Summary. It has been postulated that radiation induces breast cancers in atomic bomb survivors. Oncogene amplification is an important mechanism during breast carcinogenesis and also serves as an indicator of genomic instability (GIN). The aim of this study is to clarify the association of oncogene amplification in breast cancer in atomic bomb survivors with radiation exposure. A total of 593 breast cancers were identified in atomic bomb survivors from 1968 to 1999, and the association between breast cancer incidence and atomic bomb radiation was evaluated. Invasive ductal cancers from 67 survivors and 30 nonsurvivors were analyzed for amplification of the *HER2* and c-*Myc* genes by fluorescence in situ hybridization and expression of hormone receptors by immunostaining. The incidence rate significantly increased as exposure distance decreased from the hypocenter [hazard ratio (HR) per 1.0-km decrement, 1.47; 95% confidence interval (CI), 1.30–1.66]. The incidence of *HER2* and c-*Myc* amplification was significantly increased in the order of control, distal, and proximal groups ($P = 0.0238$ and 0.0128, respectively). Multivariate analyses revealed that distance was a risk factor for co-amplification of *HER2* and c-*Myc* in breast cancer in survivors (odds ratio per 1.0-km increment, 0.17; 95% CI, 0.01–0.63]. The histological grading of breast cancers became significantly higher in the order of control, distal, and proximal groups, and was associated with oncogene amplifications. This study suggested that atomic bomb radiation may affect the development of oncogene amplification by inducing GIN and may be associated with a higher histological grade in breast cancer found in survivors.

---

[1] Department of Tumor and Diagnostic Pathology, Atomic Bomb Disease Institute, Nagasaki University Graduate School of Biomedical Sciences, 1-12-4 Sakamoto, Nagasaki 852-8523, Japan
[2] Tissue and Histopathology Section, Division of Scientific Data Registry, Atomic Bomb Disease Institute, Nagasaki University Graduate School of Biomedical Sciences, Nagasaki, Japan
[3] Biostatistics Section, Division of Scientific Data Registry, Atomic Bomb Disease Institute, Nagasaki University Graduate School of Biomedical Sciences, Nagasaki, Japan
[4] Department of Pathology, National Hospital Organization Nagasaki Medical Center, Nagasaki, Japan
[5] Department of Pathology, Nagasaki University Hospital, Nagasaki, Japan
[6] Department of Epidemiology, Radiation Effects Research Foundation, Nagasaki, Japan

Key words Breast cancer · Atomic bomb survivors · Radiation · Gene amplification · Genomic instability

Introduction

Sixty-two years have now elapsed since two atomic bombs were exploded on Hiroshima and Nagasaki, Japan, on August 6 and 9, 1945, respectively. The incidence of several types of leukemia peaked during the 5- to 10-year period after the atomic bomb explosions. Meanwhile, an increased risk of cancer has continued for decades, and the incidence of certain types of cancer is still higher than in controlled populations [1–3]. Thus, although a long-lasting radiation effect is suggested to contribute to tumorigenesis in atomic bomb survivors, the molecular mechanisms that are involved are not yet fully understood.

Recently, we detected amplification of the *RET* oncogene in human thyroid cancers [4]. Gene amplification is a term used to indicate the production of multiple copies of a specific gene [5]; it is associated with genomic instability (GIN), the main characteristic of solid tumors, and it frequently involves proto-oncogenes [6]. In thyroid cancers, *RET* oncogene amplification has been shown to correlate with radiation-induced and high-grade malignancy, providing further evidence for the involvement of GIN in tumor progression [4].

In addition to thyroid cancer, the incidence of breast cancer was also reported to be elevated in atomic bomb survivors, suggesting a radiation etiology in breast carcinogenesis as well [4]. Both *HER2* and c-*Myc* oncogene amplifications are well-known molecular alterations observed in breast cancer and correlate with a poor prognosis for patients [7,8]. In the present study, to determine the significance of oncogene amplifications in the occurrence of breast cancer in atomic bomb survivors, we analyzed the *HER2* and c-*Myc* oncogenes by fluorescence in situ hybridization (FISH) on paraffin-embedded tissue. We describe here the higher incidence of *HER2* and c-*Myc* oncogene amplifications in breast cancers from survivors who were exposed at a proximal site from the hypocenter than in breast cancers from those who were exposed at a distal site from the hypocenter or from nonexposed control patients. Thus, a higher frequency of oncogene amplifications found in cancer cells from survivors may be associated with atomic bomb radiation exposure.

Material and Methods

Identification of Breast Cancer in Atomic Bomb Survivors

A series of clinical data were available on 91 890 atomic bomb survivors registered since 1968 at the Division of Scientific Data Registry, Atomic Bomb Disease Institute, Nagasaki University Graduate School of Biomedical Sciences. The population used in this study was confined to residents of the city of Nagasaki who were directly exposed to the atomic bomb. To identify breast cancer cases in survivors, we used a database compiled by the Nagasaki Tumor Tissue Registries (NTTR), which includes 301 673 pathological reports of patients living in south Nagasaki Prefecture, including the city of Nagasaki, collected from 1961 to 1999. The database includes patient age, gender, tumor site, histological diagnosis, and date of diagnosis.

Evaluation of the Association Between Breast Cancer and Atomic Bomb Radiation

An event of breast cancer in each survivor was considered to occur with a pathological diagnosis. Person-years (PY) of observation were cumulated from the date on which an individual survivor's data were registered in our database, beginning in 1968 and continuing until either diagnosis of breast cancer, time of death, termination of follow-up (emigration from the city of Nagasaki), or the end of study (December 31, 1999). Then, the incidence rate (IR) of breast cancer per 100 000 PY among atomic bomb survivors was calculated with stratification by the distance from the hypocenter (0–1.0, 1.1–1.5, 1.6–2.0, 2.1–2.5, 2.6–3.0, >3.0 km) and age at the time of bombing (ATB) (0–9, 10–19, 20–29, 30–39, ≥40 years).

Subjects

This study included 67 cases of invasive ductal carcinomas surgically resected from atomic bomb survivors, which were archived in pathological records at the Nagasaki University Hospital. These breast cancer cases were divided into two different distance groups: individuals exposed at or less than 1.5 km from (proximal) and those exposed more than 1.5 km from (distal) the hypocenter. The proximal distance group included 35 cases (mean age, 58.5 years; range, 42–82 years) and the distal distance group included 32 cases (mean age, 66.8 years; range, 41–84 years). Diagnosis was reviewed, and the histological grade was determined according to the modified Bloom–Richardson histological grading system [9]. All samples were formalin-fixed and paraffin-embedded tissues. As control subjects, 30 cases of invasive ductal carcinoma from calendar year-matched patients (mean age, 58.8 years; range, 43–80 years), who were not exposed to the atomic bomb, were also analyzed.

Dual-Color Interphase FISH

For *HER2* hybridization, LSI *HER2/CEP17* probes (Vysis, Downers Grove, IL, USA) were used according to the manufacturer's instructions. For c-*Myc* hybridization, a cocktail containing an LSI c-*Myc* probe labeled with Spectrum Orange (Vysis) and a *CEP8* probe labeled with Spectrum Green (Vysis) was used. Deparaffinized sections were heated by microwave in 0.01 M citrate buffer (pH 6.0) and pretreated with 0.3% pepsin. Subsequently, slides were immersed in 0.1% NP-40 and denatured by heating in 70% formamide/2× SSC. The mixture of probes was denatured and applied to the pretreated tissue. After hybridization, slides were washed, counterstained with 4,6-diamidino-2-phenylindole dihydrochloride (DAPI; Vysis), and photographed using a fluorescence microscope. Signals were analyzed in approximately 500 nuclei per case at 1000-fold magnification. A minimum 2-fold increase in *HER2*/c-*Myc* signals over *CEP17*/*CEP8* signals in cancer cells was considered as positive for gene amplification.

Immunohistochemistry

After immersion in 0.3% H_2O_2/methanol, sections were preincubated with 10% normal goat serum. After antigen retrieval, tissues were incubated overnight at 4°C with anti-HER2 (DakoCytomation, Glostrup, Denmark) at a 1:300 dilution, anti-estrogen receptor (ER) (Novocanstra Laboratory, Newcastle, UK) at a 1:80 dilution, or antiprogesterone receptor (PgR) (Novocanstra Laboratory, Newcastle, UK) monoclonal antibodies at a 1:200 dilution. The slides were subsequently incubated with biotinylated goat antirabbit or antimouse IgG antibody for 1 h at room temperature and then with avidin-peroxidase, and visualized with diaminobenzidine (DAB).

Statistical Analyses

The effects of exposure distance and ATB on the IR of breast cancer in atomic bomb survivors were measured as hazard ratio (HR) with 95% confidence interval (CI) using a multivariate Cox proportional hazard model. The Jonckheere–Terpstra test was used to assess differences in pathological factors of breast cancer, such as the tumor size, score of histological grading, and level of nodal metastasis among the three different exposure distance groups. The Cochran–Armitage trend test was used to evaluate the association between the *HER2*/c-*Myc* amplifications and exposure distance groups. Associations between the presence of oncogene amplifications (none, single, and co-amplification), or immunohistochemical results (−, 1+, and 2+) and exposure distance groups were assessed by the Jonckheere–Terpstra test. Furthermore, associations between exposure distance, ATB, age at the time of diagnosis (ATD), tumor size, or histological grading and the incidence of oncogene amplification were evaluated as odds ratio (OR) with 95% CI using a multivariate logistic regression model.

Results

The IR of Breast Cancer and Its Association with Atomic Bomb Radiation

Overall, 91 890 atomic bomb survivors have been followed for 1 095 486 PY, during which 593 breast cancer cases have been confirmed. The crude IR of breast cancer was 54.1 per 100 000 PY in the overall study population. The IR of breast cancer significantly increased as the distance from the hypocenter decreased (HR per 1.0-km decrement, 1.47; 95% CI, 1.30–1.66). In addition, an age effect was observed, as evidenced by a significant decrease in the IR of breast cancer in older subjects ATB based on the ATD (HR per 1-year increment in the overall study population, 0.96; 95% CI, 0.95–0.97).

Comparison of Pathological Profiles of Breast Cancers Between Exposure Distance Groups

The mean of tumor size was 21.8, 20.3, and 30.5 mm in the proximal distance, distal distance, and control groups, respectively. Statistical analyses revealed no significant difference in tumor size between the three groups ($P = 0.647$). Histological scores of histological grading became significantly higher in the order of the control, distal distance, and proximal distance groups ($P = 0.0022$). With regard to the factors of histological grading, the scores of nuclear size ($P < 0.001$) and mitotic counts ($P = 0.0184$), but not tubule formation ($P = 0.398$), were significantly associated with exposure distance. The level of nodal metastasis was not significantly associated with exposure distance ($P = 0.881$).

Comparisons of HER2 and c-Myc Amplifications Detected by FISH Among Exposure Distance Groups

FISH analyses for *HER2* and c-*Myc* in 97 cases showed that 68 (70.1%) and 61 (62.9%) samples, respectively, showed clear hybridization signals, which confirmed the presence of oncogene amplifications. Among them, the incidence of both *HER2* and c-*Myc* amplifications became significantly increased in the order of control, distal distance, and proximal distance groups ($P = 0.0238$ and 0.0128, respectively). The incidence of co-amplification was 42.1% (8 of 19 cases) in the proximal distance group, 6.3% (1 of 16 cases) in the distal distance group, and 4.8% (1 of 21 cases) in the control group. Furthermore, the presence of oncogene amplifications (none, single, and co-amplification) became significantly higher in the order of the control, distal distance, and proximal distance groups (*P* = 0.0028).

Comparison of HER2, ER, and PgR Expressions by Immunohistochemistry Among Exposure Distance Groups

HER2 immunoreactivity was detected in 14 (40%) of 35 cases from the proximal distance group, 14 (34.4%) of 32 cases from the distal distance group, and 8 (26.7%) of 30 cases from the control group. ER immunoreactivity was detected in 18 (51.4%) of 35 cases from the proximal distance group, 12 (37.5%) of 32 cases from the distal distance group, and 19 (63.3%) of 30 cases from the control group. PgR immunoreactivity was detected in 18 (51.4%) of 35 cases from the proximal distance group, 14 (43.8%) of 32 cases from the distal distance group, and 19 (63.3%) of 30 cases from the control group. Statistical analyses revealed no significant associations between immunoreactivity of HER2, ER, or PgR expression and exposure distance (*P* = 0.432, 0.294, and 0.274, respectively).

Associations Between Exposure Distance, ATB, ATD, Tumor Size, or Histological Grading and the Incidence of Oncogene Amplifications in Breast Cancer

In breast cancers from atomic bomb survivors, the incidence of *HER2* amplifications tended to decrease as the distance increased from the hypocenter (OR per 1.0-km increment, 0.71; 95% CI, 0.38–1.15), although this decrease was not statistically significant. Furthermore, detection of c-*Myc* amplifications and co-amplification with *HER2* in breast cancer from atomic bomb survivors significantly decreased as the distance from the hypocenter increased (OR per 1.0-km increment, 0.59 and 0.17; 95% CI, 0.28–0.99 and 0.01–0.63). Among incidences of *HER2*, c-*Myc* amplification, and co-amplification, OR per 1.0-km increment for the incidence of co-amplification was lowest. This result indicates that the distance effect is most strongly associated with the occurrence of oncogene co-amplification in breast cancer. However, ATB did not significantly affect the incidence of either *HER2* or c-*Myc* amplification and co-amplification in the breast cancer samples analyzed.

Collective analysis of the entire study group used in FISH revealed that the incidence of *HER2* amplification decreased with older ATD, although this association was not statistically significant (OR per 1-year increment, 0.92; 95% CI, 0.82–1.01). Furthermore, the incidences of both c-*Myc* amplification and co-amplification significantly decreased as ATD increased (OR per 1-year increment, 0.89 and 0.79; 95% CI, 0.78–0.99 and 0.58–0.96). Among incidences of *HER2*, c-*Myc* amplification, and co-amplification, the OR per 1.0-year increment for the incidence of co-amplification was lowest. This finding indicates that the ATD effect is most strongly associated with the occurrence of co-amplification in breast cancer. The incidence of both *HER2* and c-*Myc* amplification significantly increased as the histological scores increased (OR per 1-score increment, 1.78 and 1.99; 95% CI, 1.06–3.37 and 1.07–4.61, respectively). Moreover, the incidence of co-amplification also showed a positive correlation with histological grading, and its OR exceeded those of *HER2* or c-*Myc* amplification (OR per 1-score increment, 8.63; 95% CI, 1.77–147). However, tumor size did not correlate with *HER2*, c-*Myc*, or co-amplification in breast cancer.

Discussion

Our retrospective search using two independent databases identified a total of 593 patients of breast cancer patients, tracked from 1968 to 1999, who were directly exposed to the Nagasaki atomic bomb radiation. Among these patients, an increased risk for development of breast cancer is hypothesized to occur in the survivors who were exposed at a closer distance and a younger age. This study correlates with other reports, such as the Life Span Study (LSS) by the Radiation Effects Research Foundation, and provide further evidence that atomic bomb radiation is significantly associated with the occurrence of breast cancer [10]. Furthermore, our histopathological analyses revealed a higher histological grading, including larger nuclear size and higher mitotic counts, in breast cancers in the survivors who were exposed to atomic bomb radiation at a closer distance.

FISH technology has high sensitivity and great accuracy in detection of *HER2* amplification [11]. Our FISH analyses demonstrated 31.6%/29.4% and 18.5%/14.3% of *HER2*/c-*Myc* amplification in cases from the distal distance group and controls, respectively. These results are comparable to those in previous reports, in which *HER2* gene amplification and/or protein overexpression was identified in 10% to 34% of invasive breast cancers [12]. Another study using the FISH technique found *HER2* amplification in 22% (24 of 110 patients) of invasive ductal carcinomas in Japanese women [13]. c-*Myc* has been reported to be amplified in 20% to 30% of clinical breast cancers [14]. A recent meta-analysis reported that, on average, 15.5% of breast cancers bear c-*Myc* amplification [15]. However, in contrast to other reports, results of the current analyses revealed a higher incidence of both *HER2* and c-*Myc* amplifications in invasive ductal carcinomas from atomic bomb survivors of the proximal distance group.

Our multivariate statistical analyses revealed that exposure distance can be a strong risk factor for the development of co-amplification of c-*Myc* and *HER2* in breast cancers in atomic bomb survivors. c-*Myc* amplification was significantly associated with *HER2* amplification in breast cancers among all of our subjects ($P = 0.0132$). The concept of concurrent amplification of multiple oncogenes in breast cancers is not novel. Frequent co-amplification of c-*Myc* and *HER2* in breast cancer has been reported by others performing FISH analysis on conventional tissue section, with 40% to 60% of c-*Myc* amplifications being associated with *HER2* co-amplification [16]. In the present study, among the proximal distance group, co-amplification was detected in 8 (42.1%) of 19 breast cancer cases that showed clear hybridization signals for both *HER2* and c-*Myc* status. A higher incidence of co-amplification of multiple oncogenes suggests the presence of increased GIN in breast cancer arising in survivors who were exposed proximally to the hypocenter.

In summary, this study demonstrated a higher incidence of oncogene amplification in breast cancers in atomic bomb survivors who were exposed at a distance proximal to the hypocenter. Atomic bomb radiation may affect the development of oncogene amplification by inducing a higher level of GIN and is associated with a higher histological grade, characterized by a larger nuclear size and increased mitotic counts, in breast cancer found in atomic bomb survivors who were exposed proximally to the hypocenter.

References

1. Preston DL, Shimizu Y, Pierce DA, et al (2003) Studies of mortality of atomic bomb survivors. Report 13: Solid cancer and noncancer disease mortality: 1950–1997. Radiat Res 160:381–407
2. Ron E, Lubin JH, Shore RE, et al (1995) Thyroid cancer after exposure to external radiation: a pooled analysis of seven studies. Radiat Res 141:259–277
3. Carmichael A, Sami AS, Dixon JM (2003) Breast cancer risk among the survivors of atomic bomb and patients exposed to therapeutic ionising radiation. Eur J Surg Oncol 29:475–479
4. Nakashima M, Takamura N, Namba H, et al (2007) RET oncogene amplification in thyroid cancer: correlations with radiation-associated and high-grade malignancy. Hum Pathol 38:621–628
5. Brown DD, Dawid IB (1968) Specific gene amplification in oocytes. Oocyte nuclei contain extrachromosomal replicas of the genes for ribosomal RNA. Science 160:272–280
6. Zimonjic DB, Zhang H, Shan Z, et al (2001) DNA amplification associated with double minutes originating from chromosome 19 in mouse hepatocellular carcinoma. Cytogenet Cell Genet 93:114–116
7. Slamon DJ, Clark GM, Wong SG, et al (1987) Human breast cancer: correlation of relapse and survival with amplification of the HER-2/neu oncogene. Science 235:177–182
8. Slamon DJ, Godolphin W, Jones LA, et al (1989) Studies of the HER-2/neu proto-oncogene in human breast and ovarian cancer. Science 244:707–712
9. Robbins P, Pinder S, de Klerk N, et al (1995) Histological grading of breast carcinomas: a study of interobserver agreement. Hum Pathol 26:873–879
10. Land CE, Tokunaga M, Koyama K, et al (2003) Incidence of female breast cancer among atomic bomb survivors, Hiroshima and Nagasaki, 1950–1990. Radiat Res 160:707–717
11. Press MF, Slamon DJ, Flom KJ, et al (2002) Evaluation of HER-2/neu gene amplification and overexpression: comparison of frequently used assay methods in a molecularly characterized cohort of breast cancer specimens. J Clin Oncol 20:3095–3105
12. Ross JS, Fletcher JA, Linette GP, et al (2003) The HER-2/neu gene and protein in breast cancer 2003: biomarker and target of therapy. Oncologist 8:307–325
13. Ogura H, Akiyama F, Kasumi F, et al (2003) Evaluation of HER-2 status in breast carcinoma by fluorescence in situ hybridization and immunohistochemistry. Breast Cancer 10:234–240

14. Schlotter CM, Vogt U, Bosse U, et al (2003) c-Myc, not HER2/neu, can predict recurrence and mortality of patients with node-negative breast cancer. Breast Cancer Res 5:R30–R36
15. Liao DJ, Dickson RB (2000) c-Myc in breast cancer. Endocr Relat Cancer 7:143–164
16. Park K, Kwak K, Kim J, et al (2005) c-Myc amplification is associated with HER2 amplification and closely linked with cell proliferation in tissue microarray of nonselected breast cancers. Hum Pathol 36:634–639

Paracrine Interactions Between Normal, but Not Cancer, Epithelial and Normal Mesenchymal Cells Attenuate Radiation-Induced DNA Damage

Vladimir A. Saenko[1], Yuka Nakazawa[2], Tatiana I. Rogounovitch[2], Keiji Suzuki[2], Norisato Mitsutake[2], Michiko Matsuse[2], Yasuyoshi Oka, and Shunichi Yamashita[1,2]

Summary. Developmentally, every tissue accommodates different types of cells, for example, epitheliocytes and stromal cells of mesenchymal origin in parenchymal organs. To gain insights into the particulars of radiation response, it is essential to evaluate possible cross talk between different cellular components of a tissue. This work addressed the reciprocal influence of normal human epithelial/mesenchymal cells interactions on the extent of radiation-induced DNA damage in comparison with epithelial cancer/normal mesenchymal cells. Individual or mixed epithelial/mesenchymal cell cultures, including primary human thyrocytes (PT), normal diploid fibroblasts, normal mammary epithelial or endothelial cells, and several human thyroid and breast cancer cell lines, or cell cultures after conditioned medium transfer, were tested for the number of γ-H2AX foci as a measure of double-strand DNA breaks following exposure to gamma rays. In the mixed PT/fibroblast cultures, the number of γ-H2AX foci was significantly lower in both types of cells as compared to individual cultures. Reciprocal conditioned medium transfer to individual counterpart cells before irradiation also resulted in the reduction in the number of γ-H2AX foci in both PT and fibroblasts. The reciprocal DNA-protective effect was likewise observed in the endothelial cell/fibroblast but not in the epithelial cell/endotheliocyte systems. In contrast to medium conditioned on PT cells, conditioned medium collected from cancer cell lines did not establish a DNA-protected state in normal fibroblasts and vice versa. The results imply the existence of a soluble factor-mediated network of reciprocal interactions between normal epithelial and some types of mesenchymal cells that act in a paracrine manner to protect DNA from genotoxic stress.

---

[1]Department of International Health and Radiation Research, Nagasaki University Graduate School of Biomedical Sciences, 1-12-4 Sakamoto, Nagasaki 852-8523, Japan
[2]Department of Molecular Medicine, Atomic Bomb Disease Institute, Nagasaki University Graduate School of Biomedical Sciences, Nagasaki, Japan

Key words Radiation · DNA damage · γ-H2AX foci · Intercellular interactions

Introduction

Ionizing radiation induces a variety of DNA lesions such as nucleotide base modifications, abasic sites, strand cross-linking, DNA adducts, and single- and double-strand DNA breaks (DSBs). Although all these types of lesions may potentially result in gene mutations, DSBs are considered to be the most significant for chromosomal aberrations, mutagenesis, genetic instability, and carcinogenesis. The multiplicity of DNA damage induced by radiation is thought to be one of the reasons for the diversity in biological consequences of exposure.

Evaluation of radiation response in complex systems, such as tissues, is a difficult challenge. Naturally, every human organ accommodates different types of cells, for example, epithelial cells and stromal cells of mesenchymal origin in parenchymal organs. Interactions between the stroma whose cellular component includes different mesenchymal cells and epithelium determine tissue homeostasis and performance through reciprocal endocrine and paracrine interactions. Stroma plays an essential role in the development, differentiation, growth, and regeneration of epithelial cells. At the same time, the role of epithelial–stromal cell interactions in radiation response is poorly understood.

Most previous studies have assessed this problem in cancer cell lines/normal stromal cells (fibroblasts or endotheliocytes) models. The results of these works suggested that intercellular cross talk can either increase or decrease radiation sensitivity. The issue of modulation of radiation response by interactions between normal epithelial and stromal cells has remained rather unexplored despite its substantial biological, medical, and public health importance.

In this study, we tested primary human thyrocytes (PT) and a normal mammary epithelial cell strain as proxies of epithelial tissue components, and several lines of human diploid fibroblasts and endothelial cells as a cellular component of the stroma, in the context of radiation exposure. In addition, some thyroid and breast cancer cell lines were assayed for interaction with normal fibroblasts.

The mechanisms of intercellular interactions were addressed using cell co-culture and conditioned medium transfer methodologies. After irradiation, the extent of DNA damage was estimated as the number of γ-H2AX foci per cell, which is a well-established and a sensitive technique of DSB detection [1].

Here we report that, in mixed PT/fibroblast cultures and after reciprocal conditioned medium (CM) transfer, the number of radiation-induced γ-H2AX foci was significantly lower in both types of cells. A reciprocal DNA-protective effect was also observed after CM transfer in the endothelial cells/fibroblasts but not in the epithelial cells/endotheliocytes system. In contrast to the medium conditioned on normal epithelial cells, CM collected from cancer cell lines did not establish DNA-protected state in normal fibroblasts, and no DNA-protective effect was observed in cancer cells after CM transfer from fibroblasts.

Subjects and Methods

Cell Cultures

Primary human thyrocyte (PT) cultures were established from fresh specimens of surgically removed human thyroid tissue [2] and maintained in Dulbecco's modified Eagle's medium (DMEM):F12 (1:2) medium/3.3% fetal bovine serum (FBS). Appropriate informed consent was obtained from each patient, and study protocols were approved by the Nagasaki University Review Board. Normal human foreskin diploid fibroblasts, BJ (ATCC, USA), and human fetal lung fibroblast lines MRC-5 and WI-38 (JCRB, Japan) were cultured in DMEM/10% FBS. A normal human endothelial cell line, HUV-EC-C (HSRRB, Japan), was maintained in EGM-2 medium (Cambrex, walkersville, MD, USA) supplemented with 2% FBS. Normal human mammary epithelial cells (HMEC; Cambrex), were cultured in HEGM-2 medium (Cambrex) according to the supplier's instructions. Human thyroid carcinoma cell lines TPC-1, NPA, FRO, and ARO, and the MCF-7 breast cancer cell line, were grown in RPMI-1640/5% FBS.

Individual Cell Cultures, Co-Cultures, and Conditioned Medium Transfer

One hundred thousand cells were seeded onto sterilized glass coverslips in 12-well plates (1×10^5/well) to form confluent individual cultures. In co-cultures, PT and BJ cells were mixed at a ratio of 1:1 and kept in either PT or fibroblast medium. To distinguish PT and BJ under the fluorescent microscope in co-cultures, BJ cells were pre-loaded with 500 nM Mito Tracker Red 580 (Molecular Probes, Eugene, OR, USA).

To make conditioned medium (CM), fresh medium was added to each confluent cell culture and incubated overnight. On the next day, recipient cells were washed three times with phosphate-buffered saline (PBS), and CM was transferred and incubated overnight before irradiation.

Irradiation and Detection of γ-H2AX Foci by Immunofluorescence

Cells were γ-irradiated using a ^{137}Cs source (PS-3100SB; Pony, Osaka, Japan) at a dose rate of 1 Gy/min and incubated at 37°C for 30 min before fixation. Fixation (10% PBS-buffered formalin) and immunostaining for γ-H2AX foci were done as described previously [3]. Images were acquired with a LSM510 confocal laser scanning microscope (Carl Zeiss, Oberkochen, Germany). γ-H2AX foci in at least 100 nonoverlapping nuclei were counted for each data point.

Statistical Analysis

Significance of difference between the groups was estimated with analysis of variance (ANOVA). A *P* value not exceeding 0.05 was considered statistically significant.

Results

Extent of DNA Damage in Individual Cultures, in Co-Cultures, and After Conditioned Medium Transfer

The number of γ-H2AX foci in irradiated PT/BJ co-cultures, as compared to individual PT and BJ fibroblast cultures, appeared to be significantly lower (Fig. 1A). After conditioned medium (CM) transfer, the DNA-protective effect of heterologous CM (i.e., medium conditioned on heterologous cells) was even stronger (Fig. 1B), whereas no significant changes in the number of γ-H2AX foci were observed after cell incubation with fresh heterologous medium, ruling out influence of the medium components. In additional experiments it was found that neither cell co-culture nor CM transfer alters DNA repair kinetics in any type of cells (data not shown).

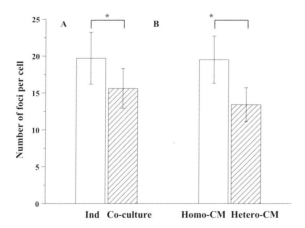

Fig. 1. Number of γ-H2AX foci in primary thyrocytes 30 min after irradiation with 1 Gy γ-rays in (**A**) individual cultures (Ind., *open bar*) and co-cultures (Co-culture, *hatched bar*), and (**B**) after homologous (Homo-CM, *open bar*) or heterologous (Hetero-CM, *hatched bar*) conditioned medium (CM) transfer. Similar results were obtained for BJ fibroblasts. Co-cultures displayed an approximately 25% reduction in the number of radiation-induced γ-H2AX foci whereas in the cells that received heterologous conditioned medium the reduction was about 35%. Results are shown as mean ± SD, *$P < 0.01$. Data are representative of at least ten reproduced experiments

Conditioned Medium Transfer Between Various Normal Human Cell Lines, and Between Cancer Cell Lines and Normal Fibroblasts

As summarized in Fig. 2 (left part), the DNA-protected state was observed in PT and HMEC cells after CM transfer from any fibroblast cell line tested and vice versa. Also, there was a well-pronounced reciprocal DNA-protective effect in the fibroblast/endothelial cell systems. In contrast, a DNA-protective effect could not be detected in the epithelial (either PT or HMEC)/endothelial cell systems.

The DNA-protected state could not be established in any type of cells after CM transfer for any combination of normal fibroblasts and epithelial cancer cells tested (Fig. 2, right part).

Mechanisms of DNA-Protective Effect

The high confluence of cultures used in our experiments might enable gap junction intercellular communications (GJIC) between adjacent cells. To examine the involvement of this type of cell-to-cell interaction in the DNA-protective effect, GJIC in individual and mixed cultures of PT and BJ fibroblasts was blocked with lindane. Presence of the chemical in the medium led to an even increase in the number of radiation-induced γ-H2AX foci in any type of cells, in both monocultures and co-cultures. However, the number of γ-H2AX foci in co-culture did not reach the

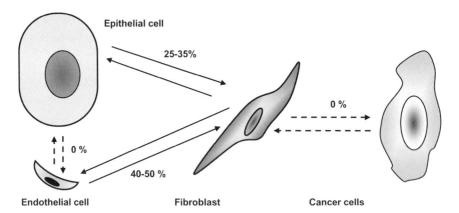

Fig. 2. The DNA-protective effect of conditioned medium transfer between different types of cells. Extent of γ-H2AX foci reduction (%) after irradiation with 1 Gy γ-rays is shown for each combination tested. Note that only paracrine interactions between certain types of normal cells resulted in the establishment of the DNA-protected state whereas epithelial cancer cells reciprocally failed to do so in normal fibroblasts. Fresh heterologous medium was used as a compulsory control for each cell combination; there was no DNA-protective effect for any nonconditioned medium

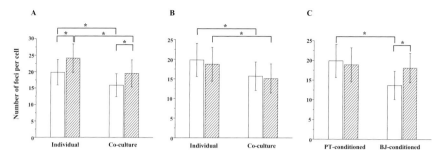

Fig. 3. Influence of gap junction intercellular communications (GJIC) (**A**), nitric oxide (**B**), and thermal inactivation of conditioned medium (**C**) on the DNA-protective effect in the PT/BJ cell system. **A** Nuclear γ-H2AX foci were counted in PT cells 30 min after irradiation with 1 Gy γ-rays in individual PT cultures or in PT/BJ co-cultures not treated (*open bars*) or treated (*hatched bars*) with lindane. **B** γ-H2AX foci were counted in PT cells in individual PT cultures or in PT/BJ co-cultures not treated (*open bars*) or treated (*hatched bars*) with PTIO. **C** γ-H2AX foci were counted in PT cells after the transfer of medium conditioned on PT or BJ cells; before the transfer, conditioned medium was incubated for 30 min at 37°C (*open bars*) or 56°C (*hatched bars*). Similar results were obtained when BJ fibroblasts were used as target cells. PT, primary human thyrocytes. Results are shown as mean ± SD, *$P < 0.01$. Data are representative of three experiments

values observed in the control and lindane-treated irradiated monocultures (Fig. 3A). These results implied that functional GJIC can partly diminish the extent of radiation-induced DNA damage but it was unlikely involved in the DNA-protective effect arising from interactions between epithelial and mesenchymal cells.

Nitric oxide (NO) influences multiple pathways in the cell, including DNA protection from genotoxic agents. We therefore examined its role in irradiated mono- and co-cultures. Addition to the medium of a NO scavenger, PTIO, did not change the number of radiation-induced γ-H2AX foci in any type of cells in both monocultures and PT/BJ co-cultures (Fig. 3B).

Because the results of CM transfer experiments suggested the involvement of soluble factors, CM was subjected to heat treatment to elucidate whether these factors were thermosensitive. After CM was exposed to heat, its capacity to establish the DNA-protected state in recipient cells was significantly reduced, implying that the factors are thermolabile (Fig. 3C). Perhaps this finding may point to the protein nature of those factors.

Discussion

Here we investigated whether cross talk between normal epithelial and mesenchymal cells could influence the extent of DNA damage after irradiation. Of note, in the experiments we used confluent cultures that recreated conditions of postmitotic tissue. Primary thyrocytes initially divide several times in vitro but then stop growing under the culture conditions used. Also, at high cell densities, proliferation of normal fibroblasts is suppressed through contact inhibition. Thereby, the proportion of S-phase cells that may form γ-H2AX foci without a certain kind of external genotoxic challenge [4] or display an elevated number of foci after irradiation [3] was exceedingly low. Thus, in all experiments, involving either individual normal cell cultures or co-cultures, data were obtained for densely seeded quiescent diploid human cells.

Evaluation of DNA damage in irradiated co-cultures and after CM transfer demonstrated its decrease, as compared to respective controls, suggestive of possible intercellular interactions between different types of cells leading to the establishment of the DNA-protected state. In particular, CM transfer experiments, taken together with the unaltered DNA repair kinetics, implied that the effect was the result of soluble paracrine factors secreted into the medium by corresponding cells. At the moment it is difficult to identify such factor(s) and clarify the mechanism involved, although one may speculate that the latter may be somewhat similar to that of radioprotectors.

The DNA-protected state was documented not only for the thyrocyte/fibroblast cell system but also for other combinations of normal cells of different origin. This reproducibility might be indicative of the universality of the protective effect of normal epithelial–stromal cell interaction. At the same time, not all types of mesenchymal cells could protect epithelial cells. For example, the DNA-protective effect was not observed after reciprocal CM transfer between epitheliocytes and endotheliocytes, which may imply its cell type specificity.

An interesting and important finding was a lack of DNA-protective interactions between fibroblasts and cancer cells. It is tempting to speculate that metabolic and gene expression changes in transformed cells may result in a loss of their ability to produce factors protecting normal stromal cells or to sense or react on paracrine protective factors. Genetic alterations of stromal cells have been reported to be a frequent event in human cancers [5]. Absence of protective signals from cancerous epithelium might possibly contribute to mutagenesis of stromal cells, thereby promoting a permissive tumor microenvironment.

Our attempts to elucidate some details of the mechanisms underlying the DNA-protective effect in the thyrocyte/fibroblast system demonstrated that GJIC and nitric oxide (NO) were unlikely to be involved. At low radiation doses, GJIC potentiate radiation damage in exposed and bystander cells while at higher doses they may exert a protective effect [6]. Our observations correspond well with the latter observations, once again emphasizing the importance of functional GJIC in cellular resistance to an unfavorable environment causing genotoxic stress. However, the extent of changes produced by a GJIC blocker in irradiated individual cell cultures and co-cultures did not support possible protective role of GJIC in epithelial–mesenchymal cell cooperation. Also, the effect of nitric oxide appeared to be sparse. NO can radiosensitize or protect cells from radiation damage. Thus, our findings are at variance with these reports as well as with those documenting the role of NO in the bystander effect [7]. CM thermolability, which could be considered as a manifestation of the protein nature of soluble factors that cause the DNA-protected state, indirectly supports the idea that the observed DNA-protective effect was not caused by secreted small molecules such as NO or others whose effect is mediated by GJIC.

In conclusion, our work demonstrated that normal epithelial and stromal cells principally differ from cancer cells in terms of their ability to protect each other from DNA damage. It is attractive to propose that such selectivity, once its mechanisms are understood, may be used for protection of normal tissues surrounding the tumor during radiation therapy or other circumstances associated with anticipated radiation exposure.

References

1. Rogakou EP, Pilch DR, Orr AH, et al (1998) DNA double-stranded breaks induce histone H2AX phosphorylation on serine 139. J Biol Chem 273:5858–5868
2. Kawabe Y, Eguchi K, Shimomura C, et al (1989) Interleukin-1 production and action in thyroid tissue. J Clin Endocrinol Metab 68:1174–1183
3. Suzuki K, Okada H, Yamauchi M, et al (2006) Qualitative and quantitative analysis of phosphorylated ATM foci induced by low-dose ionizing radiation. Radiat Res 165:499–504
4. MacPhail SH, Banath JP, Yu Y, et al (2003) Cell cycle-dependent expression of phosphorylated histone H2AX: reduced expression in unirradiated but not X-irradiated G_1-phase cells. Radiat Res 159:759–767
5. Kurose K, Hoshaw-Woodard S, Adeyinka A, et al (2001) Genetic model of multi-step breast carcinogenesis involving the epithelium and stroma: clues to tumour–microenvironment interactions. Hum Mol Genet 10:1907–1913
6. Hei TK, Persaud R, Zhou H, et al (2004) Genotoxicity in the eyes of bystander cells. Mutat Res 568:111–120
7. Sokolov MV, Smilenov LB, Hall EJ, et al (2005) Ionizing radiation induces DNA double-strand breaks in bystander primary human fibroblasts. Oncogene 24:7257–7265

Chernobyl and Semipalatinsk Nuclear Test Sites: Related Issues

Thyroid Cancer in Ukraine After the Chernobyl Accident: Incidence, Pathology, Treatment, and Molecular Biology

Mykola Tronko[1], Tetyana Bogdanova[1], Ilya Likhtarev[2], Ihor Komisarenko[1], Andriy Kovalenko[1], Valentyn Markov[1], Valery Tereshchenko[1], Larysa Voskoboynyk[1], Lyudmyla Zurnadzhy[1], Victor Shpak[1], Lyudmyla Gulak[3], Rossella Elisei[4], Cristina Romei[4], and Aldo Pinchera[4]

Summary. The number of thyroid cancer cases in those who were children and adolescents at the time of the Chernobyl accident is steadily increasing in Ukraine, and 466 newly diagnosed cases were observed in 2006. An estimation of the Clinical-Morphological Register data by age at the time of the accident shows that, for the post-Chernobyl period (1986–2006), 4369 cases of thyroid cancer have been registered in this age group, among which 3170 (72.6%) were children aged 0 to 14 years and 1199 (27.4%) were adolescents aged 15 to 18 years at the time of the accident. As well as in previous years, also in 2005–2006 the highest thyroid cancer incidence was registered in the six most contaminated northern regions of Ukraine. In the cohort of those born in 1968–1986 and operated on in 2005–2006, thyroid cancer was observed only in young adults 19–38 years of age, and more than 90% of these cancers were represented by papillary carcinoma. These tumours were mainly of papillary or papillary-follicular structure and presented with low levels of regional and/or distant metastases. Thyroid cancer incidence among children and adolescents born after the accident was much lower than in appropriate control patients born before the accident. Nevertheless, the pathological features of papillary carcinomas in both groups were similar. Molecular-biological studies showed that RET/PTC1, RET/PTC3 rearrangements and BRAF^{V600E} mutations were detected only in papillary thyroid carcinomas. Unknown RET/PTC rearrangements (RET/PTCX) were observed in both malignant (papillary carcinomas) and benign (follicular adenomas) thyroid tumours. Papillary carcinomas with RET/PTC rearrangements were characterized by more prominent aggressiveness with respect to tumours with BRAF mutation or without any genetic alterations.

---

[1]Institute of Endocrinology and Metabolism of Academy of Medical Sciences of Ukraine, ul. Vyshgorodskaya 69, 04114 Kyiv, Ukraine
[2]Research Center for Radiation Medicine of Academy of Medical Sciences of Ukraine, Kyiv, Ukraine
[3]Institute of Oncology and Radiology of Academy of Medical Sciences of Ukraine, Kyiv, Ukraine
[4]Department of Endocrinology, Pisa University, Pisa, Italy

Key words Chernobyl accident · Thyroid cancer incidence · Pathology · Treatment · Latency · Molecular biology

Introduction

At 22 years after the Chernobyl nuclear accident, the number of thyroid cancer cases is steadily increasing in the cohort of those who were children and adolescents at the time of the accident. In this chapter, we describe the epidemiology of thyroid cancer in Ukraine with particular regard to the relationship between the thyroid cancer incidence and gender, age, and place of residence of subjects aged 0 to 18 years at the time of the Chernobyl accident and diagnosed in 2005–2006. We also describe the pathological features and the degree of extension of these thyroid tumours. The results of comparison with our previous reported data [1,2] are also included. This report includes the molecular analysis performed in a selected group of both papillary carcinomas (PTC) and follicular adenomas (FA) of genetic alterations more frequently found to be associated with thyroid cancer.

Subjects and Methods

Statistical data were obtained from the Clinical-Morphological Register of the Institute of Endocrinology and Metabolism of the Academy of Medical Sciences of Ukraine [1].

The pathological study group was represented by 358 patients who were 19 to 38 years old at the time of diagnosis and born before the Chernobyl accident and by 51 patients who were 11 to 18 years old at the time of diagnosis and born after the accident. All patients were treated at the Hospital of the Institute of Endocrinology during 2005–2006. These cases were analyzed together with 1342 cases of thyroid carcinomas belonging to patients who were 4 to 36 years old at the time of surgery and born before the accident, and 87 cases of thyroid carcinomas belonging to children and adolescents who were born after the accident and described in our previous article [2].

The pathological diagnosis was made according to the WHO Histological Classification [3]. Most of the cases were additionally reviewed by the International Pathology Panel, established in the framework of the Tissue Bank Project [4]. The diagnosis of thyroid carcinoma was confirmed in all cases.

Fifty-nine cases (35 PTC and 24 FA) were also studied by molecular biology. In particular, total RNA was extracted from the frozen thyroid tumours and/or normal tissues, obtained from Chernobyl Tissue Bank (http://www.chernobyltissuebank.com). The mean age at surgery of this selected group of patients was 21 ± 5 years for PTC and 23 ± 7 years for FA. The mean latency period (14 ± 1 year) was similar in the groups of benign and malignant tumours.

For RET/PTC analysis, reverse transcriptase-polymerase chain reaction (RT-PCR) and Southern blot were used as previously described [5]. BRAF^{V600E} mutations were studied by direct sequencing of exon 15 [6]. The real-time RT-PCR method was used to measure the expression levels of the tyrosine kinase domain (TK) and extracellular domain (EC) of the RET gene [7]. Target gene mRNA levels were expressed as $2^{-\Delta Ct}$, where $\Delta Ct = C_{t\ of\ target\ gene} - C_{t\ of\ reference\ gene}$ [6]. The ratio TK/EC was calculated for all studied samples. The value of TK/EC values higher than 2 suggested the presence of an RET/PTC rearrangement.

Results and Discussion

Epidemiology and Statistics

In Ukraine, 466 newly diagnosed thyroid cancer cases were reported in 2006. An estimation of registered data by age at the time of the accident shows that, for the post-Chernobyl period (1986–2006), 4369 cases of thyroid cancer have been registered in the above age group, among which 3170 (72.6%) were children aged 0 to 14 years at the time of the accident, and 1199 (27.4%) were adolescents aged 15 to 18 years (Tables 1, 2).

Undoubtedly, this steady increase in thyroid cancer cases may be to some extent associated with a gradual increase in the age of the cohort under study for the period 1986–2006. At the same time, a comparison between the thyroid cancer incidence rates in the six more highly contaminated regions of Ukraine and in the other regions of Ukraine shows the most significant difference between the rates for the last 5 years of follow-up, which confirms that a direct relationship is still present between the rise in thyroid cancer incidence and the post-Chernobyl radiation exposure.

A total of 4369 patients who were 4 to 38 years old at surgery (461 children, 546 adolescents, and 3362 adults) and who were born before 1987 are included in the Register. Another 203 cases (108 children, 90 adolescents, and 5 adults) detected among patients born after the accident have been added (Tables 3–5). Thus, a total of 4572 cases have been included in the Register for the period of 1986–2006. Most cases in the last years have been detected in young adults having been operated on at the age of 19 years and older.

The incidence per 100 000 of the appropriate age population (children, adolescents, or adults) shows a tendency to steady growth only in the group of young adults. In patients having been operated on as children and adolescents, the incidence decreasing beginning from 1996, and in 2005–2006 the indicators were represented only by cases, revealed in such age groups, born after the accident (see Tables 3, 4).

At the same time, if we consider the incidence among children born before and after the Chernobyl accident separately, it appears that in children born before the

Table 1. Number of thyroid cancer cases and incidence per 100 000 population of children in 1986[a] by year, sex, and region

	Year																				
	1986	1987	1988	1989	1990	1991	1992	1993	1994	1995	1996	1997	1998	1999	2000	2001	2002	2003	2004	2005	2006
Number of females	4	9	7	18	24	32	61	54	80	92	100	106	135	162	149	231	211	193	240	248	299
Number of males	4	2	4	8	17	15	27	30	29	33	43	31	38	59	38	55	52	52	48	64	66
Total number	8	11	11	26	41	47	88	84	109	125	143	137	173	221	187	286	263	245	288	312	365
Incidence	0.07	0.10	0.10	0.23	0.37	0.42	0.79	0.75	0.97	1.12	1.28	1.22	1.54	1.97	1.67	2.55	2.35	2.19	2.57	2.79	3.26
Incidence in 6 regions	0.14	0.00	0.14	0.38	0.76	1.10	2.38	2.10	2.62	2.90	3.33	2.76	3.81	5.14	4.86	6.81	6.19	5.10	5.43	6.14	7.52
Incidence in 21 regions	0.05	0.12	0.09	0.20	0.27	0.27	0.42	0.44	0.59	0.70	0.80	0.87	1.02	1.24	0.92	1.57	1.45	1.52	1.91	2.01	2.27

[a]Those aged 0–14 years at the time of the Chernobyl accident

Table 2. Number of thyroid cancer cases and incidence per 100000 population of adolescents in 1986[a] by year, sex, and region

	Year																				
	1986	1987	1988	1989	1990	1991	1992	1993	1994	1995	1996	1997	1998	1999	2000	2001	2002	2003	2004	2005	2006
Number of females	9	9	10	9	19	19	26	42	37	60	46	51	70	61	56	74	71	75	79	95	84
Number of males	2	6	2	4	2	4	9	7	9	8	10	11	11	9	14	15	22	13	9	13	17
Total number	11	15	12	13	21	23	35	49	46	68	56	62	81	70	70	89	93	88	88	108	101
Incidence	0.42	0.57	0.45	0.49	0.79	0.87	1.32	1.85	1.74	2.57	2.11	2.34	3.06	2.64	2.64	3.36	3.51	3.32	3.32	4.08	3.81
Incidence, 6 regions	0.19	1.15	0.00	0.58	1.15	1.54	1.92	1.92	2.12	4.23	2.69	3.65	5.38	3.27	5.00	6.15	6.73	6.73	5.58	7.88	8.27
Incidence, 21 regions	0.47	0.42	0.56	0.47	0.70	0.70	1.17	1.83	1.64	2.16	1.97	2.02	2.49	2.49	2.07	2.68	2.72	2.49	2.77	3.15	2.72

[a]Those aged 15–18 years at the time of the Chernobyl accident

Table 3. Number of thyroid cancer cases[a] and incidence per 100000 population of children by year, year of birth, sex, and region

	Year																				
	1986	1987	1988	1989	1990	1991	1992	1993	1994	1995	1996	1997	1998	1999	2000	2001	2002	2003	2004	2005	2006
Born before 1987																					
Number of females	4	8	6	7	14	17	36	29	28	33	34	29	30	14	9	0	0	0	0	0	0
Number of males	4	2	3	5	12	7	21	19	20	13	21	7	11	9	7	2	0	0	0	0	0
Total number	8	10	9	12	26	24	57	48	48	46	55	36	41	23	16	2	0	0	0	0	0
Incidence	0.07	0.10	0.09	0.13	0.32	0.32	0.83	0.79	0.77	0.99	1.41	1.15	1.75	1.48	2.04	0.53	0	0	0	0	0
Incidence, 6 regions	0.14	0	0.11	0.23	0.69	0.96	2.97	2.60	2.78	3.65	4.74	4.24	5.69	4.95	5.21	1.37	0	0	0	0	0
Incidence, 21 regions	0.06	0.12	0.09	0.11	0.23	0.17	0.31	0.35	0.42	0.35	0.61	0.40	0.80	0.64	1.27	0.33	0	0	0	0	0
Born in 1987 and later[b]																					
Number of females	NA[c]									1	—	1	1	2	9	8	20	6	5	18	6
Number of males	NA									0	2	0	1	3	1	7	6	3	4	3	1
Total number	NA									1	2	1	2	5	10	15	26	9	9	21	7
Incidence	NA									0.02	0.03	0.02	0.02	0.11	0.13	0.20	0.34	0.14	0.13	0.30	0.1
Incidence, 6 regions	NA									0	0	0.08	0.0	0.14	0.13	0.40	0.71	0.20	0.15	0.28	0.22
Incidence, 21 regions	NA									0.02	0.04	0	0.03	0.10	0.13	0.15	0.24	0.11	0.12	0.30	0.07

NA, not available
[a]Those aged 0–14 years at the time of surgery
[b]There was no case from 1987 to 1994

Table 4. Number of thyroid cancer cases[a] and incidence per 100000 population of adolescents by year, year of birth, sex, and region

	Year																				
	1986	1987	1988	1989	1990	1991	1992	1993	1994	1995	1996	1997	1998	1999	2000	2001	2002	2003	2004	2005	2006
Born before 1987																					
Number of females	9	6	6	15	10	15	18	16	24	23	23	17	22	41	31	38	30	23	13	4	0
Number of males	2	5	2	3	5	6	3	6	8	8	10	8	17	18	11	17	15	11	5	2	0
Total number	11	11	8	18	15	21	21	22	32	31	33	25	39	59	42	55	45	34	18	6	0
Incidence	0.69	0.39	0.27	0.60	0.50	0.70	0.70	0.74	1.08	1.05	1.12	0.85	1.32	1.96	1.38	1.77	1.92	2.2	2.3	2.3	0
Incidence, 6 regions	0.18	0.76	0.17	0.73	0.91	1.27	1.27	1.65	3.48	1.48	2.22	2.4	3.12	5.41	5.71	5.76	6.29	7.02	3.47	8.32	0
Incidence, 21 regions	0.45	0.30	0.3	0.58	0.41	0.57	0.57	0.54	0.54	0.96	0.88	0.5	0.91	1.18	0.40	0.87	0.91	1.11	2.03	0.94	0
Born in 1987 and later[b]																					
Number of females	NA[c]																1	11	11	27	22
Number of males	NA																3	0	5	3	7
Total number	NA																4	11	16	30	29
Incidence	NA																0.58	0.79	0.71	1.08	1.01
Incidence, 6 regions.	NA																0.78	1.10	0.48	1.77	1.69
Incidence, 21 regions	NA																0.53	0.73	0.76	0.93	0.85

NA, not available
[a]Those aged 15–18 years at the time of surgery
[b]There was no case from 1987 to 2001

Table 5. Number of thyroid cancer cases[a] and incidence per 100000 appropriate population by year, year of birth, sex, and region

	Year																				
	1986	1987	1988	1989	1990	1991	1992	1993	1994	1995	1996	1997	1998	1999	2000	2001	2002	2003	2004	2005	2006
Born before 1987																					
Number of females	NA[c]	4	5	5	19	19	33	51	65	96	89	111	153	168	165	267	252	245	306	338	383
Number of males	NA	1	1	4	2	6	12	12	10	20	22	27	21	41	34	51	59	54	52	76	83
Total number	NA	5	6	9	21	25	45	63	75	116	111	138	174	209	199	318	311	299	358	414	466
Incidence	NA	0.75	0.46	0.44	0.76	0.71	1.05	1.25	1.30	1.79	1.56	1.77	2.04	2.27	2.0	2.99	2.73	2.46	2.77	3.03	3.42
Incidence, 6 regions	NA	1.51	0	0.76	1.10	1.44	1.54	1.41	1.49	3.30	2.49	2.53	3.87	4.40	4.54	6.78	6.16	5.09	5.42	6.16	7.53
Incidence, 21 regions	NA	0.56	0.57	0.37	0.67	0.53	0.93	1.21	1.25	1.42	1.33	1.58	1.59	1.74	1.38	2.06	1.89	1.81	2.12	2.26	2.41
Born in 1987 and later																					
Number of females	NA[c]																				4
Number of males	NA																				1
Total number	NA																				5
Incidence	NA																				0.4
Incidence, 6 regions	NA																				0
Incidence, 21 regions	NA																				0.5

NA, not available
[a]Those aged 19–38 years at the time of surgery
[b]There was no case from 1987 to 2005

accident and operated on at the age of 15 years, the incidence remained high until 2000. Beginning from 2001, these children have gone over to the category of adolescents. At the same time, the indices of incidence in children born after the accident were and remain much lower (e.g., −0.10 in 2006).

A rise in the incidence among children operated on at the age of 15 years and born before the accident has also been reported, mainly in the 6 most exposed northern regions of Ukraine, as clearly demonstrated by indicators of comparison with the other 21 regions of Ukraine (see Table 4). A similar tendency was also noted when comparing the incidence in young adult patients operated on at the age of 19 to 38 years, but it should be stressed that the difference in rates in this group becomes significant only since 1998, and the greatest difference was observed in 2006 (see Table 5). It is worthy of note that the group of those diagnosed in 2006 and aged 19 to 38 years at the time of surgery is represented by those who were 0 to 18 years at the time of the accident; thus, these data represent additional evidence of a direct relationship between the Chernobyl accident and thyroid cancer development, at least in those who were aged up to 18 years at the time of the nuclear accident.

Pathology

The histological examination of thyroid carcinomas diagnosed between 2002 and 2006 showed that 90.6% of cases were represented by PTC. It is of interest that the percentage of follicular carcinomas (FTC) increased from 3.0% in cases diagnosed in 1990–1995 to 7.4% in those diagnosed in 2002–2006. This finding suggests that FTC incidence might be related both to an older age at diagnosis and to a longer latency period of development when compared to PTC. However, the relatively small number of FTC does not allow any definitive conclusions on this matter.

The ratio of PTC subtypes in young adults during the period of 2002–2006 confirmed an inverse relationship between the latency period and the prevalence of more aggressive variants (i.e., solid variant). In this regard, also in the Ukrainian series we observed a decrease in the percentage of solid variant from 21.4% in 1990–1995 to 4.5% in 2002–2006, and an increase in the percentage of typical papillary and mixed variants from 21.4% in 1990–1995 to 40.4% in 2002–2006 and from 21.4% in 1990–1995 to 37.9% in 2002–2006, respectively. The structural combinations of mixed variant have also changed over time: the percentage of tumours with solid-follicular structure has considerably decreased while the percentage of tumours with papillary-follicular structure has increased from 16.7% in 1990–1995 to 58.5% in 2002–2006.

An analysis of invasive properties of PTC has revealed two main relationships: age and time dependence. Extrathyroid tumour spreading to soft tissues adjacent to the thyroid, which allowed referring such a tumour to category T4 according to the 5th edition of TNM classification, and to category T3 according to the 6th edition, was more often detected among children compared to adolescents, and especially young adults (64.8%, 38.9%, and 29.0%, respectively). However, when we pool together all age groups, a marked decrease in the percentage of tumours with extrathyroid tumoral spreading is observed in those cases with a longer latency period, varying from 61.8% in cases diagnosed in 1990–1995 to 27.2% in those diagnosed in 2002–2006. A similar change was observed when the prevalence of regional metastases to cervical lymph nodes was considered. Lymph node metastases in the neck were most often reported among children operated on at the age up to 15 years, whereas the percentage of these metastases was decreasing, with the increase of the latency period varying from 58.2% in 1990–1995 to 31.2% in 2002–2006. The analysis of cases with distant metastases to lungs has shown a similar tendency. Particular attention should be given to the fact that for the last period of follow-up (2002–2006) only 3.7% of 775 cases of PTC showed distant metastases to lungs. From our standpoint, this fact was likely favoured by the above change in the PTC structure, associated with the increase of both the patients' age and the latency period of tumour development.

Other possible reasons to explain this change of the biological behaviour of PTC might be related to two new interesting findings: (a) the significant increase in the percentage of completely encapsulated tumours found in the last years (23.5% in 2002–2006) with respect to that observed previously (7.4% in 1990–1995), and (b) the progressive increase of "small" tumours with the largest diameter less than 1 cm (micro-PTC), which is undoubtedly the result of an intensification of screening examinations and improvement of diagnostic facilities (i.e., modernization of ultrasound equipment and widespread use of fine-needle aspiration biopsy) [8,9].

A comparison of different histotypes of thyroid carcinomas in children and adolescents born before and after the Chernobyl accident shows that in both groups the PTC was the prevalent histotype (93.0% and 80.4%, respectively). However, it should be noted that in patients born after the accident (i.e., in 1987 and later) the percentage of FTC was notably higher (4.6% and 15.2%, respectively).

Invasive properties of PTC are similar in both groups, when considering either extrathyroid spreading or the presence of regional lymph node metastases. The percentage of distant metastases to lungs (22.7% and 13.5%, respectively) is somewhat lower among patients born after the accident, but this finding might reflect early diagnosis as well as the higher percentage in this group of micro-PTC (7.6% and 15.4%, respectively).

Treatment

The main principles of our current protocol are practically identical to the American-Italian protocol [10,11], which may be explained by the use of similar modern approaches to the diagnosis and treatment of thyroid nodular pathology. At the same time, there are a number of differences, reflecting the local conditions of Ukraine as well as our own scientific and practical experience.

As it is generally known, the method of choice in the treatment of PTC and FTC is total thyroidectomy, followed by therapy with radioactive iodine and suppressive hormone therapy. Preoperative cytological diagnosis is mandatory to choose the appropriate surgical treatment. However, in the case of undetermined preoperative cytology (i.e., follicular neoplasm), the question of whether a total thyroidectomy or a hemithyroidectomy should be performed is still unresolved. An intraoperative histological examination may be performed and, if negative, hemithyroidectomy should be considered as the minimal surgical treatment. In case of a confirmed diagnosis of PTC or FTC at final histological examination, the necessity for a complete thyroidectomy is determined by tumour size, localization, and invasive properties.

Molecular Biological Study

Molecular biological investigations have been carried out in collaboration with the University of Pisa (Italy). RET/PTC rearrangements (mainly RET/PTC1 and RET/PTC3, and RET/PTCX) and BRAF^{V600E} point mutation in exon 15 have been searched for in both PTC and FA. As shown in Table 6, RET/PTC1 and/or RET/PTC3 rearrangements were detected only in PTC. RET/PTC1 and/or RET/PTC3 were present in 11 of 35 (31.4 %) PTC, 1 of which showed the simultaneous expression of both RET/PTC1 and RET/PTC3. It is worth to note that in 1 case RET/PTC3 was present in association with the BRAF mutation. When the prevalence of the two types of RET rearrangements was analysed, we found that RET/PTC3 was more frequent than RET/PTC1 [7/35 (20%) vs. 4/35 (11.4%), respectively].

At variance to RET/PTC1 and RET/PTC3, unknown RET/PTCX were detected in both PTC and FA, but not in normal thyroid (NT). It should be noted that the prevalence of RET/PTCX in FA (25%) was slightly higher with respect to PTC (17.1%). The BRAF^{V600E} point mutation was found in PTC (6/25, 24.0%) but in neither FA nor NT (see Table 6).

Table 6. Gene alterations in post-Chernobyl thyroid tumours

	PTC, % (n = 35)	FA, % (n = 24)
RET/PTC rearrangements	51.4 (18/35)	25.0 (6/24)
RET/PTC1[a]	11.4 (4/35)	0
RET/PTC3[a]	17.1 (6/35)	0
RET/PTCX	17.1 (6/35)	25.0 (6/24)
BRAF + RET/PTC3	2.9 (1/35)	0
BRAF^{V600E} mutation	24.0 (6/25)	0
Totals	68.6 (24/35)	25.0 (6/24)

[a]In one papillary carcinoma (PTC), both RET/PTC1 and RET/PTC 3 were present simultaneously

Comparison of molecular and pathological features showed that extrathyroid extension and multifocality were present mainly in PTC with RET/PTC rearrangements (29.4% and 35.3%, respectively) whereas they were absent in tumours with BRAF^{V600E} mutation. Moreover, BRAF-positive tumours had a lower percentage of node metastasis with respect to PTC, and distant metastasis (eight cases) was present only in tumours harbouring a RET rearrangement. On the basis of these observations, it appears that PTC with any RET/PTC has a more aggressive behaviour when compared to both BRAF-positive tumours and PTC without gene alterations; however, the relatively small number of cases does not allow drawing any final conclusion.

Acknowledgments. The authors gratefully acknowledge the confirmation of diagnosis provided by the International Pathology Panel of the Chernobyl Tissue Bank: Dr A. Abrosimov, Professor T. Bogdanova, Professor M. Ito, Professor V. LiVolsi, Professor J. Rosai, and Professor E.D. Williams.

References

1. Tronko M, Bogdanova T, Likhtarev I, et al (2007) Thyroid gland and radiation (fundamental and applied aspects): 20 years after the Chernobyl accident. In: Shibata Y, Namba H, Suzuki K, Tomonaga M (eds) Radiation risk perspectives. Elsevier, Amsterdam, pp 46–53
2. Bogdanova T, Zurnadzhy L, Tronko M, et al (2007) Pathology of thyroid cancer in children and adolescents of Ukraine having been exposed as a result of the Chernobyl accident. In: Shibata Y, Namba H, Suzuki K, Tomonaga M (eds) Radiation risk perspectives. Elsevier, Amsterdam, pp 256–270
3. DeLelis R, Lloyd R, Heitz PH, Eng CH (eds) (2004) Pathology and genetics of tumors of endocrine organs. WHO classification of tumors. IARC Press, Lyon
4. Thomas GA, Williams ED, Becker DV, et al (2000) Thyroid tumor banks. Science 289:29
5. Elisei R, Romei C, Vorontsova T, et al (2001) RET/PTC rearrangements in thyroid nodules: studies in irradiated and not irradiated, malignant and benign thyroid lesions in children and adults. J Clin Endocrinol Metab 86:3211–3216
6. Fugazzola L, Puxeddu E, Avenia N, et al (2006) Correlation between B-RAFV600E mutation and clinico-pathologic parameters in papillary thyroid carcinoma: data from a multicentric Italian study and review of the literature. Endocrinol Relat Cancer 13:455–464
7. Rhoden KJ, Johnson C, Brandao G, et al (2004) Real-time quantitative RT-PCR identifies distinct c-RET, RET/PTC1 and RET/PTC3 expression patterns in papillary thyroid carcinoma. Lab Invest 84:1557–1570
8. Gulcelik MA, Gulcelik NE, Kuru B, et al (2007) Prognostic factors determining survival in differentiated thyroid cancer. J Surg Oncol 96:598–604
9. Davies L, Welch HG (2006) Increasing incidence of thyroid cancer in the United States, 1973–2002. JAMA 295:2164–2167
10. Pacini F, Schlumberger M, Dralle H, et al (2006) European Thyroid Cancer Taskforce European consensus for the management of patients with differentiated thyroid carcinoma of the follicular epithelium. Eur J Endocrinol 154:787–803
11. Cooper DS, Doherty GM, Haugen BR, et al (2006) The American Thyroid Association Guidelines Taskforce. Management guidelines for patients with thyroid nodules and differentiated thyroid cancer. Thyroid 16:109–142

Current Trends in Incidence and Mortality from Thyroid Cancer in Belarus

Pavel I. Bespalchuk[1], **Yuri E. Demidchik**[1,2], **Eugene P. Demidchik**[1,2], **Vladimir A. Saenko**[3,4], and **Shunichi Yamashita**[3,5]

Summary. During the period from January 1, 1985 to December 31, 2006, 14 147 primary patients with pathologically proven thyroid cancer underwent therapy and were followed up in the Thyroid Cancer Center (Minsk, Belarus). The standard incidence of thyroid cancer during these 22 years increased from 1.3 to 8.8 per 100 000 individuals, with the mortality rate remaining stable and low. These observations demonstrate that the number of patients treated for thyroid malignancies is growing in the Belarusian population. Current trends in the incidence of and mortality resulting from thyroid cancer imply this disease comprises a considerable medical problem in the country.

Key words Thyroid carcinoma · Incidence

Introduction

At present, most of the primary thyroid carcinomas in Belarus are likely to be promoted by radionuclide incorporation at the time of Chernobyl Power Plant disaster [1–4]. As it has been demonstrated earlier, these malignances are no longer confined within the southern areas of the country that are located closer to the Chernobyl Power Plant. Disease incidence tends to increase in five of six regions of Belarus, including those considered minimally affected by the radioiodine fallout in 1986 [5]. This finding suggests that the threshold of the absorbed dose for radiogenic thyroid carcinomas may be extremely low, and that the risk of cancer after radioiodine exposure may depend on patient age at the time of accident. According to

---

[1]Belarusian State Medical University, 83 Dzerzhinsky Av., 220116 Minsk, Belarus
[2]Thyroid Cancer Center, Minsk, Belarus
[3]Department of International Health and Radiation Research, Atomic Bomb Disease Institute, Nagasaki University Graduate School of Biomedical Sciences, Nagasaki, Japan
[4]Medical Radiological Research Center RAMS, Obninsk, Russian Federation
[5]Department of Molecular Medicine, Atomic Bomb Disease Institute, Nagasaki University Graduate School of Biomedical Sciences, Nagasaki, Japan

Table 1. Patients with thyroid carcinomas for the period from 1985 to 2006 (residents at Chernobyl disaster)

Region of Belarus	Age group (years)					
	0–15	16–18	19–35	36–45	46+	Total
Brest	217	91	363	340	922	1 933
Vitebsk	22	22	254	369	1 155	1 822
Gomel	431	154	656	548	1 266	3 055
Grodno	64	20	171	156	417	828
Minsk (city)	94	38	470	618	1 583	2 803
Minsk	78	33	269	329	968	1 677
Mogilev	54	29	334	497	1 115	2 029
Total	960	387	2 517	2 857	7 426	14 147

the previously reported data, the greatest number of cases of thyroid carcinoma in childhood patients occurred after a 9- to 10-year period between exposure and diagnosis (a significant increase was first registered 4 years after the Chernobyl disaster), whereas in adolescents most tumors developed after a 14- to 15-year latency. Hitherto, no definite peak in incidence rate is recognized in adults.

This chapter reports current trends in incidence and mortality from thyroid carcinomas in Belarus for the period from 1985 to 2006.

Patients and Methods

Data for the analysis were retrieved from the Thyroid Cancer Center database (Minsk, Belarus). During the period from January 1, 1985 to December 31, 2006, 14 147 consecutive primary patients with pathologically proven thyroid cancer underwent therapy and were followed up in the Thyroid Cancer Canter (Table 1).

Results and Discussion

During 22 years of observations, the standard incidence of thyroid cancer increased from 1.3 to 8.8 per 100 000 individuals. The mortality rate was stable and very low, ranging from 0.1 to 0.7 per 100 000 (Fig. 1). The number of patients treated for thyroid malignancies is clearly growing in the Belarusian population. These individuals in most cases have lost their thyroid glands as a consequence of surgery and need to receive lifelong maintenance therapy with frequent control of hormonal status and, if necessary, isotope therapy or repeated surgical interventions for local or regional relapse.

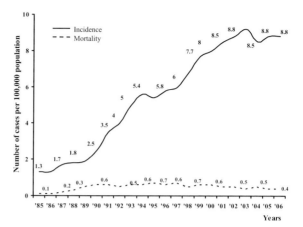

Fig. 1. Overall thyroid cancer incidence and mortality in Belarus during the period from 1985 to 2006

The current distinctive features of thyroid carcinomas in Belarus are the high proportion of small solitary intrathyroid nodules (47.9%) and the prevalence of papillary carcinoma (95.4%) among all histological types of thyroid malignancies. By now, the frequency of advanced cancers with extraglandular spread does not exceed 8.7%, and efficient screening methods allow detecting microcarcinomas in 35.3% of all primary cases.

Within the first decade after the Chernobyl accident, a high prevalence of childhood papillary carcinomas in two southern regions (Gomel region and Pinsk district of Brest region) was the main peculiarity of thyroid malignancies in Belarus, with the peak incidence in 1995–1996. After that, the number of primary childhood cases gradually decreased, while the incidence in adolescents was growing, until 2001. In both age groups (children and adolescents), the observed mortality was extremely low (12 cases; Fig. 2). Thus far, cause-specific fatal outcomes in the age group under 19 years old were registered in 9 patients, mostly with medullary carcinomas; only 2 pediatric patients died of advanced papillary carcinoma.

Within the past 3 years, the number of primary cases in patients aged 19 to 45 years did not grow significantly, with very low annual mortality (Fig. 3). In contrast, patients more than 46 years of age still demonstrate increasing incidence associated with more frequent fatal outcomes, as compared with the younger groups (Fig. 4).

Data presented here are in line with the well-known fact that favorable prognosis of thyroid cancer is associated with young age at diagnosis and therapy [6,7]. In our opinion, the higher mortality in individuals aged more than 46 years may be, in part, the result of the higher frequency of aggressive types of thyroid cancer (medullary, poorly differentiated, or anaplastic) that are uncommon in children, adolescents, or young adults. It is also possible that the poorer survival of older patients reflects the insufficiency of screening methods in this group. Therefore, the efficacy of age-specific early primary diagnosis requires special detailed studies.

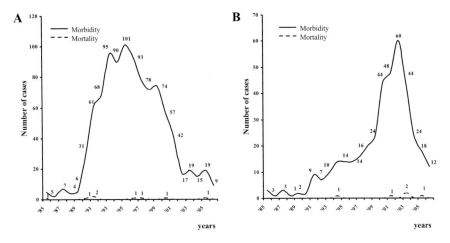

Fig. 2. Incidence of and observed mortality (absolute number of cases) caused by thyroid cancer in children (**A**) and adolescents (**B**)

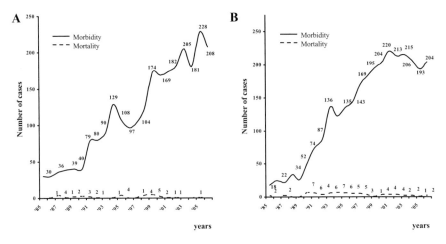

Fig. 3. Incidence of and observed mortality caused by thyroid cancer in the age group 19–35 years old (**A**) and 36–45 years old (**B**)

Thyroid malignancies other than papillary carcinoma in adults can strongly affect life expectation. Our estimates demonstrate that median survival in patients with anaplastic carcinomas is only 5.04 months, and that 2-year survival is only 5.2%, despite therapy. This highly aggressive type of carcinoma has never been diagnosed in patients younger than 45 years old. Five-year survival for widely invasive poorly differentiated carcinomas does not exceed 51.2%, whereas in patients with medullary cancer, 5- and 10-year survival rates are 74.0% and 53.9%, respectively.

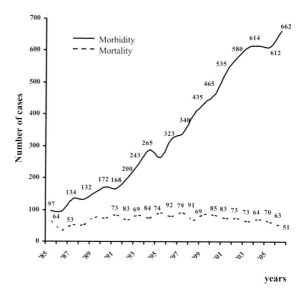

Fig. 4. Observed primary cases and mortality caused by thyroid cancer in the age group 46+ years

In conclusion, current trends in the incidence of and mortality from thyroid cancer demonstrate that this disease is an important medical problem in Belarus.

References

1. Cardis E, Kesminiene A, Ivanov V, et al (2005) Risk of thyroid cancer after exposure to ^{131}I in childhood. J Natl Cancer Inst 97:724–732
2. Cardis E, Howe J, Ron E, et al (2006) Cancer consequences of the Chernobyl accident: 20 years on. J Radiol Prot 26:127–140
3. Jacob P, Bogdanova TI, Buglova E, et al (2006) Thyroid cancer risk in areas of Ukraine and Belarus affected by the Chernobyl accident. Radiat Res 165:1–8
4. Jacob P, Bogdanova TI, Buglova E, et al (2006) Thyroid cancer among Ukrainians and Belarusians who were children or adolescents at the time of the Chernobyl accident. J Radiol Prot 26:51–67
5. Bespalchuk PI, Demidchik YE, Demidchik EP, et al (2007) Thyroid cancer in Belarus after Chernobyl. In: Shibata Y, Namba H, Suzuki K, Tomonaga M (eds) Radiation risk perspectives. Elsevier, Amsterdam, pp 27–31
6. Demidchik YE, Demidchik EP, Reiners C, et al (2006) Comprehensive clinical assessment of 740 cases of surgically treated thyroid cancer in children of Belarus. Ann Surg 243:525–532
7. Demidchik YE, Saenko VA, Yamashita S (2007) Childhood thyroid cancer in Belarus, Russia, and Ukraine after Chernobyl and at present. Arq Bras Endocrinol Metab 51:748–762

The Health Status of the Population in the Semey Region and Scientifically Proven Measures to Improve It

Tolebay K. Rakhypbekov

Summary. We analyzed the state of health of the general population in the eastern Kazakhstan area, which showed a continuing high level of radiation-related diseases such as cancers. The affected region has been also characterized by high figures for mental disorder diseases and drug addiction. In comparison to the rest of Kazakhstan, our region has had the highest rates for cancer pathology and mortality from cancer, even exceeding the rate for the rest of the country in thyroid and breast cancer by 1.5 fold. In 2007, in the Semey region there were 1347 registered new cases of malignant neoplasia. From that number, 827 (61.4%) cases were in the city of Semey and 520 (38.6%) new cases were among rural inhabitants. By comparison, in 2006, the total number of known malignant neoplasms was 1291. The need for improvement of the state of health of the population in the Semey region demands a working out of further scientifically proven measures. Some of these measures are, to consistently decrease the level of socially significant diseases, to decrease the number of malignant neoplasms, and to facilitate systemic transition to international standards, new technologies, modern methods of treatment, and modern health services.

Key words Semipalatinsk Nuclear Test Site · Radiation · Thyroid cancer · Breast cancer · Screening · Population health

Introduction

August 21, 1947, was a "rainy day" in the history of Kazakhstan: the decision to create the Semey nuclear test site was accepted. As a result of the long-term activity of this test site, from 1949 to 1989 there were more than 470 air, ground, and underground explosions. Nuclear radiation polluted a significant area of Kazakhstan and even beyond its borders. More than 1 million hectares of ground have been destroyed over these many years. Many of the people living in the surrounding territory were exposed to ionizing radiation [1–3]. The general capacity of all

---

Semey State Medical Academy, Abai 103 Street, Republic of Kazakhstan

explosions comprised 17 420 kilotons, and the affected range of the area was 18 500 km² [4].

There has been no place on our planet similar to the Semey region where so many people have been intentionally exposed to combined external and internal radiation in doses of 100 Bq (1 Gy, 1000 mSv) [5]. The situation is unique in that in Hiroshima and Nagasaki the radiation was mainly external, and in the population in the Chernobyl region the radiation doses were incomparably lower. The majority of the population received about 30 mSv. In the Semey region, the effects of the radiation have lasted for more than 40 years.

The consequences of the tests in the Semipalatinsk nuclear test site have been the destruction of natural ecological systems, the deterioration of the surrounding testing area, the unfitness of reservoirs for industrial and agricultural usage, the high levels of disability and mortality rates among the affected population, the wide prevalence of oncological pathology and disorders of the blood circulation system, and the development of congenital defects [6].

The Japanese government was one of the first that rendered real help to the medical institutions in the city of Semey, and gave a grant for the project "Improvement of Medical Services in the Semey Region" in the sum of 648 million Japanese yen (6 million dollars). During the realization of the project, various modern diagnostic equipment was acquired, including endoscopy tools. The Medical Center of the Semey State Medical Academy was gratuitously given equipment for telemedicine with the Japanese Government in the value of 0.5 million dollars.

The aim of this study was to determine the health status of the population in the Semey region and to suggest scientifically proven interventions to improve it.

Material and Methods

Census data for years 2003 to 2007 were obtained from the National Census Bureau [7], and data on the number of malignant neoplasia were obtained from the annual reports of the Regional Eastern Kazakhstan Oncological Centre [8]. Data on numbers of infant and maternal mortalities and numbers of narcological and mental disorders for the year 2007 were obtained from the Department of Statistics, Ministry of Health, Kazakhstan [9]. The research was performed as a retrospective cross-sectional observational study. At the stage of study preparation, approval from the Semey State Medical Academy's Ethical Committee was obtained. All data were analyzed by the statistical package EpiInfo Version 6.04.

Results

The rate of cancer pathologies for the 5-year period in the Semey region (2003–2007) ranged from 0.227% to 0.221%. Comparison with the average Kazakhstan Republic levels is shown in Table 1.

Table 1. Rate (%) of malignant neoplasms in the Semey region and Kazakhstan Republic, 2003–2007

	2003	2004	2005	2006	2007
Semey region	0.227	0.228	0.207	0.211	0.221
Kazakhstan Republic	0.194	0.194	0.192	0.192	0.193

Table 2. Distribution of the most frequent new cases of malignant neoplasia in the Semey region in 2007

Rank	Type of malignant tumor	No. of new cases	Percent (%)
1	Trachea, bronchial, and lung tumors	175	13
2	Breast cancer	151	11.2
3	Stomach cancer	144	10.6
4	Skin cancer	119	8.8
5	Cervical cancer	72	5.3
6	Esophagus cancer	53	3.9
7	Pancreas cancer	52	3.8
8	Thyroid cancer	49	3.6
9	Kidney cancer	45	3.3
10	Rectal cancer	42	3.1

In comparison to the rest of Kazakhstan, our region has had the highest rates for cancer pathology and cancer mortality, even exceeding the rate for the rest of the country in thyroid and breast cancer by 1.5 fold [7,9].

In 2007, in the Semey region there were 1347 registered new cases of malignant neoplasms. From that number, 827 (61.4%) cases were in the city of Semey and 520 (38.6%) new cases were among rural inhabitants. By comparison, in 2006, the total number of known malignant neoplasia was 1291. The most frequent disorder in 2007 in the Semey region was malignant neoplasm of the trachea, bronchi and lung, comprising 175 patients, or 13%. Then, the next most frequent incidences were breast cancer, 151 patients (11.2%); stomach cancer, 144 patients (10.6%); skin cancer, 119 patients (8.8%); cervical cancer, 72 patients (5.3%); esophageal cancer, 53 patients (3.9%); pancreas cancer, 52 patients (3.8%); thyroid gland cancer, 49 patients (3.6%); kidney cancer, 45 patients (3.3%); and rectal cancer, 42 patients (3.1%). The 2007 statistics of new cases of malignant neoplasia are presented in Table 2. Tables 3 and 4 demonstrate the 2007 gender distributions of different types of malignant tumors in newly diagnosed patients.

Nowadays it is considered to be a well-known fact that malignant tumors of the thyroid gland show the strongest correlation with exposure to ionizing radiation [10]. The rate of thyroid cancers in the Semey region was 0.027%, 0.166%, and 0.445% in 1966–1976, 1977–1986, and 1987–2007, respectively.

The proportion of patients with the early stages of cancer (stage I–II) has decreased in 2007 as compared to 2006 (47.0% and 48.8%, respectively). At the

Health Status of the Semey Region Population

Table 3. Distribution of the most common types of malignancy in males of the Semey region in 2007

Rank	Type of malignant tumor	No. of new cases	Percent (%)
1	Trachea, bronchial, and lung tumors	152	23.4
2	Stomach cancer	101	15.6
3	Skin cancer	48	7.4
4	Prostate cancer	34	5.3
5	Esophagus cancer	33	5.1
7	Larynx cancer	17	2.6
8	Liver cancer	16	2.5

Table 4. The distribution of the most common types of malignancy in females of the Semey region in 2007

Rank	Type of malignant tumor	No. of new cases	Percent (%)
1	Breast cancer	151	22
2	Cervical cancer	72	10.3
3	Skin cancer	71	10.1
4	Ovarian cancer	52	7.4
5	Thyroid cancer	44	6.3
6	Stomach cancer	43	6.1
7	Endometrial cancer	28	4

Table 5. The rate (%) of different cancer stages in the Semey region in 2006–2007

	Stages I–II	Stage III	Stage IV	No stage
2006	48.8	24.1	17.2	9.8
2007	47.0	28.2	18.7	6.3

same time, the percentage of more advanced cancer stages (stages III and IV) increased (see Table 5).

Morphological verification for 2007 in the Semey region was performed for 1138 patients (85% of all new cancer cases). Overdue diagnostics were registered in 341 cases, 25.3% [as compared to 2006: 309 (23.9%)] in 2007 in the Semey region.

The reasons for neglect were the following:

- Latent current status: 195 cases, 57.2% (2006: 151, 48.9%)
- Untimely referral for medical aid: 136 cases, 40% (2006: 146, 47.2%)
- Incomplete examination of patients: 5 cases, 1.5% (2006: 12, 3.9%)
- Mistakes in diagnosis: 5 cases, 1.5% (2006: not available)

The death rate from malignant neoplasia in 2007 in the Semey region was equal to 824 people, or 0.135%. In comparison, in 2006 there were 804 registered deaths from malignant tumors [8].

We also analyzed the state of health of the general population in the eastern Kazakhstan area and found it showed continuing high levels of infant and maternal mortality. The affected region has been characterized by high figures for mental disorder diseases and drug addiction. According to the statistical facts, maternal mortality per 100 live births in eastern Kazakhstan is 0.0497; the same statistic for all the Republic of Kazakhstan is 0.0421%. Infant mortality per 100 live births in eastern Kazakhstan is 0.17; the same statistic for all the Republic of Kazakhstan is 0.15. The rate of diseases of narcological and mental disorders per 100 people in eastern Kazakhstan is 0.592; the same statistic for the entire Republic of Kazakhstan is 0.425%.

Discussion

In our study we attempted to investigate the health status of the population in the Semey region and to suggest scientifically proven interventions to improve it. Unfortunately, the current public health statistics shows a high prevalence of cancer in the population in the Semey region, which is especially true for thyroid cancers. The unfavorable ecological situation in the Semey region affects the status of the whole population. The prolonged influence of small doses of radiation as a result of prolonged nuclear tests has caused a disturbance in the immune, endocrine, and genetic systems and has resulted in the continual growth of malignant tumors. The need for the improvement of the state of health of the population in the Semey region demands a working out of further scientifically proven measures. Among these measures is included—to consistently decrease the level of socially significant diseases, to decrease the number of malignant neoplasms, and to facilitate systemic transition to international standards, new technologies, modern methods of treatment, and modern health services.

It is of utmost importance to solve the existing medical, social, and environmental problems in the region:

- The first issue is the screening and monitoring of the health status of those affected by the radiation by the use of modern technical and medical equipment.
- The second issue is to perform detailed genetic investigations on those affected by the radiation.
- The third issue is to exactly define the dose of reconstruction of radiation received from internal and external sources.
- The fourth issue is to carry out epidemiological research using the obtained given doses of reconstruction of radiation.
- The fifth issue is to introduce and use the international standards of investigation, education, and clinical practice.
- The sixth issue is to apply modern technologies of treatment for certain localizations of cancer and to use programs for early detection, and then to estimate and facilitate the decrease of the death rate from cancer.

References

1. Nugent RW, Zhumadilov ZS, Hoshi M, Gusev BI et al (2000) Health effects of radiation associated with nuclear weapons testing at the Semipalatinsk Test Site. New York-Semipalatinsk-Hiroshima
2. Takada J, Hoshi M, Rozenson R, et al (1997) Environmental radiation dose in Semipalatinsk area near nuclear test site. Health Phys 73:524–527
3. Kerber RA, Till JE, Simon SL, et al (1992) A cohort study thyroid disease in relation to fallout from nuclear weapons testing. JAMA 270:2076–2082
4. Shapiro CS, Kiselev VI, Zaitsev EV (eds) (1998) Nuclear tests, long-term consequences in the Semipalatinsk/Altai region. NATO/SCOPE RADTEST Advanced Research Workshop, 5–9 September 1994. NATO ASI Series, SERS E-N (Partnership Subseries, SERS E-N; Partnership Subseries). 2. Environment, vol 36. Springer-Verlag, Heidelberg
5. Hill P, Hille R, Bouisset P, et al (1996) Radiological assessment of long-term effects at the Semipalatinsk Test Site. NATO-Semipalatinsk Project 1995/1996 Jul-3325, December
6. Takada J, Hoshi M, Nagatomo T, et al (1999) External doses for residents near Semipalatinsk Nuclear Test Site. J Radiat Res 40:337–344
7. Annual Bulletin of the National Agency on Statistics, Kazakhstan, 2003–2007
8. Annual Reports (2003–2007) The Regional Eastern Kazakhstan Oncological Centre, Semey
9. The 2007 Report of the Department of Statistics. Ministry of Health, Kazakhstan
10. Shore RE (1992) Issues and epidemiological evidence regarding radiation-induced thyroid cancer. Radiat Res 131:98–111

Nuclear Explosions and Public Health Development

Aikan Akanov[1], **Serik Meirmanov**[2], **Arslan Indershiev**[1], **Aigul Musahanova**[3], **and Shunichi Yamashita**[4]

Summary. More than 60 years ago, on August 6 and 9, two atomic bombs destroyed two Japanese cities: Hiroshima and Nagasaki. It was the first time in history that a single weapon caused such enormous casualties in a population. About 120 000 and 75 000 people of Hiroshima and Nagasaki, respectively, most of whom were civilians, died instantaneously. Doctors and scientists had to contend with a new kind of unknown effect: irradiation. The public health system of Japan, as concerns atomic bomb survivors, has passed several stages of development: from individual dose evaluation to well-organized health care. This unique experience may be applied to other areas, such as cancer screening and elderly care. Over 40 years the USSR has tested nuclear bombs more than 450 times at the Semipalatinsk Nuclear Test Site (SNTS), Kazakhstan. There are many villages and larger settlements, including the city of Semey (distance from SNTS, about 150 km) in the vicinity of the test site. It is believed that hundreds of thousands of inhabitants were more or less exposed to long-term radiation fallout. The government of the Republic of Kazakhstan and the international community, including the government of Japan, have implemented several steps toward research on the influence of radioactive fallout and the support of health care of the Semey region inhabitants. However, research and health care concerning the people of the Semey region still needs improvement. For this purpose, the experience of the Japanese public health system may be useful.

Key words Public health · Nuclear explosion · Radiation · Hiroshima · Nagasaki · Semipalatinsk Nuclear Test Site (SNTS)

---

[1]Institute of Public Health, Almaty, Kazakhstan
[2]Tissue and Histopathology Section, Division of Scientific Data Registry, Atomic Bomb Disease Institute, Nagasaki University Graduate School of Biomedical Sciences, 1-12-4 Sakamoto, Nagasaki 852-8523, Japan
[3]Semey Oncology Center, Semey, Kazakhstan
[4]Department of Molecular Medicine, Atomic Bomb Disease Institute, Nagasaki University Graduate School of Biomedical Sciences, Nagasaki, Japan

Nuclear Explosions and Public Health Development in Japan

Introduction

The atomic bombs dropped on Hiroshima on August 6, 1945 and on Nagasaki on August 9, 1945 killed as many as 220 000 people by the end of 1945. Since then, thousands more have died of burns, radiation, and related diseases, aggravated by lack of medical resources. Nuclear explosions produce both immediate and delayed destructive effects. Blast, thermal radiation, and immediate ionizing radiation cause significant destruction within seconds or minutes of a nuclear detonation. The delayed effects, such as radioactive fallout and other environmental impacts, inflict damage over an extended period ranging from hours to decades. These nuclear explosions produced new challenges for public health that had never happened before.

Investigations into the aftermath of the bombing began immediately after the nuclear explosions, because Japanese scientists were aware within a few days that the weapon was a new atomic device [1,2]. The main events in the development of health care for atomic bomb survivors in Japan are shown in Table 1.

To define atomic bomb survivors, the Relief Law defines these survivors as (1) people who were exposed directly (within the former city area and surrounding towns and villages); (2) persons who entered the city within approximately 2 km of the hypocenter within 2 weeks of the explosion; (3) those who were engaged in disposal of the dead or in relief work; and (4) children of survivors certified in categories 1 through 3 who were in utero at the time of the bombing.

On March 31, 2007, there were 251 834 atomic bomb survivors recognized by the Japanese government, including about 47 000 in the city of Nagasaki and about 80 000 in the city of Hiroshima.

Table 1. Main events of social and health care development for atomic bomb survivors in Japan

Year	Events
1945	August 6 and 9: nuclear explosions in Hiroshima and Nagasaki
1947	ABCC (predecessor of RERF) established (in 1948, JNIH of the Ministry of Health and Welfare joined the studies)
1953	"Free" medical examination started
1954	U.S. hydrogen bomb tested on Bikini, exposing Japanese fishermen
1957	The Law for Atomic Bomb Survivors, including medical treatment, enacted
1961	"General" medical examination started
1968	Hibakusha Special Welfare Law enacted
1971	"Further" medical examination started
1988	Screening for cancers (stomach, lung, and multiple myeloma) started
1994	Screening for uterus and breast cancer started
1995	Hibakusha Relief Law (combining 1957 and 1968 laws)

ABCC, Atomic Bomb Casualty Comission
RERF, Radiation Effect Research Foundation
JNIH, Japan National Institute of Health

Social Protection and Health Support for the Population Suffering from Exposure to Nuclear Explosions in Japan

Politics in support of the atomic bomb survivors in Japan has a sufficient legislative base. In 1957, a law related to the medical service of *Hibakusha* was brought into existence according to which medical examinations and medical service were provided by the government. In 1968, the law about special measures for the support of atomic bomb survivors was accepted, and in 1995 these two laws were united to form the existing law in support of atomic bomb survivors (Table 1).

Social protection comes in the form of the following activities.

Health examinations:

- Atomic bomb survivors are entitled to receive health examinations regularly twice a year.
- Two additional examinations are available on request. One of the additional examinations can be for cancer, if desired.
- To encourage survivors to come in for health examinations, those who participate are provided with transportation expenses.

Provision of medical services:

- All expenses for the medical treatment of injuries and diseases that have been designated by the Minister of Health, Labor and Welfare to be attributable to the atomic bombing or to exposure to atomic bomb radiation are to be provided for those who are certified as atomic bomb survivors [3].
- Additional medical expenses beyond those covered by the National Health Insurance will be provided for the treatment of injuries and diseases other than those designated as caused by the atomic bomb.

Financial assistance:

- Financial assistance in the form of special allowances is to be provided to promote the welfare of atomic bomb survivors suffering from ill health conditions resulting from atomic bomb effects (Table 2).

Table 2. Financial allowance for atomic bomb survivors

Types of benefits	Amount of money paid monthly[a]
1. Special medical allowance	137 430 yen ($1153)
2. Special allowance	50 750 yen ($426)
3. Microcephaly allowance	47 300 yen ($397)
4. Health care allowance	33 800 yen ($284)
5. Health promotion allowance	16 950 yen ($142) or 33 800 yen ($284)
6. Nursing allowance	104 590 yen ($884) or 69 720 yen ($589)
7. Funeral service allowance	199 000 yen ($1575)

[a] U.S. dollars given in parentheses

Nuclear Explosions and Public Health 331

Table 3. Japanese national government expenditures for atomic bomb survivors

Year	2001	2002	2003	2004	2005	2006	2007
$\times 10^8$ yen	1632	1586	1571	1566	1566	1536	1536

- The total Japanese government expenditures for atomic bomb survivors are shown in Table 3. Financial support to atomic bomb survivors is also essential, meaning not only medical but also social help for this category of the population.

Results of 50 Years of National Social and Health Support for Atomic Bomb Survivors

The following points of the Japanese model of public health have proved to reduce atomic bomb effects:

- Establishing of individual dose
- Long-term cohort screening of the population
- Database of atomic bomb survivors
- Personalized social service for exposed people
- Development of effective treatment and prevention programs
- Development and application of long-term research programs on population needs assessment (atomic bomb long-term effects)

The existing governmental program to support survivors is presented as a logical and precisely calculated project that can be a good example of competent organization of medical help to the population in general.

Social Protection and Public Health Development in Kazakhstan

Introduction

The Semipalatinsk Nuclear Test Site (SNTS) is located in the northeast of Kazakhstan, only 150 km from the city of Semipalatinsk with a population of about 350000 people. Over 40 years beginning in 1949, 458 nuclear tests including 116 air and ground tests were conducted on SNTS [4]. Basic infringements of the radioactive safety of the population during the conduct of nuclear weapon tests were as follows: (1) 65% of ground and atmospheric nuclear explosions were unreasonably conducted in unfavorable meteorological conditions such as rain and strong wind; and (2) 80% of surface nuclear tests were conducted in the months of August through November at the time of harvesting crops.

Social Protection for the Population of SNTS

The main steps in developing social protection for the population of SNTS region are as follows [5]:

- 1991: Official closing of SNTS
- 1992: Law of Social Protection of People Around SNTS
- 1997: Program of medical rehabilitation of population who suffered from nuclear tests in SNTS in 1949–1990
- 2000–2005: Japan International Cooperation Agency (JICA) Medical Assistance Project in Semey

Although several efforts in developing social protection for the population of the SNTS region have already taken place, there remain some difficulties [6,7], such as the lack of clear data about individual dose and the lack of a total database of inhabitants with periodic health evaluations. Certainly, these people receive free-of-charge medical aid and a small social benefit; however, the level of support of the population needs to be improved. Another important problem is the absence of a full and authentic database on all who suffered from nuclear explosions in this territory of Kazakhstan. Considering aspects of the Japanese model of public health services, we offer our own model of the organization of medical and social help to the Semipalatinsk area (Fig. 1). The presented scheme means frequent screenings in regions, creation of a uniform information databank on all victims, and fast and

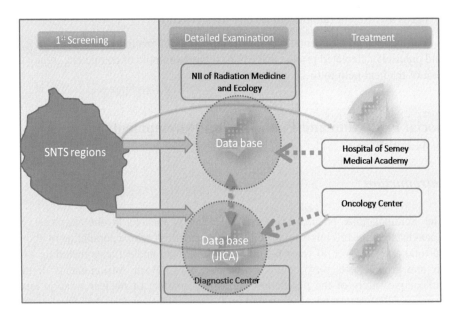

Fig. 1. Schematic representation of database accumulation for Semipalatinsk region inhabitants. *SNTS*, Semipalatinsk Nuclear Test Site; *NII*, Scientific Research Institute; *JICA*, Japan International Cooperation Agency

open data exchange between hospitals, scientific centers, partner organizations and the government of the country.

We certainly understand that the creation of a similar structure demands a great deal of financing and a long period of time; however, the results of this project would be quality medical aid and social protection for the persons who have really suffered from nuclear weapons tests on SNTS. A database and more financial support could be helpful in the case of SNTS residents, in addition to measurements of their radiation dosage.

Conclusion

The model of public health in Japan has proved to be effective for the health care of atomic bomb survivors. The experience gained with this model could be applied to other fields of medicine, such as oncology and elderly care. A database and more financial support could be helpful in the case of SNTS residents, in addition to determining their individual radiation dosage.

References

1. Bennett B (2005) Radiation effects studies of RERF. Acta Med Nagasaki 50:5–9
2. Kodama K, Mabuchi K, Shigematsu I (1996) A long-term cohort study of the atomic-bomb survivors. J Epidemiol 6:S95–S105
3. Sasaki Y (2005) Activities at the Atomic Bomb Survivors Health Care Commission. Acta Med Nagasaki 50:11–13
4. Atchabarov B (2000) Features of diseases caused by A-bomb test in Semipalatinsk. Hygiene, epidemiology and immunology. The Congress of Antinuclear Alliance, Astana
5. Akanov A, Meirmanov S, Indershiev A, et al (2008) Nuclear explosions and public health development. Nagasaki-Almaty
6. Boikov L (1999) The problems of Semipalatinsk Nuclear Test Site, 50 years after. Herald of East-Kazakhstan Technical University, pp 98–104
7. Institute of Pathology of Kazakh Academy of Science. The reports of scientific expedition of bio-medical research in the area of Semipalatinsk Nuclear Test Site, 1957–1960. Alma-Ata

Subject Index

A_L cells   136
ACTION   94
active mutagenic pathway   128
acute radiation
— injury   26
— syndrome (ARS)   256
adaptive
— mutation   129
— response   136, 137, 140, 141, 218
adipogenesis   68
AKT   207
alcohol and substance abuse   265
alkylguanine alkyltransferase   230
allelic loss   237
α (alpha)-particle   129, 136
amplification   286, 288, 291
aneuploidy   212, 214
APC   204, 205
apoptosis   235
array CGH   39
as low as reasonably achievable   16
ataxia-telangiectasia mutated protein (ATM)   184, 193, 195
atomic bomb   23, 63, 277, 279, 281, 285–292, 328
— dosimetry system   59
— radiation   220
— survivor   3, 4, 43, 51, 70, 81, 85, 105, 329
   children of —   58
   offspring of —   57
Atomic Bomb Casualty Commission/ Radiation Effects Research Foundation   57
Atomic Bomb Health Law   267
Atomic Energy Basic Law   244
ATR   195
autophosphorylation   202

Barker hypothesis   217
β (beta)-catenin   206
Bcl11b   232–235, 237, 238
Bcl-xL   235
BCR-ABL   47
Becquerel   255
biological samples   34
biopsychosocial   264, 269
bisphenol A   220
body mass index   64
bone marrow-derived cell 77   53
53BP1   196
BRAF   38, 315, 316
BRCA   47
breast cancer   177, 285–292, 296
bronchitis   272
BSS   244
bystander effect/response   29, 136–138, 140, 193, 195, 21

c-Myc   285–292
caloric restriction   219, 220
cancer   26, 75
— biology   91
— incidence   57
— mortality   57
— pathology   322, 324
— stage   325
— stem cell   217
cardiovascular disease/disorder   109, 272, 274
cellular response   27
centrosome   183, 187, 213
— destabilization   213
— duplication   188
chemotherapy   90, 183
   neoadjuvant —   180

335

Chernobyl   3, 268
— accident/nuclear accident   104, 306
— children   275
— emergency worker   95
   distribution of   96
— nuclear power plant   81, 82, 271
post —   40
Chernobyl Tissue Bank   9
chromatin   123
chromosomal/chromosome
— aberration(s)   44, 75, 144, 146, 148
— instability   129
— rearrangement   201
— translocation   47
Clinical-Morphological Register   306
Clinician-Administered PTSD Scale (CAPS)   267
clonal expansion   229, 236
COE   26
cohort studies   107
combined effect   227
compensatory hyperplasia   222
computed tomography (CT)   43
confounding factor   109
cross-talk   209
cyclin D1   162, 172
cyclooxygenase 2 (COX-2)   139, 140
cytoplasmic irradiation   193, 194

databank   51, 53, 322
death rate   325
depression   264
detrimental-adjusted nominal risk coefficient   45
diabetes   272, 274
dicentric   145, 146
— chromosome   213
diploid fibroblasts   296
DNA
— damage   125
— damage response (DDR)   193
— double-strand breaks (DSBs)   200
— -PKcs   200
— -protective effect   297
— repair   200
— replication stress   237
docetaxel   183
dose and dose rate effectiveness factor (DDREF)   44
dose
— constraint   13
— estimation   105
— of reconstruction   326
— response   44, 146
Drosophila   128

DS86   59
DSM   266

E-cadherin   207
ecological disasters   113
electron tracks in tissue   30
emergency
— exposure situation   15
— response   254
— worker   109
EMT   206
ENU   227, 228
epigenetic   219, 222
— toxicant   224
epithelial/mesenchymal cells interactions   294
ERK   139
errors in replication   221
ES cell   27
evacuation   104, 272
excess absolute risk (EAR)   46
excess relative risk (ERR)   46, 107
excess risks for leukemia   73
exclusion   17
exemption   17, 20
existing exposure situation   15
exposed in utero   272, 275
exposure experience   280
external exposure   105, 245

F_1 58, 128
Fanconi anemia (FA)   186, 187
fallout-related dose reconstruction   113
fatty liver   63
fear of exposure   277, 279
fibroblast/endothelial cell systems   298
fluorescence in situ hybridis(z)ation (FISH)   39, 144
   chromosome-orientation FISH (CO-FISH)   201

γ (gamma)-radiation   232
   indoor —   248
γ (gamma)-H2AX   202
— foci   193, 297
gap junction   137, 222, 298
gene expression profiling   179
General Health Questionnaire (GHQ)   110, 266
genetic
— effect   57
— marker   180
— risk   58
genistein   220
genome/genomic   25
— damage   26

Subject Index

— repair 25
— science 27
 — cross talk 131
 — instability 123, 127, 199, 218
— stability 197
Global COE Program 3, 4, 53
 University of Tokyo — 13
glucose metabolism 64
gpt 228
Great Hanshin Awaji Earthquake 263
growth inhibition 169
GSK-3β 205

Hanahan and Weinberg 233
haploinsufficient 234
Health Protection Agency (HPA) 258
HER2 285–287, 289–292
hematological malignancy 52, 70
hereditary risk 45
heterogeneous energy deposition 30
Hibakusha 4, 7
high-risk group 93
Hiroshima 74, 101, 263, 328
Hiroshima and Nagasaki 74, 101
Hiroshima University 23
HR 184
humanitarian aid 6
hypercholesterolemia 63
hypertension 66
hypertriglyceridemia 66
hyperuricemia 66

Ibaraki Prefecture 269
ICAM-1 162, 172
ICD, ICD-10 97, 266
ICL removal 183, 186
ICRP Publication 15, 22
IGF-1, IGF-1R 204, 206–209
Ikaros 230, 233, 237
IL-7 230
immunoprecipitation 158
in situ hybridisation 145
incidence 305, 308–312, 317
individual equity 16
inflammation 64
iNOS 139
insulin resistance 68
internal exposure 105
International Atomic Energy Agency (IAEA) 6, 244, 256, 268
International Commission on Radiological Protection (ICRP) 13, 44, 244
international consortium 4
intervention 17, 20
ionizing radiation (IR) 58, 123, 208

IRPA 246
ischemic heart disease (IHD) 64
 — risk factor 68

JHPS 246
JRIS 245
JRSM 247

Kazakhstan 332
 eastern — 322
Kudankulam 248
Ku70/Ku80 200

large-scale clinical trial 182
large-sized thymocytes 236
latency 37
late-onset carcinogenesis 54
leukemia 8, 108
Life Span Study (LSS) 69
lifespan expansion 220
Ligase IV 202
linear no-threshold (LNT) 29, 43, 217
linear-quadratic dose response 71
liquidation work 108
liver disorder 272, 274
LKB1 153, 155, 164–168, 173
long-term impacts 263
low-dose
 — effect 32
 — radiation 54
 — radiation risk 29
low-level radiation 224

machine learning method 181
malignant neoplasia 323
MAPK 38, 139
maternal exposure 60
MDM2 206
media literacy 111
mental and physical well-being 280
mental effect 81
mental health 277, 278
metabolic syndrome 63
microarray 179
microbeam 32, 194, 196
mitochondria 197
 — DNA-deficient cells 138
mitomycin C 184
molecular epidemiological studies 5
monoclonal gammopathy of undetermined significance (MGUS) 52
mouse chromosome-specific DNA library 144
mouse thymic lymphoma 227
Ms6hm 129

MTT Assay   159
multiple (primary) cancers   52, 74
Mustard gas   128
mutagenesis   137
mutant/mutation
— fraction   136
— frequency   229
delayed —   127
dynamic —   127, 128
untargeted —   127
"mutation theory" of carcinogenesis   213
myelodysplastic syndrome (MDS)   52

NADPH oxidase   196
Nagasaki   74, 101, 263, 328
National Institute of Radiological Sciences (NIRS)   254
natural background   30
naturally occurring radioactive material (NORM)   17
NBS   183
neglect   325
neuro-asthenia   266
neurotic disorder   272, 274
— symptoms   265
NFκB   139, 140, 207
nitric oxide   138, 299
non-DNA-targeted effect   29
non-hit cell   29
nonhomologous end-joining (NHEJ)   184, 199
nuclear
— accident   23
— education   20
— energy (sociology)   21

ophthalmologic studies   109
optimization of radiological protection   13
oxidative damage   195
— stress   216, 219

p27   235
p53   207, 234
— dependent S-phase checkpoint   131
paclitaxel   178
panic reaction   265
paracrine   294
— factor secreted into the medium   300
parental exposure   61
pre-conception   62
paternal exposure   60
permissive tumor microenvironment   300
persistence   145
— of chromosome translocations   148

personality problem   265
pink-eyed unstable allele   130
planned exposure situation   15
polonium-210 (^{210}Po)   258
population-based case-control study   106
posterior subcapsular cataract   109
PPB dot blot assay   186
predict/prediction
— patient response   181
— system   180
— of therapeutic response   182
preleukemic cell   47
prelymphoma   232, 244
premature senescence   218
primordial radionuclide   248
prevention   331
pripyat   104, 272
prophylactic
— intervention   271
— strategies   272
protein-target hypothesis   214
psychological
— distress   263
— effects   5
— support program   271
— trauma   269
psychosomatic
— effect   110
— problem   265
post-traumatic stress disorder (PTSD)   263, 278, 279
complete —   267
incomplete —   267
public health   332

Q-RT-PCR   179
Quality of Life (QOL)   267
quiescent diploid human cell   300

Rad3-related protein (ATR)   193
radiation   326, 329
— carcinogenesis   212, 214
— casualty   24
— damage   25
— dose   63, 74
— emergency   84, 85
    medicine   23, 24
— exposure   27, 113, 148
— health risk control   54, 104, 111
— -induced   5, 27
— protection supervisor   246
— response   295
— safety   13
— sensitivity   295

Subject Index

— signature 6
— therapy 301
— tracks 29
radioiodine/radioactive iodine 35, 315
radiology 13, 21
radioprotector 300
radon 248
ras gene mutation 77
reactive oxygen species (ROS) 194
reciprocal DNA-protective effect 298
recombination 132, 236
redox intracellular signaling 221
reference level 13
regenerative medicine 25, 53
regression model 98
relative risk 98, 272
Relief Law 329
replication fork stalling 195
RET 37, 154
RET/PTC 154, 159, 160, 163, 170–172, 174, 305, 315
retrospective dosimetry 144
risk 26
— assessment 7, 141
qualitative — 111
quantitative — 111
— communication 9, 111
— heterogeneity 44
— identification 111
— management 111
— transfer models 46
Rit1 233, 234
Roentgen 255
Russian National Medical and Dosimetric Registry 96
Russian psychiatrist 268

safety culture 16
scientific collaboration 6
secretory clusterin (sCLU) 204, 205, 208
selectivity 301
Semey/Semipalatinsk Nuclear Test Site (SNTS) 81, 322, 333
Semey/Semipalatinsk State Medical Academy 323
Semipalatinsk 3
signature gene 7
sister chromatid exchange (SCE) 132
social
— protection 330
— stigma 267
— target group 271
solid cancer 100
— other than thyroid cancer 108

soluble factor/mediators 137, 299
— -mediated network 294
soy isoflavone 221
spermatozoa 130
stakeholder involvement 16
standardized mortality ratio 99
STAT3 155, 159, 163, 164, 170, 172, 173
endogenous — 160
— linker domain 166, 167
Y705 phosphorylation of — 171
statistics 159, 324
stem cell
adult — 217
— theory of carcinogenesis 219
stigmatized 281
stomach disorder 272, 274
stromal–epithelial 218
subjective experience 279
supernumerary centrosomes 187
suppressive hormone therapy 315
surrogate marker 63

T65D radiation dosimetry system 59
nontarget(ed) effect 123, 213
TEL/AML1 47
telomeres 199
— -DSB fusion 201
tertiary radiation emergency hospital 23, 24
tetraploid 212, 213
TGF-β 197, 208, 209
therapeutics 177
thermolabile 299
Three Mile Island 109, 267
thymic
— atrophy 235
— lymphomas 232, 237, 238
— microenvironment 238
thyroid
— cancer/carcinoma 7, 113, 305, 308–312, 317
— cell lines 296
childhood — 9, 105
— incidence 305
— medullary 36
— papillary (PTC) 34, 154, 315
subtype 313
— disorder 272, 274
— follicular adenoma 108
— nodules 108
— non-cancer disease 108
tissue weighting factor 45
TLS 188
TNF-α 140
training course 255

transgenerational minisatellite mutation   129
translocation   144, 145
transmitted effect   32
trinucleotide (repeat) expansion   127, 128
tumo(u)r   35
— biology   40
— initiation   232
— promoter   223
— registry   60
tyrosine phosphorylation   160

UNSCEAR   244

vegetative nervous system disease/disorders
   272, 274
VEGF   162, 172
visceral fat accumulation   63

WHO   6, 244
WHO-REMPAN   256
whole-body counter (WBC)   256
Wnt   205, 208, 209

xip8   204
XP-F   188